GASTROINTESTINAL AND UROGENITAL RADIOLOGY

Gastrointestinal and Urogenital Radiology

NICER Series on Diagnostic Imaging

Edited by

Anders Lunderquist, MD

Professor Emeritus

Department of Radiology

University of Lund, Lund, Sweden

Holger Pettersson, MD

Professor and Chairman

Department of Radiology

University of Lund, Lund, Sweden

Merit Communications

ISBN 1 873413 05 X

Published by
Merit Communications
7 Salisbury Place
Langton Road
London, SW9 6UW
England

Printed by
Butler & Tanner Ltd
Frome and London

NYCOMED

Contents

Contributors

Albert L. Baert, MD
Professor and Chairman
Department of Radiology
University Hospitals
K.U. Leuven, Belgium

David O. Cosgrove, MA, MSc, FRCP, FRCR
Consultant in Nuclear Medicine and Ultrasound
Royal Marsden Hospital
Sutton, Surrey England

Frans-Thomas Fork, MD
Associate Professor of Radiology
Head of Endoscopy and Gastrointestinal Radiology
Malmö General Hospital
University of Lund
Malmö, Sweden

K. Ivancev
Visiting Associate Professor
Charles Dotter Institute of Interventional Therapy
Oregon Health Sciences University
and Associate Professor
University Hospital,
Lund Sweden

Howard M. Pollack, MD
Professor of Radiology
University of Pennsylvania School of Medicine and Section of Uroradiology, Department of Radiology
Hospital of the University of Pennsylvania
Philadelphia, PA, USA

Constantin Cope, MD
Professor of Radiology
Hospital of the University of Pennsylvania
Philadelphia, PA USA

Leif Ekelund, MD
Professor and Chairman
Department of Diagnostic Radiology
University Hospital
5–5901–85 Umeå, Sweden

Aksel Kruse, MD
Associate Professor
Head of Endoscopic Laboratory
Department of Surgical Gastroenterology, University Hospital of Aarhus
DK–8000 Aarhus C, Denmark

G. Marchal, MD
Department of Radiology
University Hospitals
K.U. Leuven, Belgium

H. Rigauts
Department of Radiology
University Hospitals
K.U. Leuven, Belgium

Josef Rösch, MD
Professor of Radiology and Director of the Charles Dotter Institute of Interventional Therapy
Oregon Health Sciences University
Portland, Oregon, USA

Preface

If you give a man a fish, he will have a meal
If you teach him to fish, he will have a living
If you are thinking a year ahead, sow seed
If you are thinking ten years ahead, plant a tree
If you are thinking one hundred years ahead, educate the people
By sowing seed once, you will harvest once
By planting a tree, you will harvest ten-fold
By educating the people, you will harvest one hundred-fold

(Chinese proverb, 400 BC)

The Chinese wisdom above has come to us from ancient times through the written word. Even today, in the era of advanced communication, the written word is the solid basis of knowledge. Therefore, the NICER program is based on a combination of courses, books, and educational newsletters, and it is with great pleasure that we here present the first NICER book – dealing with gastrointestinal and urogenital radiology. It is not our intention to cover the whole field of gastrointestinal and urogenital radiology. Instead, we present subjects that we think might be of special interest for future updating.

Barium examinations of the stomach and colon have, to a great extent, been replaced by endoscopy but they still have a role in specific circumstances. New imaging modalities of the kidney have changed the diagnostic work-up of patients with suspected renal tumours and the importance of ultrasound is stressed. Imaging of the prostate has long been a disappointment, but MRI now seems to provide better results. Catheterisation of the Fallopian tubes has proved to be an effective treatment for infertility. Percutaneous transhepatic cholangiography and drainage of jaundiced patients has mostly been replaced by endoscopic techniques and several new techniques have been introduced to remove stones from the gallbladder and bile ducts.

These subjects, and several more, are dealt with in more detail than is possible to discuss during the course. The chapters are written by leading authorities in the field. It is therefore our intention and hope that this book will work not only as a supplement to the course, but that it should also be useful for any readers wishing to update their knowledge of gastrointestinal radiology.

Anders Lunderquist
Holger Pettersson
Lund, June 1991

Carcinoma of the gastrointestinal tract

Frans-Thomas Fork
Department of Diagnostic Radiology, University of Lund, Malmö, Sweden

Introduction

The great improvement seen in the diagnosis of cancer of the gastrointestinal tract can be attributed to the discovery of X-rays. Increased knowledge and refinement of technique have reduced diagnostic delays to the histological stage of early malignant lesions. Modern fibre-endoscopic and cytological procedures have contributed to both increased knowledge and early diagnosis of malignant gastrointestinal lesions. Modern techniques reveal not only the macroscopic appearance of mucosal lesions but also any concomitant dysfunction of organ motility, as well as any alterations to the surrounding topography. This chapter examines the many techniques now available for diagnosis of carcinoma of the gastrointestinal tract.

Contrast Media

Barium Sulphate Examination

Suspensions specially designed for examining various areas of the gastrointestinal tract are now available, all optimized for mucosal coating. Due to the varying levels of acidity in the gut it is necessary that the appropriate product is selected. For air-barium studies a high density and low viscosity formula should be used while, a low density, more stable barium suspension is recommended for single-contrast examinations. Distension of the upper GI tract is achieved by gaseous expansion, using either a solid or liquid effervescent or by introduction of air through a naso-gastric tube. It is recommended that the large bowel be inflated with carbon dioxide rather than air - which often causes discomfort to the patient [1].

If motility is to be studied, anticholinergic drugs should not be administered. However, if the detail of the mucosa is of primary interest it might be helpful to stop peristalsis. Butylscopolamin is given in doses up to 40 mg i.m. or i.v. in patients who do not show tachycardia or hyperplasia of the prostate. Glucagon, an antihypoglucaemic hormone, is given in doses of 0.3 mg i.v., repeated if necessary, to patients who do not have phaeochromocytoma or insulinoma.

Water-soluble Agents

The indications for using water-soluble contrast media are few, of which spontaneous or post-operative perforation of the gut is the main one. Usually a flavoured sodium/meglumine diatrizoate, Gastrografin, is used. A small amount of Gastrografin added to a low density barium suspension, i.e. 2%, for follow-through examination in emergency patients with small bowel obstruction reduces the time of diagnosis.

Barium sulphate is the first choice even in patients who aspirate or have a fistula to the bronchi, as ionic water-soluble contrast media can lead to parenchymal destruction [2].

In patients with mediastinitis or peritonitis secondary to perforation non-ionic water-soluble contrast media are recommended.

Complications

Morbidity and mortality rates caused by barium examinations are low [3]. Frequently patients complain of transient bowel distension within the first few hours after air-contrast barium examinations. In addition, the use of excessive amounts of barium sulphate may lead to long-term constipation.

Rectal perforations are rare [4], the author's experience being one in 12,000 examinations. They may be attributed to the technique used or to diseased bowel. Spillage of barium into soft tissues results in a severe inflammatory reaction which results in fibrosis and formation of foreign body granulomas around barium crystals [5,6]. Spillage of barium into the abdominal cavity causes severe peritonitis and in the presence of faecal matter carries a 50% mortality risk [7,8].

Most patients are treated surgically, with antibiotic coverage and intravenous fluid. Intravasation of barium is reported as a rare complication with high mortality [9-11].

Radiological Techniques for the Gastrointestinal Tract

Single-contrast Barium Study

With the single-contrast examination technique, part of or the whole organ is filled with a low density barium suspension, 50-100 wt/vol%. This is then made semitranslucent at X-ray (120-140 kV). Lesions causing a protrusion sufficient to replace a major volume of the barium sulphate will present as a local radiolucency *en face* (Fig. 1a), or as a defect of the organ contour. Subtle lesions such as polyps or shallow ulcers are diagnosed by chance unless caught tangentially. *En face* these lesions are hidden by the full barium column if external compression cannot be applied. Compression reduces the thickness of the barium column and a minor protruding mucosal lesion will be seen as a radiolucency, while an ulcer will be barium-filled.

Due to the many factors which can affect the examination (barium density, organ thickness, kilovoltage, outer compression, dexterity and experience in the technique) the single-contrast barium examination has now been widely replaced by air contrast procedures.

Double-contrast Barium Study

With the air-barium or double contrast examination technique a reduced amount of a high density barium suspension, 200-250 wt/vol%, is used in order to coat the mucosa evenly [12,13]. The walls of the gut are separated by air, which then fills the organ. Any mucosal defect is outlined with a thin layer of barium and is thus reproducible in any projection. However, an intraluminal lesion on the dependent wall is again most readily detected in a shallow pool of barium, causing a defect. A dependent excavation acts on the other hand as a bowl, which fills with barium.

Superficial lesions originating from the non-dependent wall may be quite difficult to detect on vertical beam films. Turning the patient

(a)

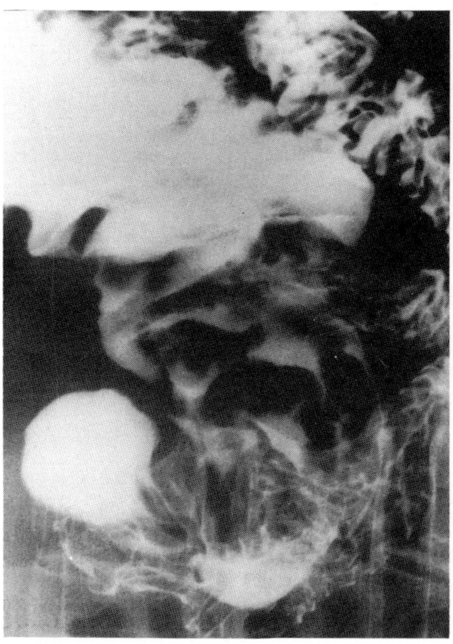

(b)

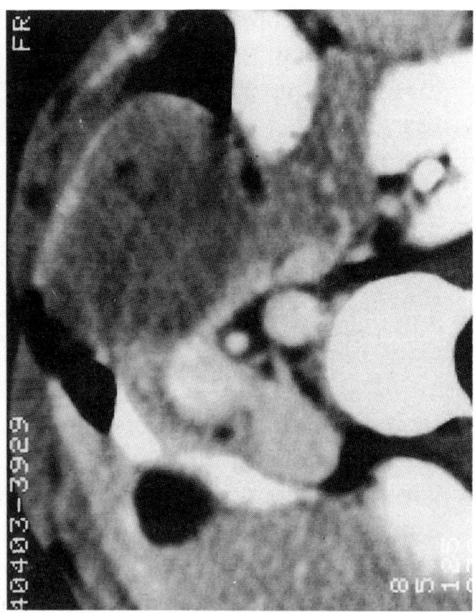

(c)

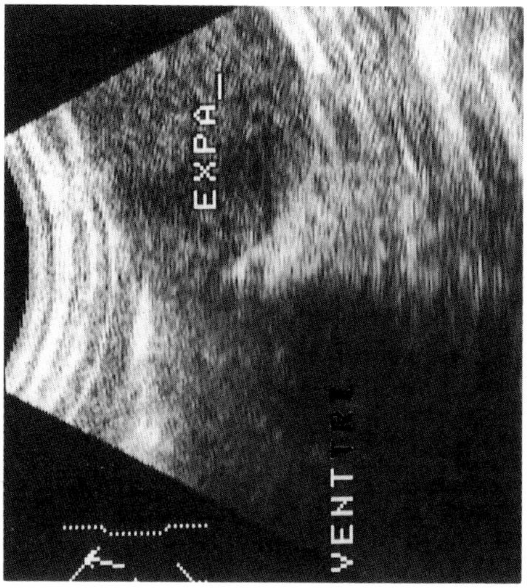

Figure 1. *(a) Deformity of the antrum caused by a large single lesion seen at CT (b) dislocating the stomach anteriorly. (c) At US the lesion was found to be attached to the gastric wall by a small pedicle only. The attenuation values and echogenicity of this leiomyoma are almost homogenous.*

counteracts this weakness and also improves the coating. Again the presence of a minute lesion is most convincingly demonstrated in profile, for instance on horizontal beam films. Double-contrast studies of the small bowel may be performed with air or methyl-cellulose for distension of the lumen [14]. Additives to the barium suspension can further increase the depiction of mucosal details [15]. The author uses a 65 wt/vol% solution for the small bowel and a 80 wt/vol% for the large bowel.

Fluoroscopy

Image intensified fluoroscopy and spot filming play an essential part in the radiographic examination of the gastrointestinal tract irrespective of barium technique chosen. Although the majority of radiologists prefer the double-contrast examination, palpation and compression studies are recommended, especially in the early phases of the examinations [16].

Gross Morphology of Gastrointestinal Cancer

Advanced tumours in spacious parts of the GI tract, viz. the stomach and proximal parts of the right hemicolon, are bulky and endophytic masses, otherwise annular 'apple-core' lesions with overhanging margins. They may also cause irregular or tubular narrowings, large craters and diffuse nodularity. Intermediate-sized tumours less than 3 cm across are usually seen as eccentric, sessile, lobulated, and sometimes ulcerated lesions. Lesions less than 1 cm are either polypoid or ulcerated. Concomitant irregularity of the surrounding mucosa is a malignant sign of infiltration. Early carcinoma is detected as an area of superficial irregularity or as a zone of decreased compliance (see below).

Acute Abdominal Survey

Patients with suspected GI obstruction are usually examined with acute abdominal plain film examination before any other study is considered. Within a few hours bowel loops proximal to an obstruction distend, while distal loops collapse. In early phases loops are mainly distended by gas while in protracted incidences increasing amounts of fluid will add. Horizontal beam films readily identify the air-fluid levels. The diaphragm and groins should always be included in radiographic abdominal survey films.

A primary tumour of the small gut seldom causes a complete obstruction whereas a large bowel one often does. Small bowel loops distend less compared to loops of the large bowel and are tube-like with closely spaced valvulae conniventes. The distended large bowel is recognized both by its scattered inter-haustral folds and its location, encircling the mid-abdominal content of small bowel and sigmoid colon.

An acute obstruction presents itself with raised air distended loops while in chronic obstruction the air-filled levels are long and the loops sometimes massively distended.

A proximal obstruction causes early vomiting and air-fluid levels are only incidentally seen. The abdomen is gas free, sometimes with fluid-filled proximal loops. With more distally located obstruction the number of air-fluid levels increases as does the duration of patient symptoms. Again distally located loops are collapsed [17].

Acute Barium Examination

If the acute abdominal survey indicates a colorectal obstruction this is verified by a limited single-contrast barium enema. Controversy exists about how to verify an acute small bowel obstruction. If the patient already has a naso-gastric tube in place it is usually possible to adjust its position to the distal duodenum or replace it by a standard type for enteroclysis under fluoroscopic control (see below). Usually the height and aetiology of the obstruction are disclosed within 30 minutes. The conventional follow-through examination after two or more cups of barium are given to the patient may take anywhere from a few hours to several days. By mixing an iodinated agent with the barium the examination is considerably speeded up. Water soluble agents are not suitable because of problems with interpretation due to hypertonicity and dilution.

Fibre-endoscopy

Where possible, upper gastrointestinal obstruction is ruled out using fibre-endoscopic procedures, mainly in order to collect biopsies from mucosal lesions and to locate a source of bleeding prior to surgery, but also because less patient co-operation is demanded and tranquilizers may be given.

Other Techniques for Evaluation of the Gut

Incidental mass lesions originating from the gut are identified by computed tomography (CT) (Fig. 1b) of the mediastinum and abdomen, and by transabdominal ultrasonography (US) (Fig. 1c). These examinations provide imaging of mural and extravisceral abnormalities, local and peripheral metastases, but give no information on the mucosa itself. Endoluminal ultrasonography (EUS) gives detailed information of the different layers of the gut wall and lesions adjacent to it, but the mucosal lining is still obscured.

These procedures should not replace the use of barium or fibre-endoscopy in the diagnosis of GI neoplasia. It is, however, important to be aware of the features of these lesions on CT and ultrasonography in order to co-ordinate the patient's management [18].

Computed Tomography (CT)

CT is routinely used for tumour-staging and is applicable to the entire gastrointestinal tract [19,20] for planning of irradiation treatment, for detection of recurrent disease, and for evaluation of spread. CT is probably the best means for distinguishing primary GI tract tumours from invasion by an adjacent malignancy and also for identification of tumour origin in cases with a palpable mass (Fig. 2) [21-24].

Local wall thickening can be evaluated when the lumen is adequately distended with an optimal amount of contrast media and enhanced by an intravenous contrast agent. By these means any local mesenteric and/or perivisceral mass or inhomogeneity will stand out more clearly [25].

Wall thickening of more than 10 mm visible in the CT scan is usually interpreted as a sign of malignancy. However, small carcinomas may not cause any such thickening, whereas benign lesions may very well be suggestive of tumour. CT is therefore unsuitable for primary diagnosis but outstanding for demonstrating extrinsic and peripheral disease [26].

All available contrast media for enteric use are compatible and may be combined. High density iodinated agents, viz. dilute, 2-3% solutions of Gastrografin or Hypaque powder are preferred by most radiologists. These agents are hardly absorbed by the gut, and are indicated in patients with suspected perforation or fistulae and immediately pre- and post-operatively. To reduce peristaltic artifacts, intravenous Glucagon 0.3-1 mg sometimes has to be given [27].

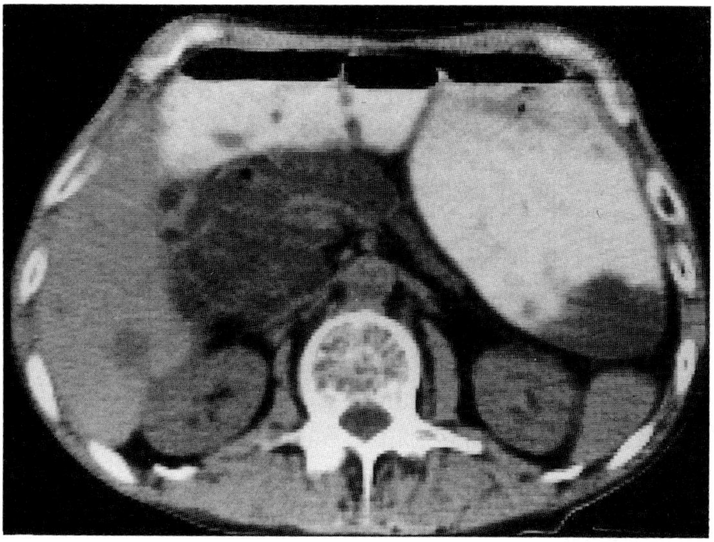

Figure 2. *Gastric retention in an old patient caused by a large carcinoma of the pancreatic head compressing the duodenal loop.*

Some radiologists prefer barium suspensions of around 2 wt/vol% as these are more palatable and do not induce diarrhoea [28,29].

With the introduction of high-resolution scanners, fat-density contrast media diluted to 12.5% emulsions are again available for abdominal CT. They provide persistent intestinal distension from the lower oesophagus downward without producing artefacts. Metoclopromide hydrochloride is usually needed to hasten gastric emptying. Precaution should be taken in using fat agents in patients with intra-abdominal inflammatory conditions. Around 1-1.5 l of a high-density contrast agent and 0.8-1 l of fat-density one have to be ingested in a two-hour period prior to scanning, in order to achieve homogeneous filling and good distension of the small gut, and during three to 12 hours for antegrade contrast filling of the colon.

Extra-intestinal tumour spread is suggested when surrounding fat planes are obliterated. However, thin patients as a rule lack these fat planes and consequently detection of spread is less likely. Furthermore, identical CT signs may be caused by scarring, inflammation and congestion. Definite invasion exists when an obvious tumour mass is involving and enveloping neighbouring organs, and probably so when a major portion of an expected fat plane is obliterated in several scans (see oesophagus and rectum) [32].

In the author's department we consider the major role of CT to be the evaluation of the paraintestinal compartments and the local lymph nodes, and not identification of the location or the size of the primary GI-tract neoplasm. Therefore we do not distend the bowel lumen but try to label the lumen of the bowel with a small amount of a 2% solution of Gastrografin.

A carcinoma of the alimentary tract may be found on CT in patients referred for other reasons. If the carcinoma has outgrown its arterial supply, low attenuation areas within the mass suggest tumour necrosis. At the same time distended bowel loops with air-fluid levels are seen proximal to the lesion. Corresponding changes are seen in the urinary tract in cases of ureteric encasement. Tumour calcification indicates a mucinous adenocarcinoma.

Lymphadenopathy is diagnosed by CT when nodes are 1 cm or more in diameter. Whether this enlargement is due to a benign or malignant cause cannot be predicted by this technique [33].

The author uses both native scans and scans after bolus intravenous contrast injection to diagnose liver metastases with CT. In spite of this combined approach, we still miss lesions up to 2 cm across which are subsequently revealed on intra-operative ultrasonography. However, therapeutic management in one out of three patients with focal abdominal mass identified by barium studies may be altered after abdominal CT, mainly because of detection of metastases [32]. CT-angiography with contrast injection directly into the hepatic artery improves detection of metastases down to 1 cm across.

Recurrent GI-tumour

After tumour resection and reanastomosis local wall thickening and surrounding scar tissue are usually present and it is not possible to distinguish these from a local recurrency. A baseline study in the post-operative recovery era is therefore recommendable, with which follow-up studies can be compared. Recurrent tumour is diagnosed when a soft tissue mass has changed or is newly appeared.

Magnetic Resonance Imaging (MRI)

Recently researchers have published series on MRI and evaluation of local tumour extent (T), lymphatic spread (N) and presence of distant metastases (M). The results of staging of gastrointestinal tumours varies depending on where the tumour is located, if cardiac and respiratory motion gating is used or not, and the size of the lesions [34]. Gastroesophageal junction tumours are located at an unfavourable site for both CT and MRI staging [35], whereas squamous cell carcinoma of the mediastinal region seems to be more suitable for staging by MRI with an accuracy of 75% [36]. Although MRI may provide information for better patient management and follow-up, it is still nor considered very effective in the TNM classification, mainly because adenopathy is identified on large nodal size only, i.e. on a diameter of 10 mm or more [37]. In patients with clinically suspected local tumour recurrence, MRI is reported to be highly accurate [38].

Transabdominal Ultrasonography (US)

Normally patients are not referred for US examination of the GI-tract but to rule out a palpable mass, metastases (Fig. 3) to local, peripheral, and remote lymph nodes, to the retroperitoneum and liver, and to guide fine needle puncture for cytology and biopsy (FNP) [39].

The GI tract is recognized during real-time scanning by its peristaltic motions, intraluminal air and content. A loop of bowel is identified by a reflecting pattern caused by hyperechoic bowel gas, often producing an acoustic shadow. The mucus itself is echogenic without shadow as is the periserosal fat, while the rim of lucency in between represents the intima, media and serosa [39-41].

If the gut wall is to be examined, the part in question has to be examined before and after distension by dearated water. By varying patient positioning the water is used as an acoustic window, displacing any air non-dependently. In order to scan intramural and intraluminal masses a smooth muscle relaxant is given [42,43].

The intestinal origin of a solid abdominal mass may be difficult to verify unless the bowel wall or its echogenic air-filled lumen is identified (Fig. 1c). In order to differentiate a large bowel loop from a pelvic mass, a water enema may be given [44]. Gastrointestinal tract involvement is assumed if a mass is in the area of the bowel [45].

The bowel wall should not measure more than 3 mm in thickness with the loop distended. Adequate distension is achieved when the stomach measures 8 cm, the small bowel 3 cm and the colon 5 cm across [46].

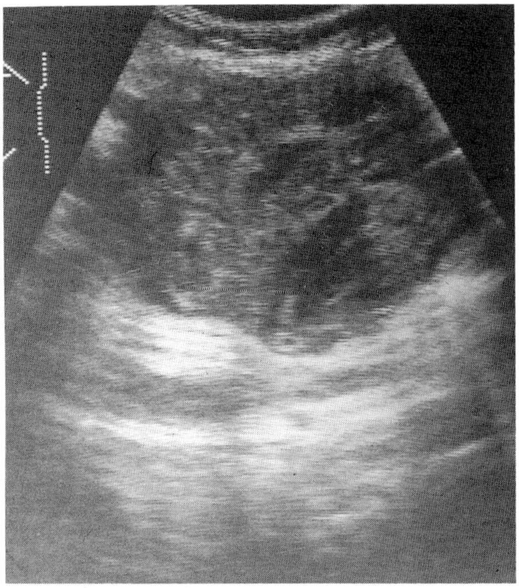

(a)

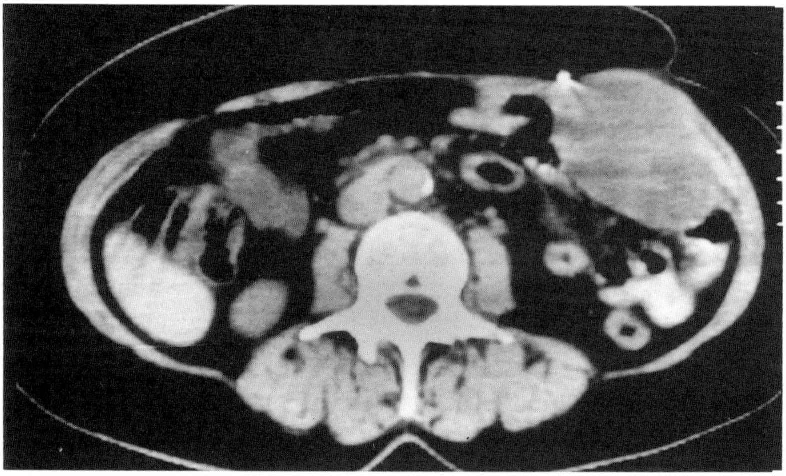

(b)

Figure 3. *Follow-up one year after removal of a colon carcinoma. (a) US with FNP of a palpable cicatricial lesion disclosed a metastasis. (b) No further lesions were found on CT.*

Divergent findings are pathologically significant in up to 90%, although histology cannot be predicted. These lesions usually resemble a target on cross sectional scans and a kidney on scans in the long axis (see Fig. 17a) [41,47].

The oesophago-gastric junction, the stomach antrum and most parts of the duodenum are usually visible by real-time US. The small bowel and colon are identified occasionally when fluid-filled by the valvulae conniventes and haustral markings, which form linear echo-densities [48].

Endoluminal Ultrasonography (EUS)

EUS is often used in conjunction with fibre-endoscopy. For exploration of the oesophageal and rectal wall a water-filled balloon covering the ultrasonic probe is used, while the exploration of the gastric and duodenal walls are performed after instillation of dearated water into these organs [49]. Due to its high resolution properties, EUS readily identifies the different layers of the gut wall (see Fig. 29), which is presently a shortcoming of transabdominal US-techniques [50].

By means of the high-frequency EUS-beam intramural tumour growth is clarified, as is the existence of spread to local lymph nodes. Thereby the evaluation of tumour resectability is facilitated [51].

Malignant mucosal lesions are hypoechoic and in most instances clearly defined [52,53]. However, small tumours may be difficult to localize due to the limited field of vision with the EUS fibre-endoscopes [54].

Recommended Sequence of Imaging Investigations

In a patient with highly suspected gastrointestinal malignancy the sequence of investigation should be considered. It is logical to start the investigation with an examination of the mucous membrane, viz. barium or fibre-endoscopic studies. However if barium contrast is retained this will cause disturbing artefacts on subsequent studies like CT, US, angiography and plain film surveys. If there are no signs of retention, the double-contrast barium examination of the colon precedes that of the oesophago-gastro-duodenum, the small bowel and the hypopharynx.

Improvement in patient survival depends on detecting gastrointestinal cancer while small and asymptomatic. This calls for the best possible examination technique, which varies between diagnostic centres. Due to the intimate relationship between the gastrointestinal tract and surrounding parenchymal organs, the former will be dislocated, constricted and infiltrated by tumour growth in the latter. Fibre-endoscopic investigation in such patients is secondary to CT and transabdominal US-techniques, which ought to be supplemented by examinations to disclose any further lesion beyond a stricture, viz. barium studies.

Malignant Lesions of the Oesophagus

Around 4% of all gastrointestinal carcinomas are confined to the oesophagus, 90% of which are squamous cell tumours, the rest being adenocarcinoma of gastric or junctional origin [55]. The abuse of tobacco and alcohol are high risk factors for oesophageal carcinoma as are mucosal lesions secondary to Barrett's oesophagus, caustic- and irradiation strictures, achalasia, etc. Oesophageal cancer is endemic in certain areas of Asia and Japan.

One fifth of all lesions are located in the upper third of the oesophagus, the rest evenly distributed [56]. The main symptom is dysphagia which brings the patient to the imaging department. Morphological investigation should be completed with video- or cine-radiography in order to disclose functional disturbances.

Oesophageal carcinoma may disappear completely after radiation therapy. However, all recur and finally occlude the lumen.

Barium Examination

The size and location of an advanced carcinoma is quickly accomplished by single-contrast examination. However, the small plaque-like and histologically early carcinoma is asymptomatic and usually hard to detect. Although good double-contrast images have the potential to depict small tumours, these are still rare findings and diagnosed by chance only [57,58].

Double-contrast images are obtained by rapid and continuous swallowing of barium contrast in erect position with the stomach distended by 500 ml gas. During gulping the oesophagus is distended mainly by eructation (Fig. 4). Limited and tiny lesions do normally not disturb peristalsis and may be recognized if the stripping movement of the oesophageal peristaltic wave is recorded on routine examination [59].

The tumour discloses itself as a medallion wagging on the stripping wave. Once located it is documented by detailed spot-films. Multiple biopsies then clarify the character of the lesion.

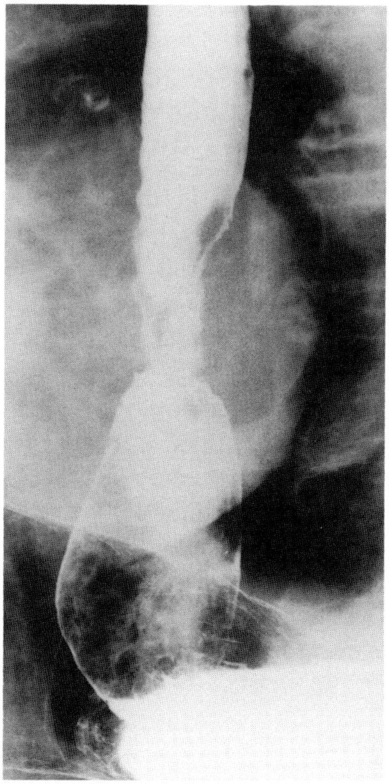

Figure 4. *Circumferential oesophageal carcinoma in a patient with a long history of gastroesophageal reflux.*

Differential Diagnoses

Lymphoma, leiomyosarcoma and invading or metastatic lung and breast carcinoma are rare diseases, reported in 3.2% of autopsy studies. Secondary neoplasms involve the oesophagus through direct invasion, via mediastinal nodes and hematogenous spread in 45%, 35% and 20% respectively [60]. Benign peptic stricture and irradiation injuries may mimic oesophageal malignancy. Fibre-endoscopy should always be performed in order to verify the radiological finding.

Achalasia is characterized by absence of or incomplete LES relaxation and defect peristalsis in the oesophageal body. The barium contrast pools in the oesophagus, which may dilate grotesquely. During fluoroscopic observation an intermittent passage of contrast is seen through the narrow sphincter region, resembling a 'rat's tail', which distinguishes the condition from a malignant condition [61].

Computed Tomography

Pre-operative staging of oesophageal cancer with CT is problematic and corresponds badly with the TNM system and patient outcome. Pre-operative CT may classify patients into different groups, to surgery for attempted cure, for palliative bypass, or to chemotherapy [62]. However there are many diagnostic pitfalls. CT criteria for diagnosing direct mediastinal invasion include both ventral displacement of the trachea and indentation from behind during inspiration of the thoracic trachea and mainstem bronchus [23].

Direct invasion of the aorta occurs in less than 2%. Since the oesophagus normally abuts the aorta and due to the normal lack of fat plane between the organs, it is difficult to prove direct invasion by CT. No tumour invasion is likely if the area of aortic contact is 45 or less of the aortic circumference (Fig. 5), but predictable if 90 or more is engaged [63].

Pericardial invasion is difficult to evaluate as intervening fat planes may or may not exist. Invasion is likely if a fat plane is obliterated at the tumour site.

Mediastinal adenopathy is diagnosed when large nodes are located outside the proper tumour. Small lymph nodes, whether benign or malignant, cannot be predicted by CT. Intra-abdominal lymph node metastases should be considered when soft tissue masses larger than 8 mm are seen around the coeliac axis and in the gastrohepatic ligament. Differentials like local varices should be considered [64]. Published data in the surgical literature show poor results with CT staging due to low success rate in detecting mediastinal invasion [65] or abdominal lymph node metastases [66]. Data summarized from six roentgenographic CT series of unquestionable methodology and statistics indicate CT to be more accurate in predicting mediastinal invasion than adenopathy [62]. The sensitivity for depicting mediastinal invasion ranged from 88-94%, and in detecting lymphadenopathy around 48%.

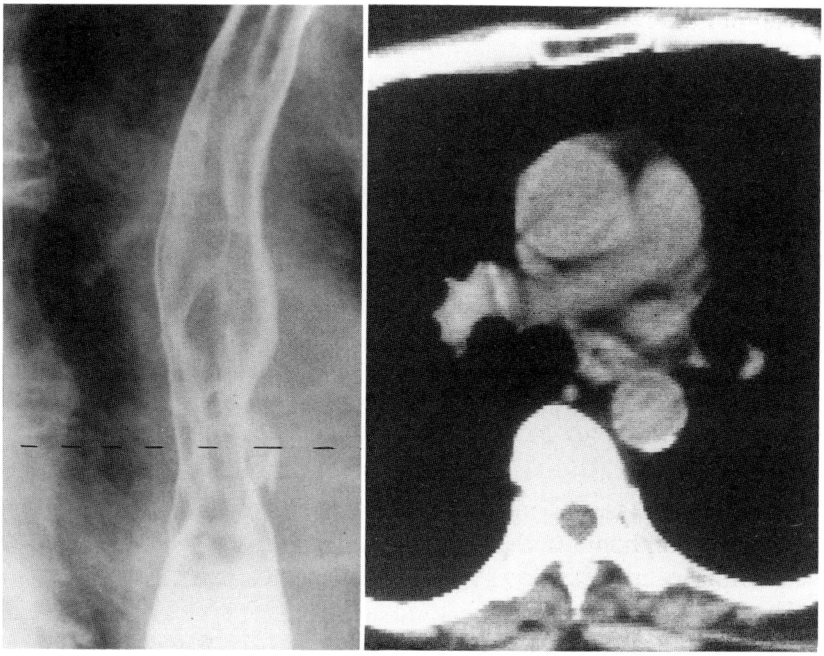

Figure 5. *Infiltrating oesophageal carcinoma with a deep ulcer. (a) The lumen is slightly narrowed and the mucosal folds broadened. (b) CT at the level indicated in (a) shows normal fat planes around the thickened oesophageal walls. Air is seen in the centre of the tumour.*

If pretreatment CT is compared with the long-term patient survival, a mean survival time of 445 days was found for patients showing no CT evidence of tumour spread to organs or nodes, compared to 127 days for patients with such spread [67].

MRI See page 9

Endoluminal Ultrasonography

EUS is performed with the balloon-contact method and although the oesophagus has no serosal layer, five layers are usually seen, the fifth being the fibrous tissue of the mediastinum. EUS compared to surgery has shown a high grade of conformity as regards resectability, local invasion and tumour growth in local lymph nodes, with an accuracy around 85% [68].

Tumour extension through the different EUS-layers of the wall was compared to histology in nine cases with an accuracy of 78% [53]. Compared to CT and histology of resected specimens, EUS is superior in evaluating depth of tumour and regional metastases in cases with early and non-resectable carcinomas, with an overall accuracy of 89% [69]. EUS in patients with occlusive disease is still difficult due to instrumentation. In others, EUS is a significant method for determining depth of tumour invasion and local adenopathy, but also a method for monitoring chemo-radiation and laser therapy.

Malignant Lesions of the Stomach

Malignant neoplasms consist of adenocarcinoma in up to 95%, with 3% being lymphoma and 2% leiomyosarcoma. In Western countries the number of afflicted patients is decreasing.

The 1962 classification of early gastric carcinoma originates from Japan where the disease is highly prevalent. By definition early carcinoma, being polypoid, flat or ulcerated (types I-III), is confined to the mucosa and submucosa, not extending beyond the muscularis propria, regardless of the macroscopic appearance, lymph nodes and distant metastases. Borrmann's classification describes advanced carcinoma:

Type 1 being a large polypoid mass lesions
Type 2 an irregular ulcer with sharply circumscribed margins, 'Carman's meniscus sign'
Type 3 a large ulcer with surrounding irregular tumour infiltration
Type 4 a diffuse infiltrated, linitis plastica type carcinoma.

Barium Examination

During the initial, erect phase of the examination the first swallows of barium stream along the gastric minor side and pool in the gastric corpus. In the supine position the barium spreads over the dorsal mucosal lining and a mucosa relief pattern is seen. Often lesions are diagnosed by these images alone.

Routinely the patient is asked to ingest another 70-100 ml of barium contrast to fill every recess. Adjusted external compression is applied so that any luminal lesion stand out as a filling defect and any ulcer as an unexpected collection of barium. Double contrast examination follows (Fig. 6), which includes images in different patient positions. In the semierect position the barium is spread out and forms a large but shallow, transparent pool, which is easily penetrated even by a minimal intraluminal lesion [70,71].

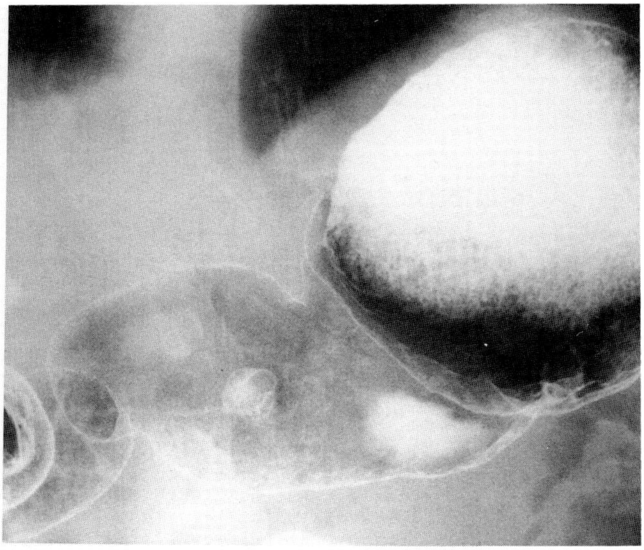

Figure 6. *Barium meal showing two 1-cm diameter gastric polyps. The base of the antral polyp is irregular and biopsies revealed severe dysplasia.*

Early Gastric Carcinoma (EGC)

Gastroparesis makes detailed analysis of the surface pattern and detection of early, flat type II malignant lesions easier. These are granular or lobular with notched contours, delineating the EGC from the normal pattern of areae gastricae (Fig. 7). Elevated early carcinoma type I is revealed on compression films, while depressed, type III early carcinoma demands analysis of converging folds on air-barium films. The shallow depression has irregular margins secondary to interruption, clubbing and fusion of mucosal folds [72].

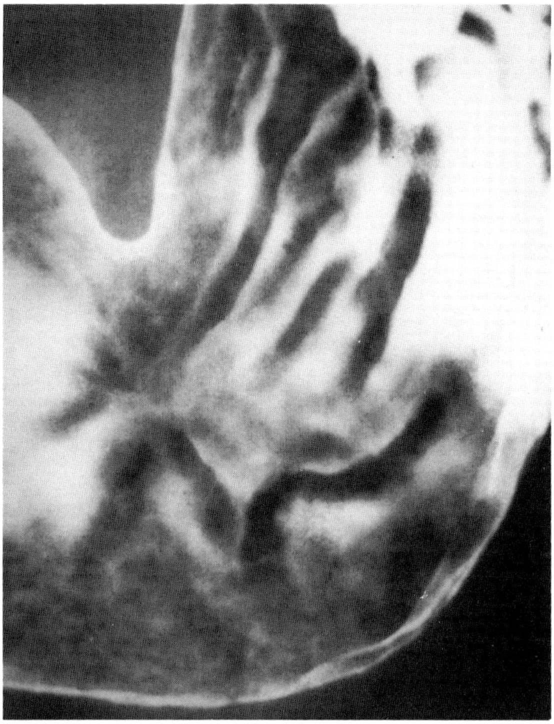

Figure 7. *Slightly elevated EGC, type IIa, with notched contours, convergence and clubbing of mucosal folds. (Courtesy of Professor A. Lunderquist, Lund).*

Again postural manoeuvres must be performed so that the barium agent does not leave the shallow depression [73].

Advanced Cancer

Histologically advanced lesions have penetrated the muscularis propria or further. Radiology of these tumours does not differ from those arising in the rest of the GI tract. However, diffuse infiltrative carcinoma typically involves the gastric antrum, which is greatly narrowed (Fig. 8). The overlying mucosa looks normal endoscopically and the stenotic lumen may be misinterpreted at endoscopy as a pyloric ring. Furthermore, the diffusely infiltrated linitis plastica type of carcinoma without a tumour edge easily passes endoscopic detection, even if shrinkage involves the stomach as a whole.

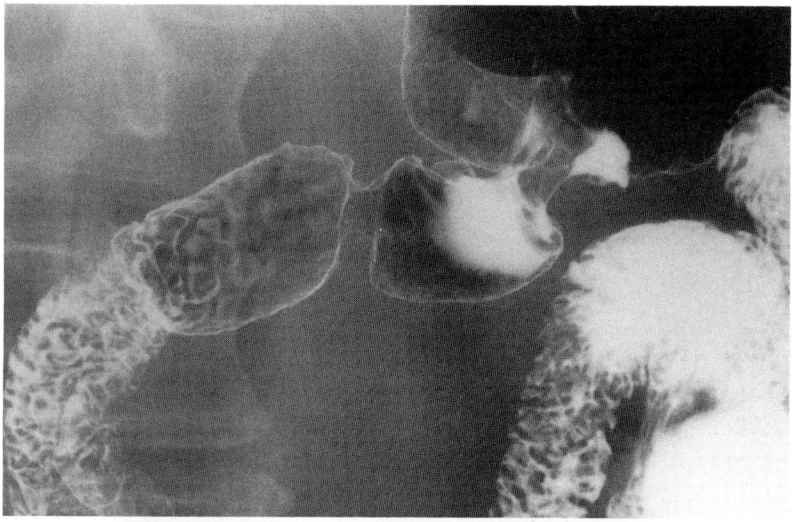

(a)

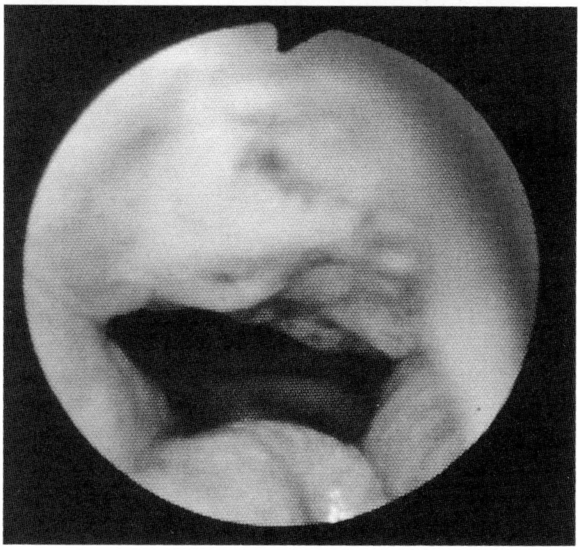

(b)

Figure 8. *Stricturing carcinoma of the gastric antrum with a large ulcer seen on both (a) double-contrast and (b) endoscopic images. In (b) The ulcer is seen at 12 o'clock.*

Computed Tomography

The depth of the cardia appears greater than the proper gastric wall due to its inclined orientation. In patients with hiatus hernia the cardiac wall thickness is still more pronounced. On transverse scans the normal oesophago-gastric junction creates a small bulge close to the cardia and should be interpreted as a normal finding.

Primary carcinoma is recognized as a mural, localized, circumferential or diffuse thickening of more than 6 mm (Fig. 9). Transmural extension is likely if the wall measures more than 2 cm [74]. CT staging in gastric cancer has proved to be of limited value with an accuracy of around 70% [75].

The sensitivity of detection of regional adenopathy with CT is around 65% with a specificity of 60. The sensitivity of diagnosing pancreatic invasion is low [76].

CT in patients with gastric cancer ought to be restricted to the detection of metastases and to follow-up after previous gastric resection [77], and is recommended in patients at bad surgical risk, where it can be a great help to decide whether or not surgery should be performed [26].

Transabdominal Ultrasonography

Depending on type and location of the lesion a large upper quadrant mass, a non-specific target sign or a local thickening of the gastric wall due to tumour (Fig. 9) and/or surrounding inflammatory changes may be observed [78,79]. When a lesion is detected by US it is normally advanced, extending through deep layers of the wall, exogastrically. Gastric retention is seen in cases with stenosis.

US may be used for tumour staging. The sensitivity for evaluating direct invasion and for detecting metastases to lymph nodes is up to 75% [81]. pre-operative US examination in order to rule out visible tumour spread to adjacent and distant organs may guide the clinician in planning the appropriate therapy.

Primary Gastric Lymphoma (PGL)

Patients with primary non-Hodgkin's lymphoma confined to the gastrointestinal tract are few [82]. Although these patients often have had symptoms for a long time, they lack palpable lymph nodes until late in the disease [83,84], and are therefore difficult to diagnose in

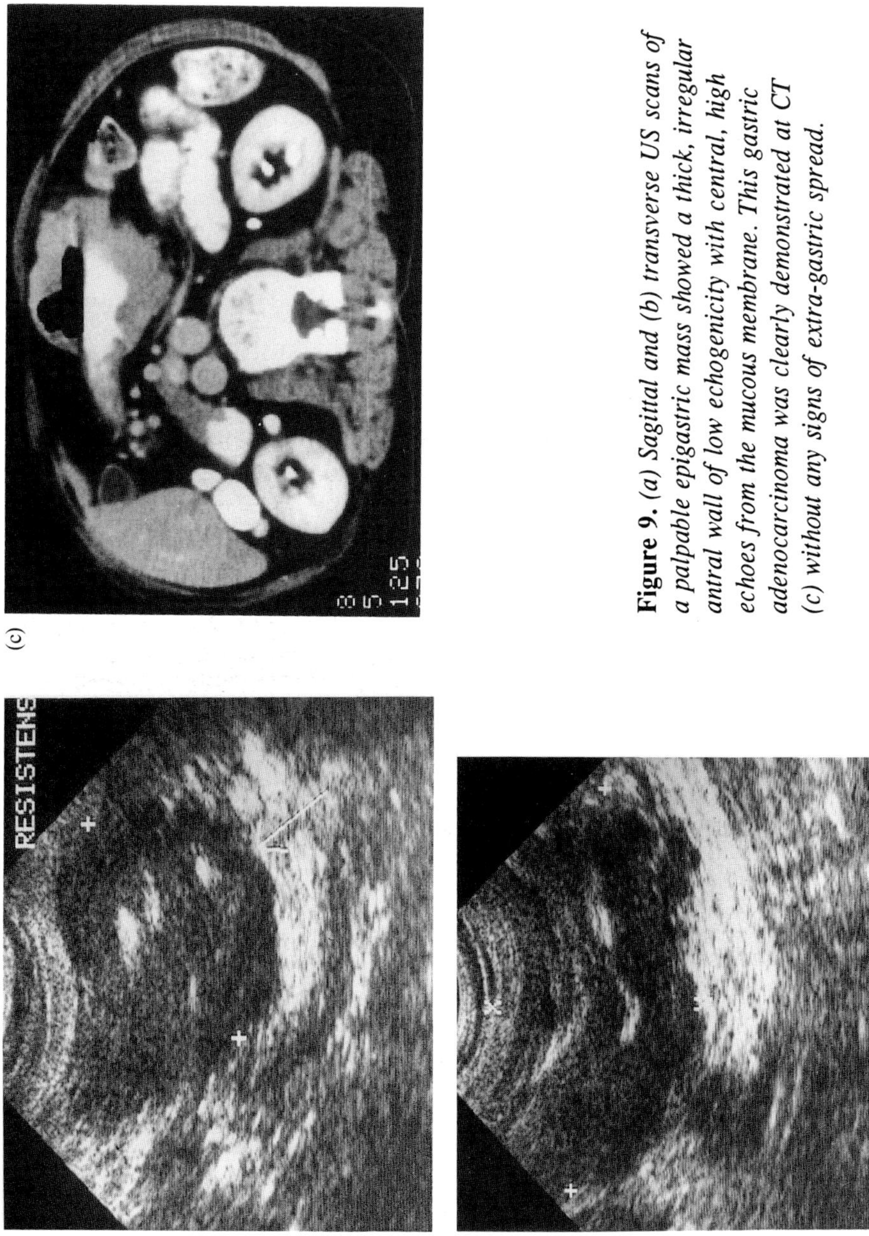

Figure 9. *(a) Sagittal and (b) transverse US scans of a palpable epigastric mass showed a thick, irregular antral wall of low echogenicity with central, high echoes from the mucous membrane. This gastric adenocarcinoma was clearly demonstrated at CT (c) without any signs of extra-gastric spread.*

early stages [85]. Barium examination of the stomach will readily disclose a lesion in these patients but fails in diagnostic accuracy. Biopsy specimens or exfoliative cytology have to be obtained to reveal the true nature of the disease [86,87].

Radiology

The radiographic signs of PGL are based on two features which are seen already in early disease, namely a mucosal elevation and multiple erosions or small ulcers [88,89].

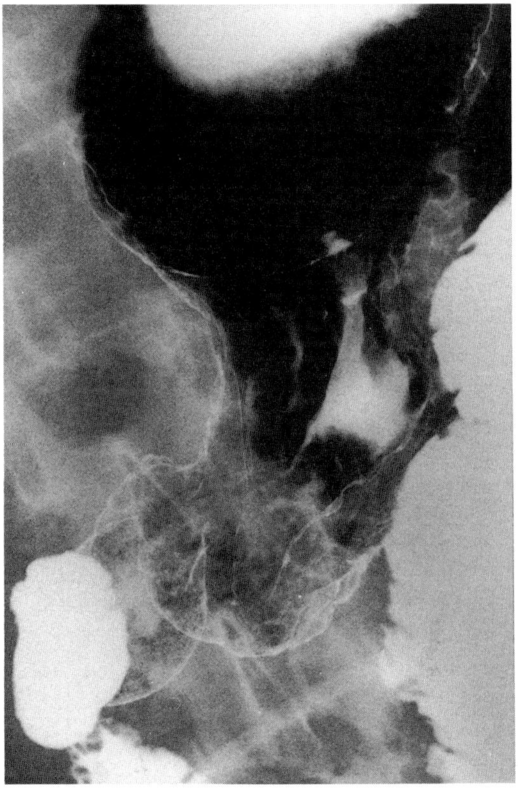

Figure 10. *Double-contrast examination showing swollen folds, multiple erosions and narrowing of the gastric corpus and antrum. The whole organ specimen revealed primary gastric lymphoma.*

In established disease there are three main radiological features adhered to its classification: Firstly, half of all lesions are infiltrative with tortuous, prominent folds resembling cobblestones (Fig. 10); secondly, one third of the lesions are mainly ulcerative, with radiating normal or thickened folds, and thirdly, a polypoid type of lesion, often with a large extragastric portion. All three types of lesions may exhibit multiple small ulcers [90,91].

The distribution of PGL when compared to gastric adenocarcinoma is somewhat more orientated towards proximal parts, while carcinomas are more often found in the antral region. PGL tends to be more extensive and bulky [92]. Sometimes a rapid reduction in tumour size after irradiation has been encountered in patients with PGL of the reticulum-cell type of sarcoma.

Computed Tomography

No specific CT sign differentiates lymphoma from other mural lesions of the stomach. However lymphoma tend to be more extensive and may cause wall thickness of more than 4 cm without concomitant infiltration of perigastric fat planes [93].

Transabdominal Ultrasound

US in gastric lymphoma is non-specific, although two signs are said to be helpful in differentiating these: a mass lesion with a spokewheel pattern, caused by the echogenic mucosal surfaces separating the tumefied gastric folds, and a homogeneously infiltrated, hypoechoic wall [94].

Leiomyosarcoma of the Stomach

Leiomyosarcoma is the most frequent submucosal tumour of the stomach and is most often found in the proximal gastric part. Leiomyosarcoma are generally irregular and huge in size and occur in the fifth and sixth decade of life. Often the blood supply is insufficient, causing tumour necrosis and cavitation (Fig. 11) [95].

Radiology

Roentgenographically leiomyosarcoma are 2-10 cm, spheric lesions and smooth when small. Frequently only a minor portion is intragastric. This part is usually ulcerated in large lesions due to tumour necrosis and may then resemble an ulcerated adenocarcinoma (Fig. 12). On CT these tumours are often large with a significant

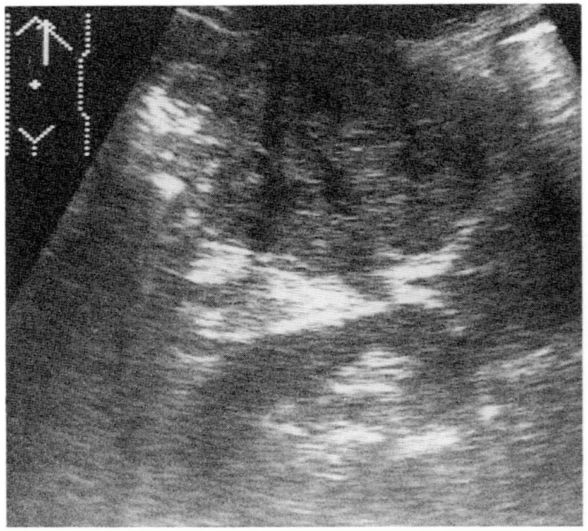

(a)

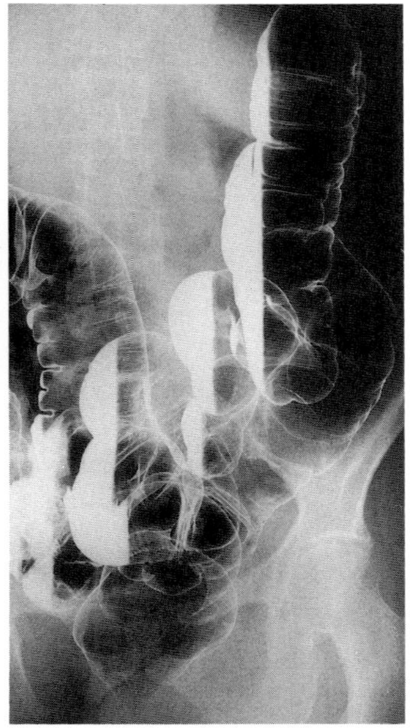

(b)

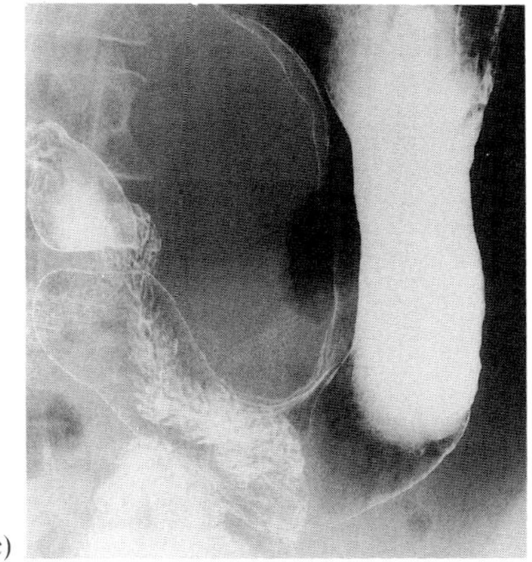

(c)

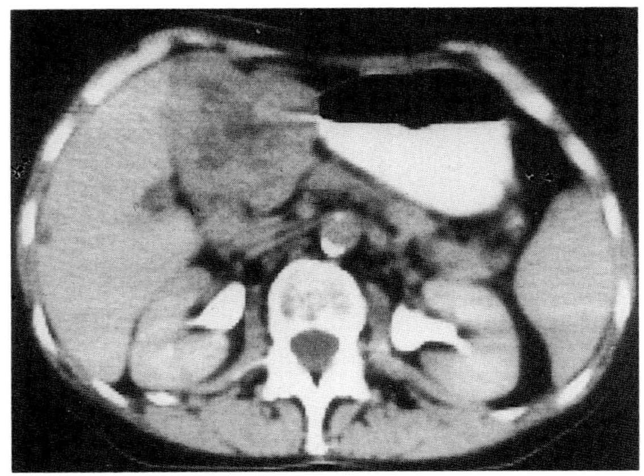

(d)

Figure 11. *(a) US of this large epigastric mass with homogenous echoes suggested a colonic origin. (b) Colonography was normal but a soft tissue mass was seen deforming the air-filled stomach, causing an indentation along the whole minor curvature (c). (d) In spite of low central attenuation values, no malignancy was found in this leiomyoma.*

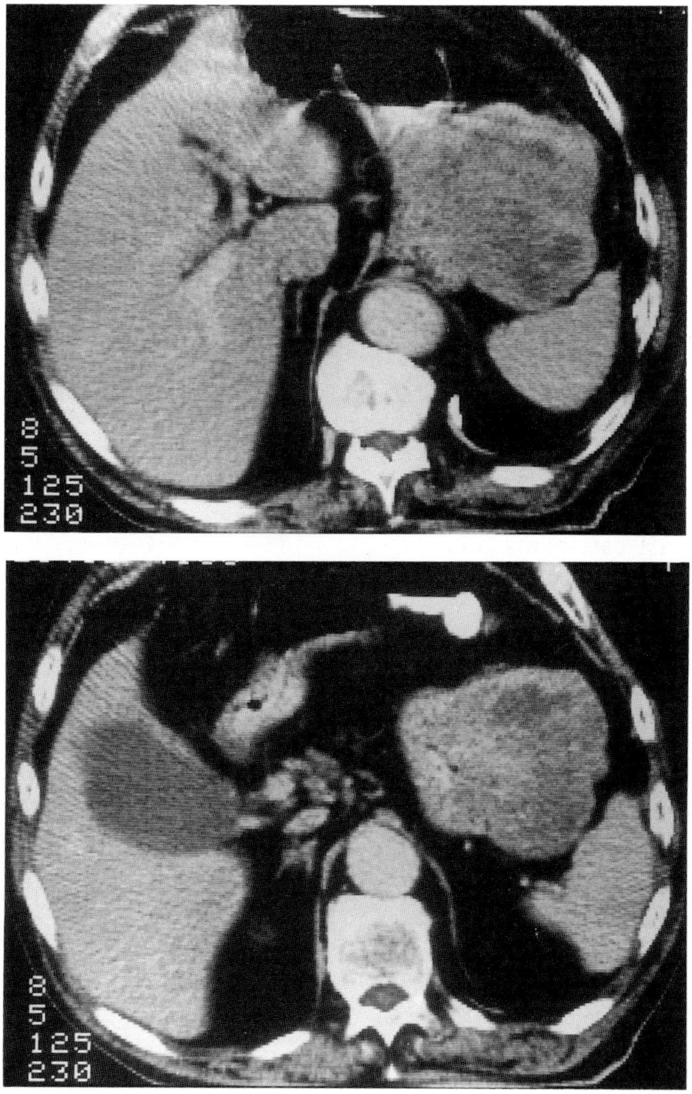

(a)

(b)

Figure 12. *Leiomyosarcoma (a) adjacent and (b) compressing the gastric corpus. Tumour size and varying low attenuation values predict malignancy.*

necrosis and may then resemble an ulcerated adenocarcinoma (Fig. 12). On CT these tumours are often large with a significant extragastric component which distinguishes them from adenocarcinoma and lymphoma. The attenuation values vary due to necrosis. The tumour attachment to the gastric wall is sometimes indistinct [96].

On US a sarcoma may be suggested if a solid mass lesion is found close to an intestinal lumen and with both hyperechoic tissue and areas of liquefficative necrosis [97]. These features at US and CT are helpful in establishing the correct differential diagnosis. Benign leiomyomas normally gives rise to homogenous echoes (Fig. 1) and attenuation values, with necrotic, malignant lesions have uneven CT values and nodular, low echoes (Fig. 12) [98].

Metastases to the Stomach

The incidence of metastases to the stomach is very low. Metastases from breast carcinoma and malignant melanoma (Fig. 13) are most

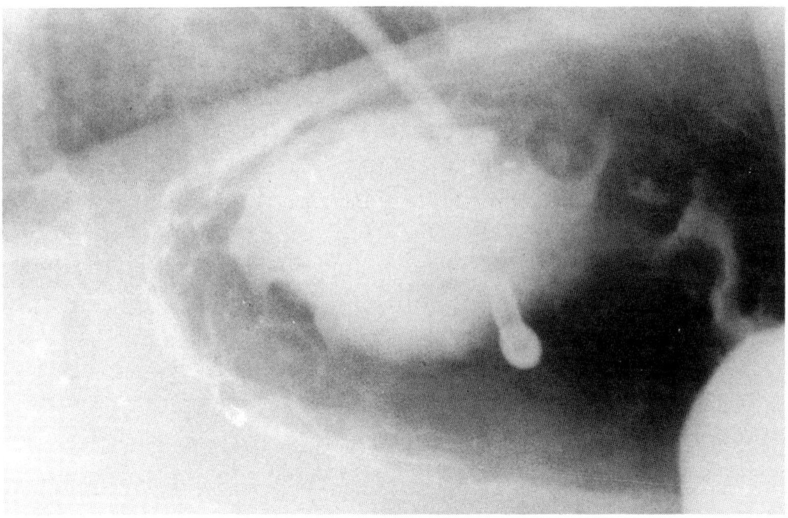

Figure 13. *'Target sign' metastases from a malignant melanoma with central ulcerations in the gastric fundus.*

often encountered. They cause multiple filling defects, located in the submucosa and eventually ulcerate when large in size, creating a target sign. This would again be identified on US. On CT a polypoid, local wall thickening may be indicative of metastasis [78].

Small Bowel Malignancy

The most frequent small bowel malignancy is the carcinoid, seen in up to 40% [99]. Carcinoma is seen in 25%, lymphoma in 20%, while 15% constitute other malignant lesions.

Carcinoid Tumour

The carcinoid can arise wherever enterochromaffin cells are normally found, usually anywhere in the GI tract. These tumours originate in the appendix, 45%, in the small bowel, 25%, and in the rectum, 15%. It causes thickening and fibrosis of the underlying muscles and finally obstruction. the malignant potential of these tumours is in direct proportion to their number and size. Some carcinoids produce bradykinin and serotonin. When these hormones are released to the systemic venous system - usually by liver metastases - they cause the carcinoid syndrome: abdominal cramps, diarrhoea, flushing, cyanosis and stenosis of the tricuspid and pulmonary values [100].

In a large review of 154 patients with carcinoid tumour radiology had limited value in detecting the primary lesion [101]. It is also of interest to mention that one-third of the patients have another, associated malignant lesion, which is more likely to cause the patients death [102].

Radiology

A carcinoid starts as a mural nodule and is incidentally found as a submucosal, sharply defined lesion in the distal ileum. It may form the leading part of an intussusception. Large lesions infiltrate the surroundings, cause bowel stricture and kinking of the loops, separated by a mesenteric mass (Fig. 14). The bowel wall may be tethered by the carcinoid, creating spicula formation of the mucosal lining and straightening of the folds. Due to ischaemic necrosis large tumours may cause intramural bleeding, seen as typical thumb-printings on barium examinations.

Small tumours are probably best depicted by enteroclysis while advanced disease is as well ruled out with single-contrast follow-through technique. Retroperitoneal fibrosis and Crohn's disease may mimic the desmoplastic reaction of a carcinoid malignancy.

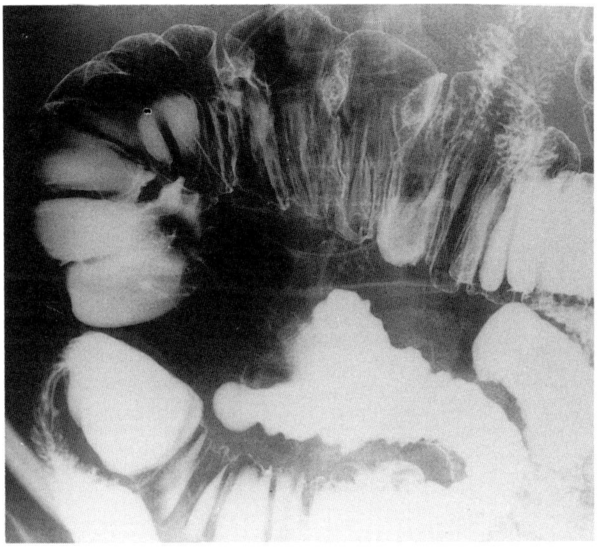

Figure 14. *Large carcinoid in the ileo-caecal region with pre-stenotic ileal dilatation and desmoplastic reaction separating bowel loops. Note the deranged mucosal folds and spicula formation (Courtesy of Dr. Olle Ekberg, Malmö)*

When the tumour is confined intramurally, CT and transabdominal US-examinations are probably normal. Tumours with calcium deposits and those which have infiltrated the mesentery and caused a desmoplastic reaction are easily recognized on CT scans [103]. Metastases to liver and pancreas are disclosed either by CT or US (Fig. 15).

Adenocarcinoma

Half of all small bowel carcinomas are found in the duodenum (Fig.

16), and less than 15% in the distal ileum. There is a slight male preponderance. Like adenocarcinomas elsewhere in the GI tract they are annular and gradually cause obstruction. They tend to metastasize early to regional lymph nodes. Duodenal tumours are frequently polypoid with late symptoms. They have often invaded the mesenteric vessels by the time of diagnosis. In rare cases adenocarcinoma of the bulb may be misinterpreted as ulcers, characterized as unresponsive to medical therapy [104]. Small bowel carcinoma is also encountered in rare cases of regional enteritis. Malignancy should be suspected if an obstruction develops after years of quiescence [105,106].

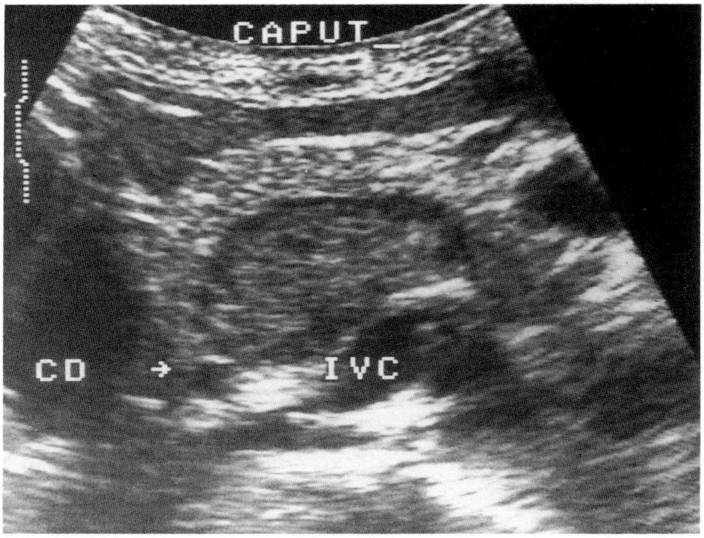

Figure 15. *Transverse US-scan of the pancreas showing a large metastasis of low echogenicity. FNP showed carcinoid cells. (IVC=inferior vena cava, CD=common bile duct).*

Radiographic features

With the enteroclysis technique an increasing number of small plaque-like lesions have been reported, as have polypoid adenocarcinomas [107]. Larger carcinomas are like those of the rest of the GI tract with well demarcated, circular or semicircular, short and irregular narrowings (Fig. 17) [108].

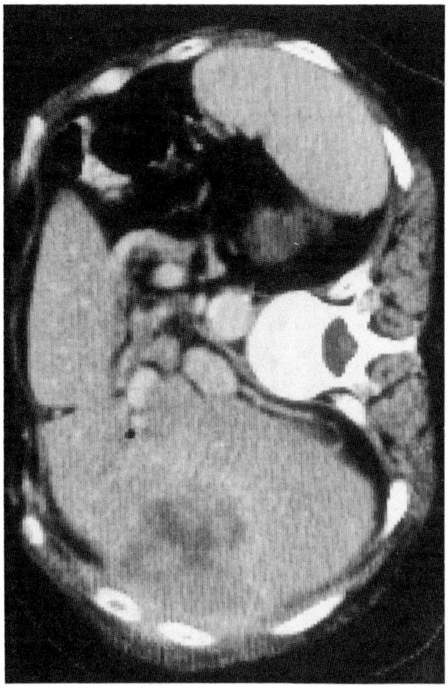

(b)

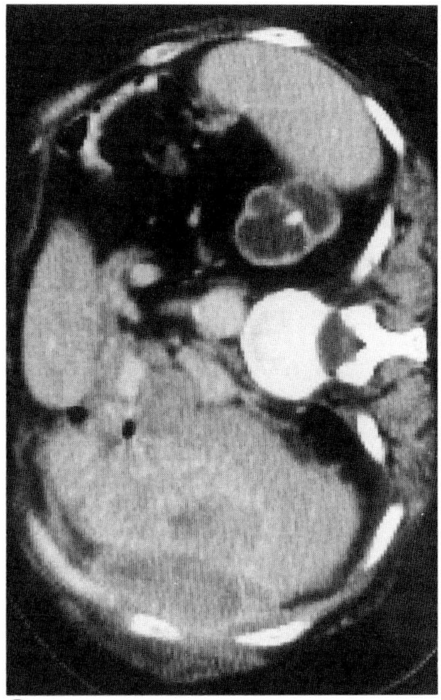

(c)

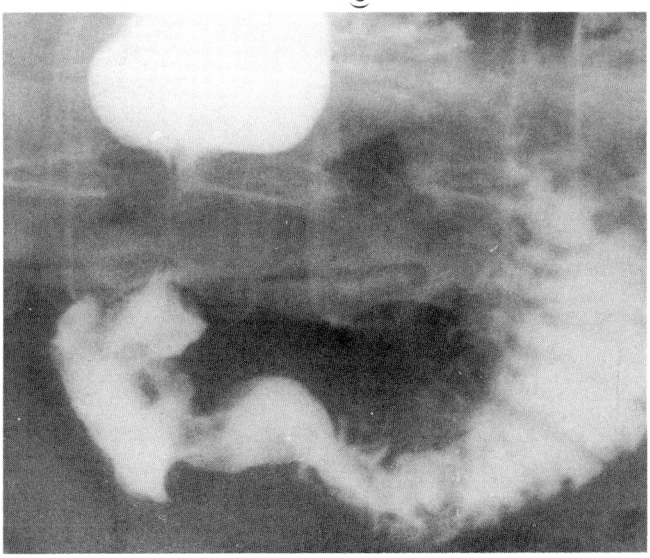

(a)

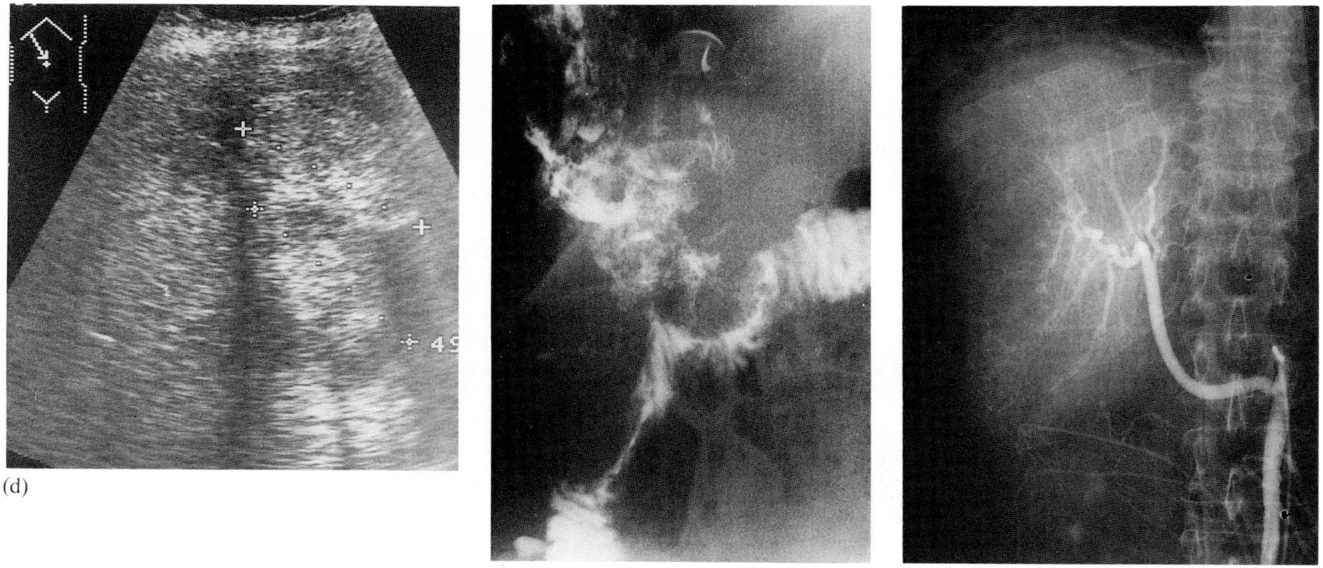

(d) (e) (f)

Figure 16. *(a) Obstructing adenocarcinoma of the descending duodenum. (b) Five years later CT of the liver showed a necrotic lesion with (c) an extrahepatic abscess involving the lateral abdominal wall. Gas is seen in the bile-ducts. (d) US showed two demarcated hepatic lesions with high echoes. Abscesses were suggested but FNP revealed the ventral lesion to be a metastasis of the duodenal carcinoma. Later a spontaneous fistula (e) was obvious. At pre-operative angiography no further lesions were seen apart from one causing deviation of intrahepatic arteries. (f) The increased distance to the lateral abdominal wall is still apparent.*

(a)

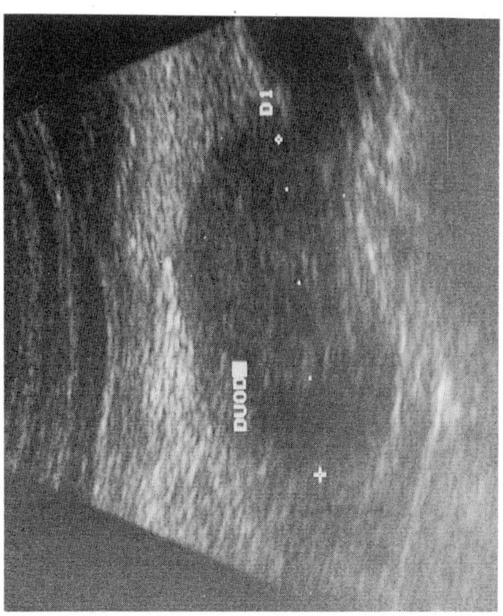

(b)

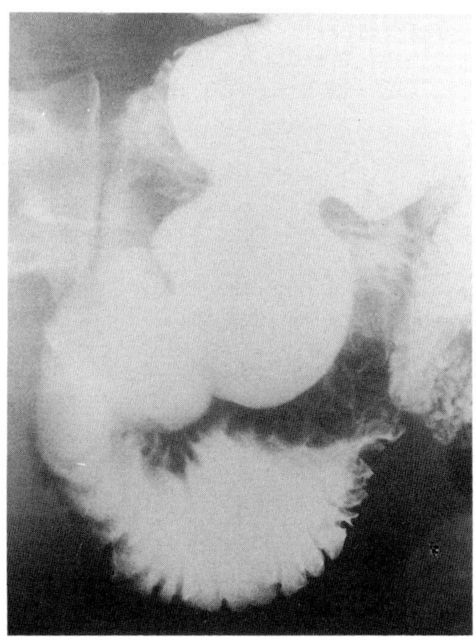

(c)

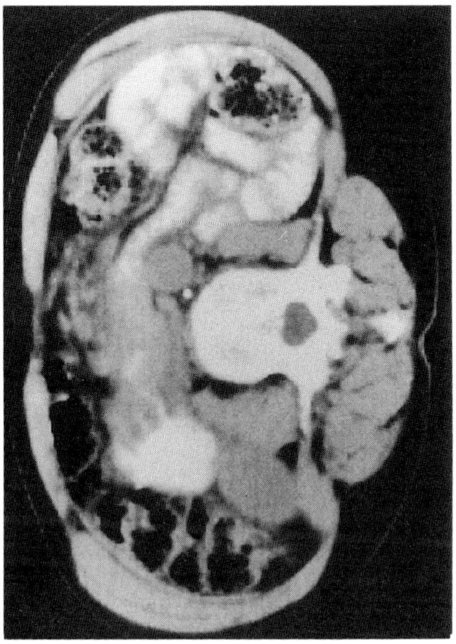

Figure 17. *(a) Transverse US scan of this palpable epigastric mass showed a kidney-like lesion. A gastrointestinal malignancy was suggested although no central, high echoes were found. (b) Follow-up examination showed a carcinoma of the duodenum, which is seen to envelope and obstruct the lumen, causing a pre-stenotic pooling of contrast (c).*

Rarely extensive bowel-wall thickening with ulceration is seen simulating lymphoma. These carcinomas may readily be shown by US and CT, but usually these modalities reveal only large lymph nodes late in the disease. At CT dilated bowel segments proximal to the tumour may indicate the site of a small, obstructing carcinoma [109].

Lymphoma

Lymphoma is the most common small bowel tumour in childhood and again seen in patients aged around 65. Lymphoma is usually part of a systemic involvement and presents with multiple submucosal nodules, mural infiltration, polypoid lesions, or as an endo/exo-enteric form with excavation and fistula [110]. Lymphoma may be secondary to long-standing coeliac disease.

The most frequent site of lymphomas is in the distal ileum. Regional lymph nodes are frequently involved and every second patient with non-Hodgkin's lymphoma have mesenteric invasion with extraluminal masses, rarely seen in those with Hodgkin's disease.

Radiology

On barium examination multiple nodules of varying size are seen as filling defects, sometimes with central ulcerations. The infiltrative form of lymphoma is seen as a narrowing of the bowel wall with thick or effaced valvulae conniventes, often in more than one area. Large, irregular collections of barium in a widened segment denote an 'aneurysmal dilatation' in a patient with the endo/exo-enteric form of intestinal lymphoma (Fig. 18). A polypoid lymphoma may act as the lead point for an intussusception and cause dynamic small bowel obstruction [111].

Computed Tomography

On CT the infiltrative form causes a non-specific thickening of the bowel wall and its mucosal folds. This thickening cannot *per se* be distinguished from other causes such as bleeding or enteritis. However, multiloculated lesions associated with enlarged lymph nodes and lesions in the liver, spleen and adrenals suggest the swollen folds and thick bowel wall to be caused by lymphoma [109]. Mesenteric infiltration is shown by CT as bulky, multilobulated masses, displacing bowel and causing obstruction. A typical sign of mesenteric involvement is the 'sandwich sign' when enlarged lymph nodes are seen embracing the mesenteric vessels [112]. Sometimes areas of low attenuation are found indicating tumour necrosis.

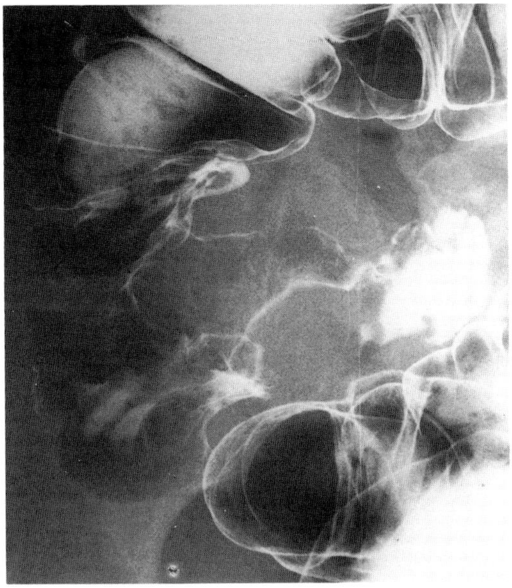

Figure 18. *Ileo-caecal lymphoma with aneurysmal dilatation, short narrowings of the ileum and mucosal ulcers.*

Transabdominal Ultrasound

Three different types of lymphomatous appearance have been reported: Small anechoic intramural or mesenteric lesions representing nodal involvement; an exo-enteric mass on the mesenteric border of the bowel; and a large mass with a target-like pattern. Often the lesion is not identified until large. It is then recognized as an irregular mass with complex echogenicity and with internal echoes due to necrosis, also reflecting dense areas of intraluminal mucus [113].

Sarcoma

The most common form arises from smooth muscle. Abdominal pain and intestinal bleeding bring the patient to the doctor, usually when the tumour is palpable and has undergone ulceration and necrosis.

Radiography

Usually the tumour appears on barium study and on CT as an extra-intestinal lesion which separates and stretches adjacent loops; when the sarcoma ulcerates, barium is collected in cavities of different sizes, and on CT necrotic masses have low attenuation values. There are no reliable radiographic signs of tumour differentiation. Large tumour size, necrosis and lymph node involvement suggest malignancy [114].

Metastases

Secondary involvement of the small intestine occurs by hematogenous spread of pulmonary and mammary carcinoma (Fig. 19) and malignant melanoma (Fig. 20), by direct invasion of neoplasms of adjacent organs and intraperitoneal seeding of tumours of gastrointestinal and ovarian origin. On barium studies metastases are evident as mural filling defects of varying size. Although annular malignancies as a rule are diagnosed as primary small bowel cancers, metastases from cancers of the colon, lungs and cervix as well as from melanoma, sarcoma, lymphoma and carcinoid tumours, may present themselves as such [115]. In dependent parts of the abdominal cavity metastases are recognized as serosal indentations. Of these the classic Blumer's shelf represents a secondary tumour deposit in the pouch of Douglas on large bowel radiograms [116].

On CT metastases may cause a diffuse bowel wall thickening and bowel encasement within a large mesenteric mass, or secondary bowel lesions in proximity to an adjacent organ neoplasm.

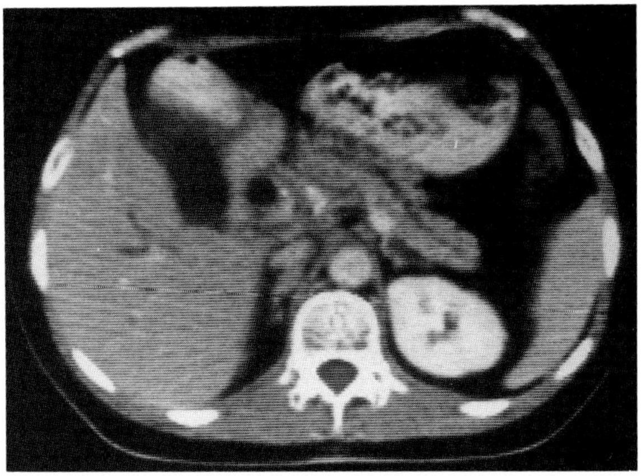

Figure 19. *Secondary dilatation of both pancreatic and bile ducts due to a mammary carcinoma metastasis to the papillary region. Gastric retention is also seen.*

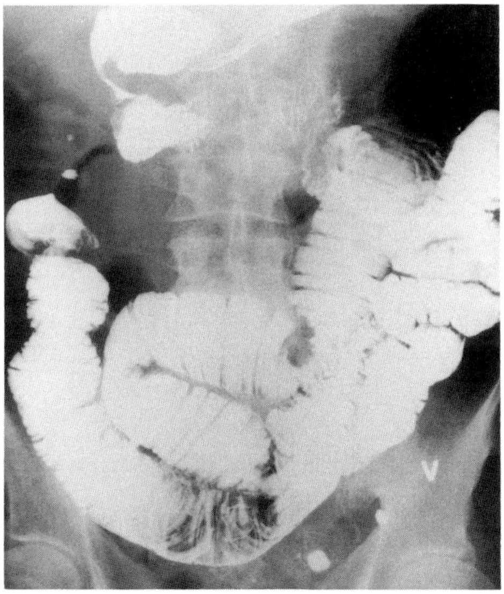

Figure 20. *Follow-up in a patient with malignant melanoma. Multiple filling defects are seen in mid and low ileal loops, as are deformities of the duodenum. A soft tissue mass indentation of the right hepatic flexure is also seen. Multiple metastases were found at autopsy. (Courtesy of Dr O. Ekberg, Malmö.)*

Malignancy of the Colorectum

Adenocarcinoma

The vast majority of large bowel neoplasms are adenocarcinomas, 75% of which occur in the recto-sigmoid region with 4-5% being multiple [117]. Contemporarily a shift in number of carcinomas towards the right hemicolon is documented [118,119] which has implications on choice of diagnostic procedure.

Also, patients with hereditary non-polyposis colorectal cancer, HNPCC, Lynch syndrome I, have site-specific cancer of the proximal colon. Usually the onset is before the age of 45 and these patients often exhibit multiple synchronous and metachronous colon tumours. Others, referred to as Lynch syndrome II, with this syndrome are susceptible to other neoplasms, especially endometrial and ovarian cancer. Approximately 6% of patients with colorectal cancer will have HNPCC, while less than 1% will belong to the familial polyposis syndrome, FAP [120-123].

If a Lymch syndrome patient is identified, regular surveillance for identification and removal of colon polyps is mandatory for proper management of the patient and recommended for his first-degree relatives. Up to 70% of polyps in these patients are also located in the right hemicolon [124].

Peak incidence of colon cancer occurs normally in the seventh decade, with less than 20% of patients diagnosed under the age of 50. At the time of diagnosis half the patients will have regional and 20% distant metastases. The incidence varies greatly with the geographic region, with high rates found in Western Europe, Canada, New Zealand, Argentina, Uruguay and the northern-eastern United States [125].

For a long time the patient with colon cancer has no symptoms before it manifests itself with pain and discharge of blood and mucus in the stools. Progressive obstruction gives rise to abdominal distension, predominantly seen in cases with carcinoma of the left hemicolon. However, dynamic ileus may be seen both in patients with a large polypoid neoplasm on the right side of the colon leading an intussusception and in whom the ileocaecal valve is involved.

It is difficult radiographically to exclude a neoplastic lesion in a segment with diverticular disease. Patients with colicky pain and fever are clinically more likely primarily to suffer from diverticulitis which, although unlikely, may hide a malignant lesion. It is therefore very important to perform a follow-up study in these patients. Transabdominal US may be helpful in these cases as inflammatory lesions tend to be axially more extensive and of lower echogenicity compared to colon carcinoma.

Radiology

The pre-malignant life of a later adenocarcinoma is roughly one decade. During this period the disease is curable through early detection, i.e. cancer prevention. Unfortunately the diagnostic shortcoming of X-ray and colonoscopy here coincide, i.e. in the regions of the sigmoid colon and caecum, where most of the neoplasms are located. Consequently the radiologist should always demand an optimal barium enema study in order to minimize pitfalls [126].

Premalignant Lesions

The natural history of untreated colonic polyps reveals a cumulative risk of cancer at the polyp site of 2.5-24% after 5-20 years respectively [127]. Histopathologically, the vast majority of pre-malignant neoplasms of the large bowel are tubular adenomas [128]. These are usually pedunculated and polypoid in shape, with histologically aggravating dysplasia. In single-contrast barium enema (SC-BE) these lesions are detected on tangential views but are hidden in the barium column on *en face* views when small. On double-contrast barium-enema (DC-BE) even a minor polyp appears as a barium coated sphere, ovoid or ring-like and as a radiolucency when dependant positioned in a pool of barium [129,130].

The head of a pedunculated polyp is usually located dependent to the wall attachment of the stalk. The polyp head moves according to the length of the stalk. On DC-BE the stalk appears as a filling defect in the pool of barium and as a tube when suspended. On tangential views the polyp with its stalk may give an impression of a broad based lesion and on vertical views as a target lesion, a bull's eye (Fig. 21) .

The incidence of carcinoma developing from a adenoma varies with type, size and duration. Malignant changes are found in approximately 5% of tubular adenomas as compared to 40% in villous ones [131]. The number of pre-malignant, villous adenomas is small. It

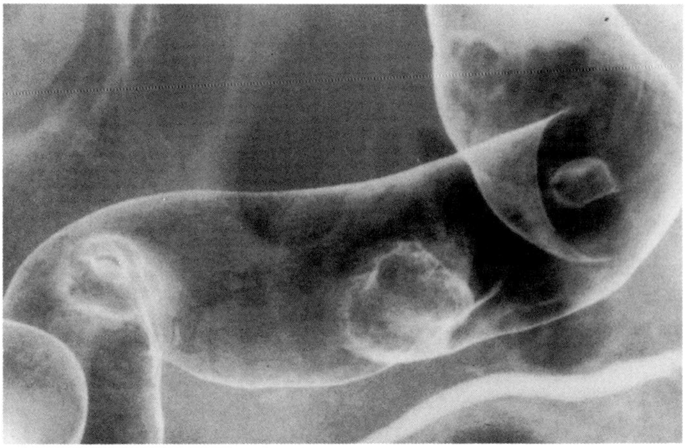

Figure 21. *Four polyps later removed colonoscopically. The proximal, stalked and the semipedunculated third polyps were adenomas, the large, irregular one an adenocarcinoma, and the flat, rectal a villous adenoma. The barium filled appendix vermiformis is seen in the right upper corner.*

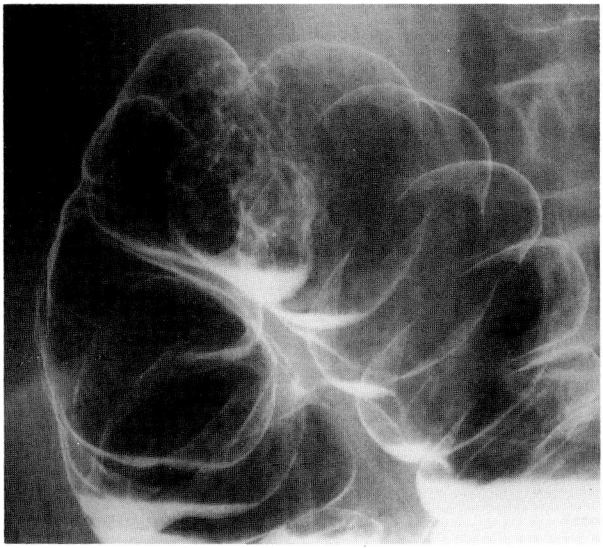

Figure 22. *Extensive, flat adenovillous carcinoma of the hepatic flexure.*

appears plaque-like, flat (Fig. 22) or as a broad-based polyp, usually in the right hemicolon or rectum [132,133].

En face flat such lesions have a mamillated, coarse reticular surface pattern with multiple rough nodules, hardly seen on SC-BE. Not until it is extensive will the tumour area appear elevated and rigid, creating a contour defect of the bowel wall [134]. The malignant potential of a villous adenoma is 10 times that of a stalked tubular adenoma, and every second lesion 2 cm^2 in size or more is a carcinoma [135].

In spite of the non-neoplastic nature of polyps in patients with Cronkhite-Canada syndrome, colorectal cancer in these has been reported [136]. The polyps are distributed in the entire gastrointestinal tract and histologically hamartoma-like, resembling broad-based juvenile polyps [137].

Hereditary Polyposis

Hereditary gastrointestinal polyposis syndrome is known since 1882 [138]. It is important that the radiologist recognizes this condition, as a strong suspicion should lead to screening for these lesions in family members. Together with Gardener's and Peutz-Jegher's syndromes, the familial polyposis syndrome is inherited in an autosomally dominant way, and shows no sexual predilection [139].

The familiar polyposis syndrome should be considered in young patients with polyps in the GI tract, although most young patients do not have a positive family history. Familial polyposis or Gardener's syndrome should also be considered in any patient with multiple polyps and in patients under the age of 40 with a colon carcinoma [140,141].

Adenocarcinoma

Radiographically four main characters of adenocarcinoma of the colon can be recognized: (1) annular constricting, (2) polypoid, (3) infiltrating and stenosing, and (4) ulcerative. Often multiple signs are present [125].

The early carcinoma is polypoid in shape (Fig. 21). Usually it ulcerates and appears then like a saddle carcinoma [106] (Fig. 23) before it grows into the most common, annular type carcinoma. It is often located in the transverse and left hemicolon. At the time of

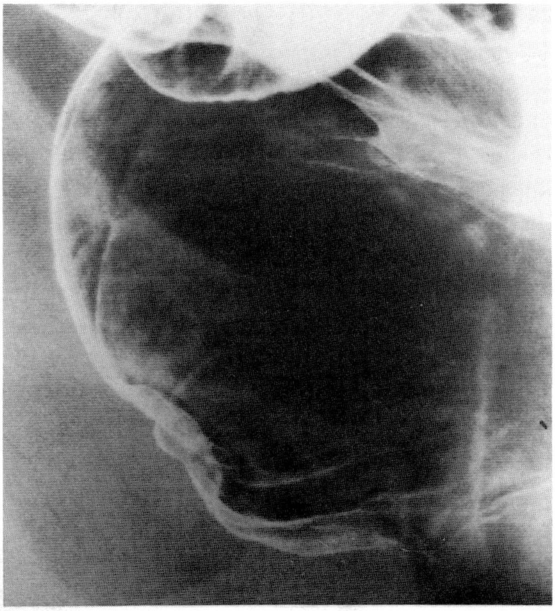

Figure 23. *Saddle carcinoma of the lower rectum causing mucosal retraction.*

diagnosis it measures around 4 cm in length, resembling an apple-core radiographically.

If the tumour predominantly grows intraluminally, it will show itself as a polypoid, bulky, cauliflower-like mass. It is often voluminous and sited in the right hemicolon. Histologically a mucoid adenocarcinoma is diagnosed. It causes the patient anemia from chronic blood loss. Faint calcifications may be recognized in the tumour itself as well as in regional metastases by CT [142].

A word of caution concerning lumen-sized caecal carcinomas. These may pass undetected when the tumour obstructs the caecal inlet. The 'missing' caecum in patients with a 'short' right hemicolon is recognized by the location of the ileo-caecal valve (Fig. 24). CT and US may be diagnostic in these cases.

Primary linitis plastica [143] is rarely encountered, and then in patients with ulcerative colitis for more than a decade. The tumour infiltrates submucosally over a considerable segment through the lymph vessels. Radiographically a rather long, tubular narrowing of the bowel lumen may be the only indication of its existence, mimicking a benign stricture. Consequently all such lesions should be considered scirrhous neoplasms until proven otherwise [144-146].

The predominantly ulcerative carcinoma of the large bowel is a rare entity. In the author's experience there is always a protruding rim of tumour tissue circumscribing the gross ulcer. Radiographically barium is collected in an excavation surrounded by a bank of tumour tissue.

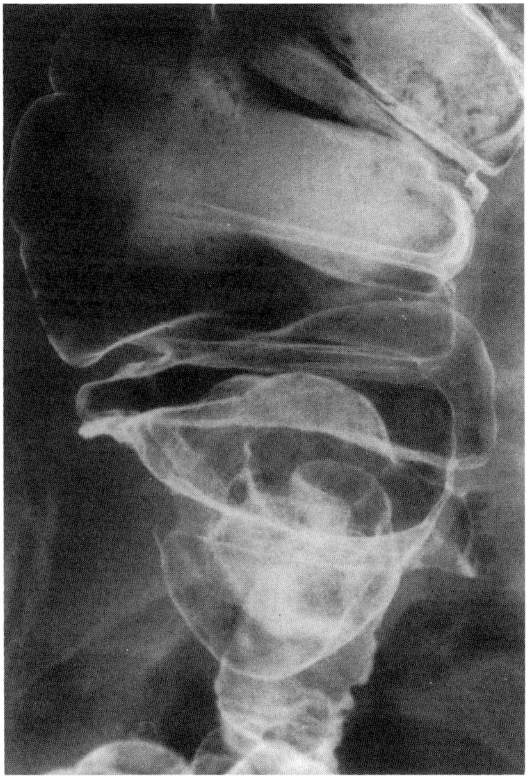

Figure 24. *Colonography fails to show the caecal lip of the Bauhinian valve due to a caecal carcinoma that almost entirely occupies the caecum.*

It is very important to look for the second, synchronous and, later on for the metachronous carcinoma, which are present in up to 6% of our patients [147].

Transabdominal Ultrasound

The normal air content of the large bowel hinders US diagnosis of neoplasms only occasionally. A voluminous and obstructive carcinoma, which causes a proximal fluid retention, is often detected. The tumour itself is hypoechoic with a central echogenic area caused by mucus or air (Fig. 25). In patients with right upper quadrant pain referred for US or CT of the liver and pancreas, we have occasionally found mass lesions from an adjacent origin: the locations of these were suggestive of their right flexure origin (Fig. 26) [148-150].

Computed Tomography

Whereas CT plays a minor role in evaluating colon carcinoma [151,152], it has proven its value in evaluating spread of rectal tumours and post-operative recurrences. Extensive tumour invasion into perirectal fat tissue and pelvic organs are reliably demonstrated as are enlarged local lymph nodes and distant metastases [20]. Limited tumour spread beyond the rectal wall is diagnosed with an accuracy of less than 70% and involvement of non-enlarged nodes is beyond the detection capabilities of CT [153-156].

In an effort to create CT-criteria comparable to the Dukes' classification, the CT stages of rectal malignancies are separated into four different staging groups: stage 1: the intraluminal mass; stage 2: the thickened rectal wall; cases with limited tumour spread to adjacent organs, stage 3a, or further spread to the sidewalls, stage 3b, and metastatic disease, stage 4 [157,158].

In early series the accuracy of CT staging of rectal tumours was reported to be very high, but when less advanced tumours of Dukes' stage A and B were included, the figures declined because microinvasion still cannot be detected with roentgen rays [153].

The perirectal fat is not always clear - even in healthy patients - due to normal vessels and nerve tissue. Usually vessels are seen when congested and areas of increased attenuations in inflammatory conditions. As a consequence, CT staging of rectal tumours of Dukes' stage C with only microscopically detectable perirectal invasion are less accurately diagnosed.

Definite invasion is diagnosed when a tumour mass is seen to extend into or to envelope adjacent pelvic organs. Then the perirectal fat planes in non-cachectic patients are obliterated and the afflicted muscles enlarged. Absence of a fat plane does, however, not signify

(a)

(b)

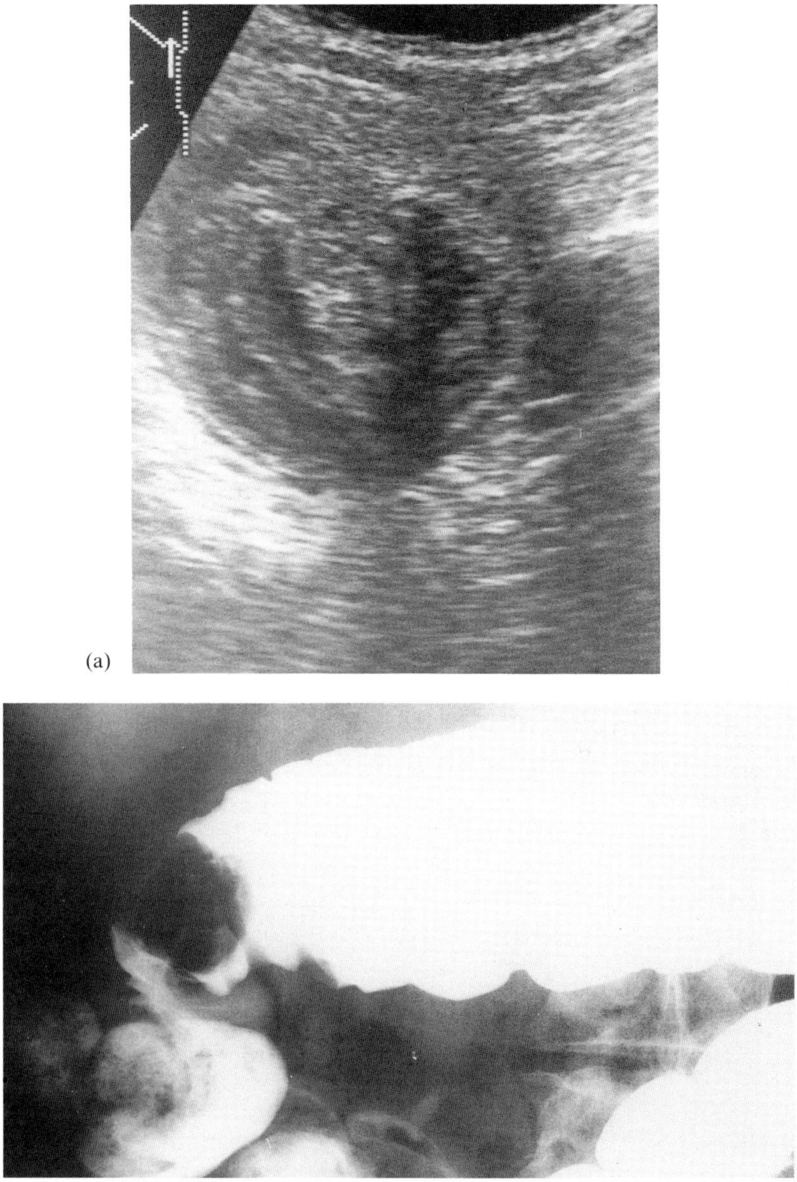

Figure 25. *(a) US in an elderly male with a palpable mass revealed a tumour with multiple layers and a colonic invagination was suggested. (b) The leading part of the invagination was a carcinoma, seen at SC-BE. (Courtesy of Dr P. Nilsson, Malmö.)*

(a)

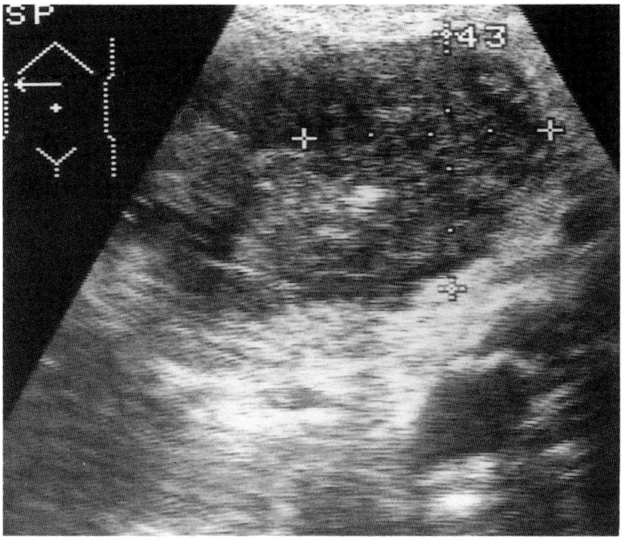

(b)

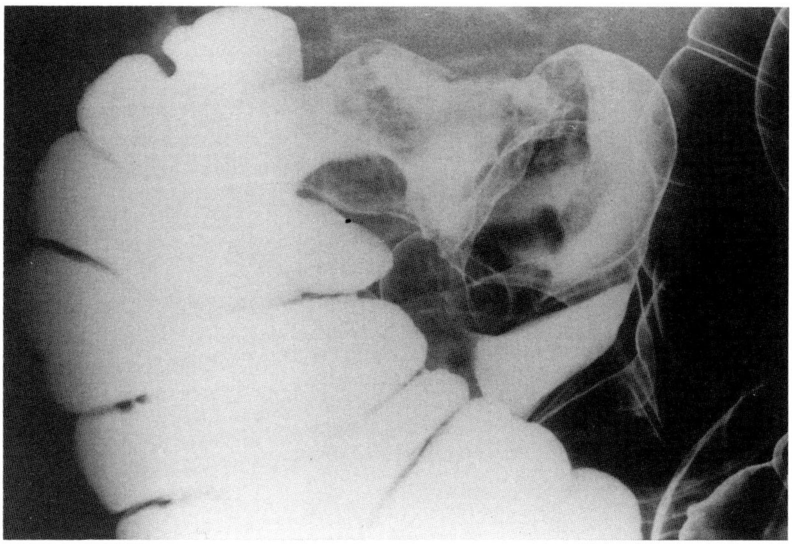

Figure 26. *(a) US in a patient with upper quadrant pain shows a thick walled intestinal loop with high luminal echoes, caused by a stricturing, 'apple-core' carcinoma (b).*

tumour extension if only seen in a short segment of an abutting area between neighbouring organs. Normally there are no fat planes between the preanal rectum, levator ani muscle, and the anal canal (Fig. 27), and may be missing towards the lower part of the prostatic gland. Endo-sonography and MRI may be helpful in these cases [159].

Advanced rectal tumours may cause obstruction of the ureters or urinary bladder seen as hydronephrosis and hydroureter on CT. Colorectal adenocarcinoma may metastasize to almost any organ, usually the liver. If larger than 2 cm across, their number and size are accurately unveiled with CT after intravenous bolus injection or hepatic CT-angiography. If less than 5 cm in size and three in number, liver resection seems to improve patients 5-year survival [160].

Sarcoma

These are rare tumours, most of which are leiomyosarcoma and found in the rectum. Their radiographic appearance does not differ from those from other sites of the GI tract, i.e. dislocation of the segment of origin and mucosal ulceration.

Lymphoma

The incidence of lymphoma of the colon is very low. Primary large bowel lymphoma is sited in the caecum and the rectum but may finally spread widely and resemble secondary lymphoma which usually involves all parts [161].

Radiology

Large bowel lymphoma presents itself as gross polypoid and ulcerated masses of the caecum together with separation and various deformities of the distal ileum (Fig. 28). In other colorectal segments lymphoma may mimic an annular stricturing carcinoma [111]. A diffuse form is reported which is very much alike benign lymphoid hyperplasia with small submucosal nodules [125].

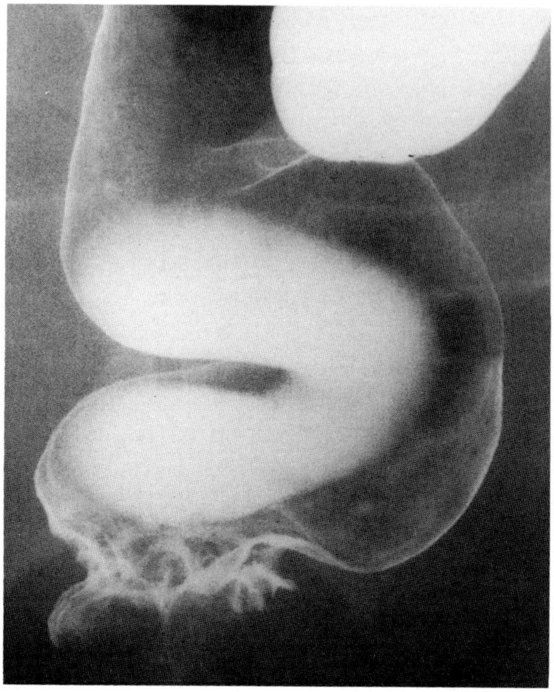

(a)

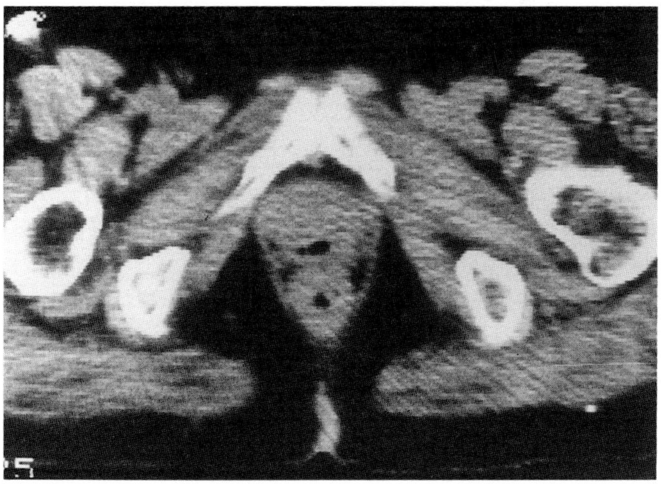

(b)

Figure 27. *(a) A low-sited rectal carcinoma abutting the vigina and levator muscles (b). Clean fat planes are seen around this Dukes' B carcinoma.*

(a)

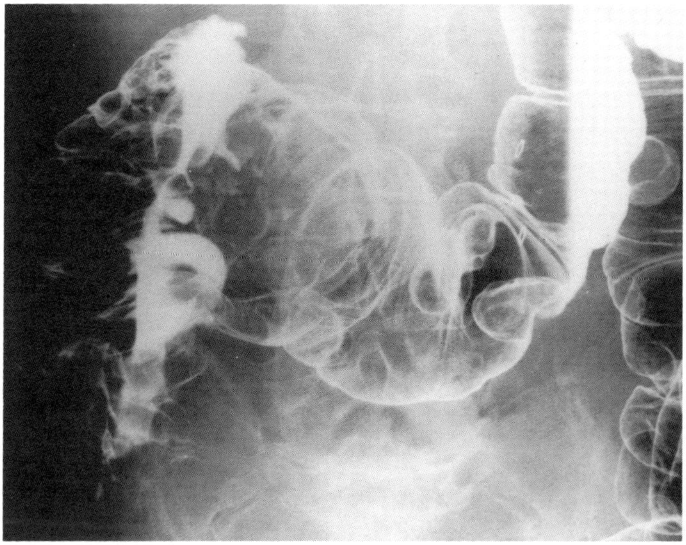

(b)

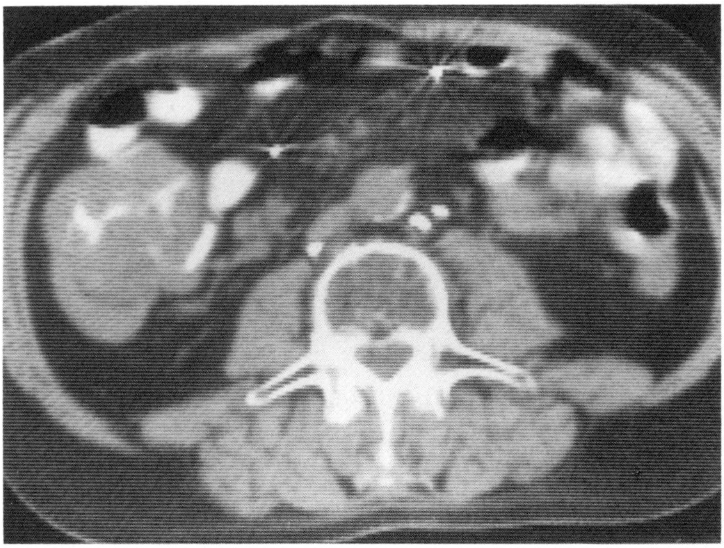

Figure 28. *(a) Primary colonic lymphoma with a cauliflower like lesion of the ascending colon and several polypoid lesions scattered in the remaining colon. (b) The thick-walled cecum is evident on the abdominal CT scan.*

Metastases

Extrinsic invasion from contiguous carcinomas originating from the urinary bladder, prostate and gynecological region is common, leading to obstruction of the colon [162]. Metastases to the colon are seen from gastric, mammary, pancreatic and female genital primaries. They spread along various pathways including intraperitoneal seeding.

Radiographically embolic metastases to the colon do not differ from those to other parts of the GI tract. Direct invasion causes bowel wall thickening and distortion while peritoneal carcinosis causes separation of loops, indentation, strictures, tethering of the colon, bellows-like spiculation of the mucosa and zigzag deformities of the lumen [163]. In these cases CT of the abdomen and pelvis will usually aid the diagnosis.

Endoluminal Ultrasonography (EUS)

Whereas barium enema and colonoscopy are accurate in detecting mucosal lesions of the colorectum, the submucosal and perirectal spaces are better assessed with CT and EUS. While CT has a low sensitivity for detecting involved nodes and minimal extrarectal spread [156,164], transrectal high-frequency ultrasound has proved itself to be more accurate in patients where the transducer can pass through the area of the tumour (Fig. 29). However, metastatic lymph nodes of normal size may still escape detection and over- as well as understaging of cancer is reported even with this technique [165-167]. Distant metastases are documented by transabdominal US and CT.

MRI

Due to the fixed position of the recto-sigmoid colon in the pelvis and the distinct differences in MR signal between various tissues, three dimensional MR imaging is well suited for assessing tumour extension into perirectal fatty compartments and pelvic organs. MR is also good for detecting both primary and recurrent pelvic tumours, as well as enlarged lymph nodes [168-170].

The author prepares patients with a small rectal clyster but does not fill the rectum in order to avoid distension and secondary compression of the perirectal compartments (Fig. 30). Others have however recommended distension of the rectum with air, water or a

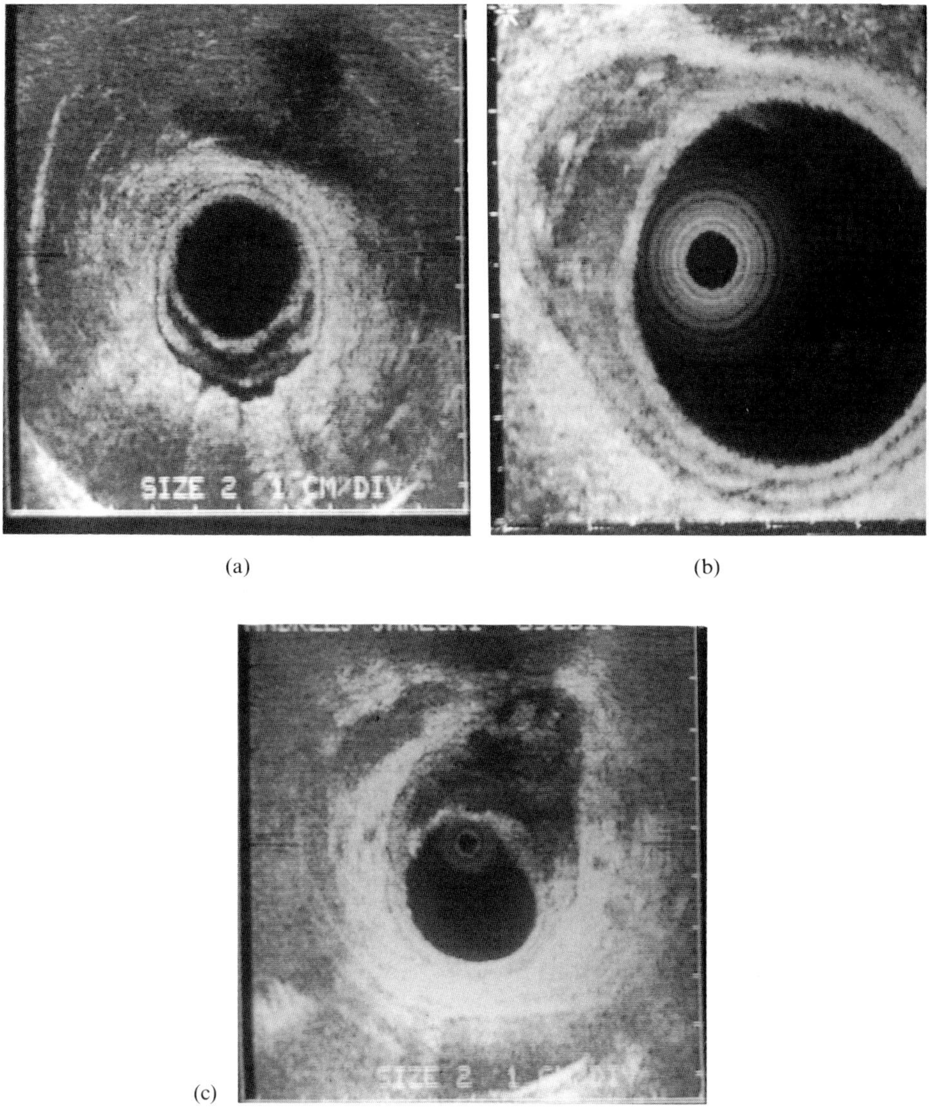

Figure 29. *Transrectal EUS of three rectal carcinomas. (a) Tumour confined to the proper muscle layer, extending up to (b) and into (c) the perirectal fat. A large lymph node is seen at 11 o'clock (c). Acoustic shadows are seen in (b). (Courtesy of Dr M. Starck, Malmö.)*

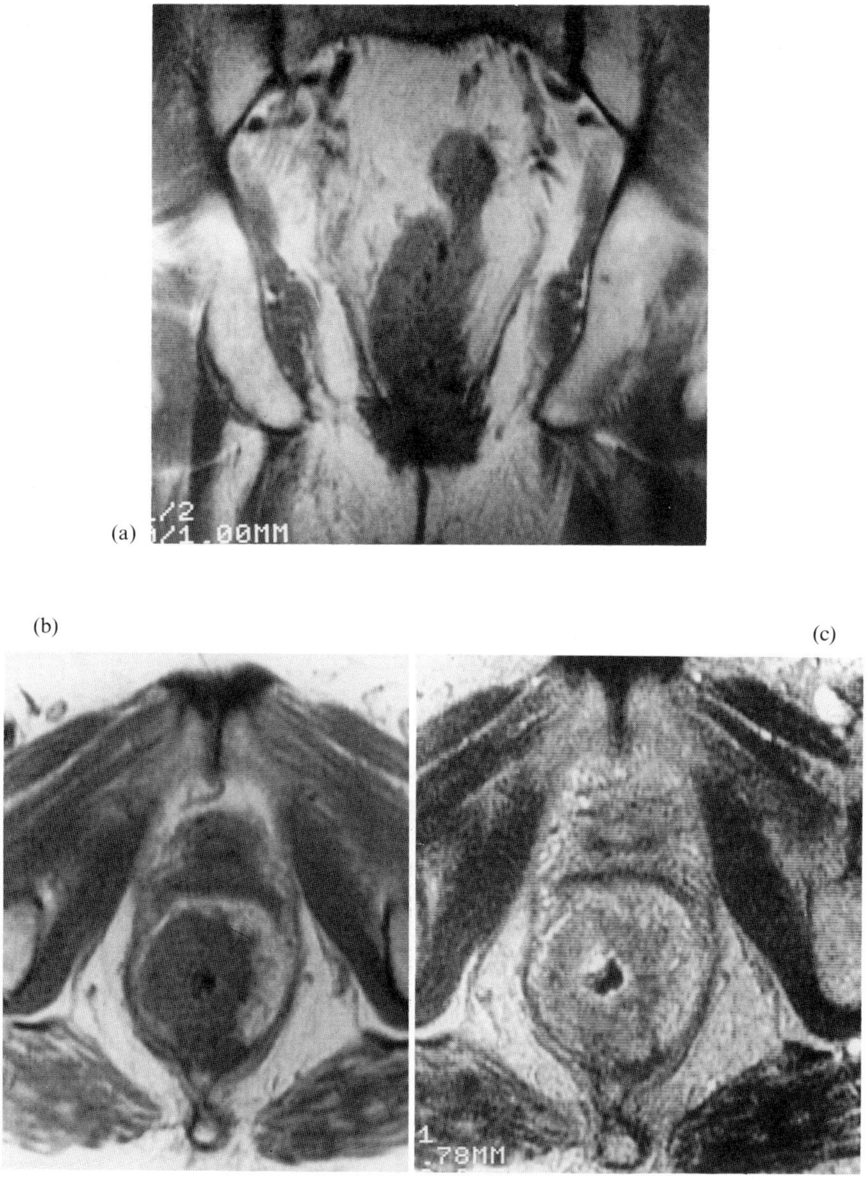

(a) (b) (c)

Figure 30. *Rectal carcinoma in (a) coronal and (b) axial T_1-weighted images and axial T_2-weighted image. (c) The tumour is circumferential with several extensions into the fatty compartments.*

paramagnetic contrast media. This probably facilitates tumour definition, but induces further inconvenience to the patient [171].

The anatomical MR definition of the pelvis is comparable to that of CT. Usually the region is covered by T_1 weighted images in three planes and two T_2 weighted sequences. The T_2 images show higher signal intensity of the tumour in comparison with normal muscle and organ tissues (Fig. 30c), while the T_1 images more readily reveal tumour extension into the perirectal fat (Fig. 30a, b) [172].

The morphological MR features of a rectal tumour are compatible with the CT ones. Consequently the same basic criteria for tumour staging are used: Tumour confined to the rectum is seen as a polypoid lesion, stage 1, or as a thickened wall, stage 2. Similarly extra rectal tumour spread is classified as stage 3a in cases of limited spread to adjacent organs, as stage 3b if further spread to the sidewalls is diagnosed, and as stage 4 if metastatic disease is seen.

As for CT, the diagnostic accuracy of MR of tumour extension just beyond the rectal wall is rather low because minor infiltrating traces are not only hard to identify but also to differentiate from inflammatory infiltrates and lymphangitis carcinomatosa [154,173].

Adenopathy is well studied on T_1 weighted spin-echo images, depicted as hypointense round or oval areas in the intense, perirectal fat, resembling contrast defects on a barium study [174].

Malignancy is suspected if the lymph nodes measure 15 mm across or more. In normal-sized nodes MR cannot differentiate between inflammatory or metastatic disease.

The main advantage of MR is the multiplanar studies in transverse, sagittal, coronal and oblique sections, where CR has a higher spatial resolution. MR, like CT, is well suited for assessing tumour spread in advanced cases, but less reliable in early, non-advanced cases and those with limited disease confined to the bowel wall.

Recurrence

After an abdominoperineal tumour resection, CT or MR has to be used in order to rule out any recurrence. After an anterior resection with an ileocolic anastomosis, endo-sonography can be useful.

Post-operative fibrosis has a very low signal on both T_1 and T_2 weighted acquisitions. Usually fibrosis is symmetrical and homogeneous and easily distinguished from a recurrence. However if not, a fine-needle puncture is needed for differential diagnosis [175].

Recurrence appears as an asymmetric mass, sometimes globar with signal heterogeneity and muscular invasion. The signal is low on T_1 weighted images and higher on T_2 ones, especially when necrotic. Still the distinction between a recurrence and a remaining, post-surgical haematoma and inflammation may be difficult.

References

1. Grant DS, Bartram CI, Heron CW. A preliminary study of the possible benefits of using carbon dioxide insufflation during double-contrast barium enema. *Br J Radiol* 1986;**59**:190-1.
2. Rust RJ, Cohen MD, Ulbright TM. Clinical, radiographic and pathologic effects of Amipaque on rabbit lung. *Acta Radiol Diagn* 1982;**23**:553.
3. Shaffer HA Jr, Eckard DA, de Lange EE, Ramakrishnan MR. Allergy to barium sulfate suspension with angioedema of the stomach and small bowel. *Gastrointest Radiol* 1988;**13**:221-3.
4. Butson ARC, D'Souza TJ, Thomson JG. Perforation of simple ulcer of the colon. *Br J Radiol* 1980;**53**:723.
5. Lewis JW Jr, Kerstein MD, Koss N. Barium granuloma of the rectum: an uncommon complication of barium enema. *Ann Surg* 1975;**181**:418.
6. Rockert H, Zettergren L. Tissue reaction to barium sulphate contrast medium. *Acta Pathol Microbiol Immunol Scand* 1963;**58**:445.
7. Nelson RL, Abcarian H, Prasad ML. Iatrogenic perforation of the colon and rectum. *Dis Colon Rectum* 1982;**25**:305.
8. Sisel RJ, Donovan A, Yellin AE. Experimental fecal peritonitis. Influence of barium sulfate or water-soluble radiographic contrast material on survival. *Arch Surg* 1972;**104**:765.
9. Juler GL, Dietrick WR, Eisenman JI. Intramesenteric perforation of sigmoid diverticulitis with non-fatal venous intravasation. *Am J Surg* 1976;**132**:653.
10. Mahboubi S, Gohel VK, Dalinka MK, Cho SY. Barium embolization following upper gastrointestinal examination. *Radiology* 1974;**111**:301.
11. Archer FH, McClennan BL. Adverse reactions to contrast material. *Br J Radiol* 1981;**54**:69.
12. Levine MS, Rubesin SE, Herlinger H, Laufer I. Double-contrast upper gastrointestinal examination: Technique and interpretation. *Radiology* 1988;**168**:593-602.
13. Kelvin RM, Maglinte DDT. Colorectal carcinoma: A radiologic clinical review *Radiology* 1987;**164**:1-8.
14. Herlinger H. A modified technique for the double-contrast small bowel enema. *Gastrointest Radiol* 1978;**3**:201-7.
15. Desaga JF. Visualization of the mucosal villi on double-contrast barium studies of the small intestine by using a high molecular fraction of Guaran. *Gastrointest Radiol* 1989;**14**:25-30.
16. Gelfand DW. The multiphasic or 'double-contrast' upper gastrointestinal examination. In Gelfand DW (ed). *Gastrointestinal Radiology*. Edinburgh: Churchill Livingstone, 1984.

17. Skucas J, Spataro RF (eds). *Radiology of the acute abdomen*. Small bowel and colon, pp 135-248. Edinburgh: Churchill Livingstone, 1986.
18. Salem S, O'Malley BP, Hiltz CW. Ultrasonographic appearance of gastrointestinal masses. *J Can Assoc Radiol* 1980;**31**:163-7.
19. Moss AA, Schnyder P, Thoeni RF. Esophageal carcinoma. Pre-therapy staging by computed tomography. *AJR* 1981;**136**:1051-6.
20. Thoeni RF, Moss AA, Schnyder P, Margulis AR. Detection and staging of primary rectal and rectosigmoid cancer by computed tomography. *Radiology* 1981;**141**:135-8.
21. Megibow AJ. Techniques of gastrointestinal computed tomography. In: Megibow AJ and Balthazar EJ (eds). *Computed Tomography of the Gastrointestinal Tract.* St Louis: CV Mosby, 1986.
22. Zerhouni EA, Fishman EK, Jones B. Principles and techniques. In: EK Fishman and B Jones (eds). *Computed Tomography of the Gastrointestinal Tract.* (New York: Churchill Livingstone, 1988.
23. Halvorsen RA, Thompson WM. Computer tomographic staging of gastrointestinal tract malignancies. Part 1: Esophagus and stomach. *Invest Radiol* 1987;**22**:2-16.
24. Halvorsen RA, Thompson WM. Computer tomographic staging of gastrointestinal tract malignancies. Part 2: The small bowel. *Invest Radiol* 1987;**22**:96-105.
25. Megibow AJ. The gastrointestinal tract. In: Haaga JR, Alfidi RJ (eds). *Computed Tomography of the Whole Body.* St Louis: CV Mosby, 1988.
26. Grosser G, Wommer B, Ruf G. Diagnostischer Wert der Computertomographie beim Magenkarzinom. *RöFo* 1985;**142**:514-9.
27 Aronberg DJ. Techniques. In JKT Lee, SS Sagel and RJ Stanley (eds). *Computed Body Tomography*, pp 9. New York: Raven Press, 1983.
28. Hatfield KD, Segal SD, Tait K. Barium sulfate for abdominal computer assisted tomography. *J Comput Assist Tomogr* 1980;**4**:570.
29. Megibow AJ, Zerhouni EA, Hulnick DH, Beranbaum ER, Balthazar EJ. Air insufflation of the colon as an adjunct to computed tomography of the pelvis. *J Comput Assist Tomogr* 1984;**8**:797-800.
30. Cronin EB, Belville JS, Tumeh SS. New low-density contrast agent for evaluation of the rectosigmoid with CT. *Radiology* 1988;**169P**:405.
31. Raptopoulos V, Davis MA, Davidoff A, Karellas A, Hays D, D'Orsi CJ, Smith EH. Fat-density oral contrast agent for abdominal CT. *Radiology* 1987;**164**:653-6.
32. Coscina WF, Arger PH, Levine MS, Herlinger H, Cohen S, Coleman BG, Mintz MC. Gastrointestinal tract focal mass lesions: Role of CT and barium evaluations. *Radiology* 1986;**158**:581-7.
33. Lee KT, Stanley RJ, Sagel SS, McClennan BL. Accuracy of CT in detecting intra-abdominal and pelvic lymph node metastases from pelvic cancers. *AJR* 1978;**131**:675-9.
34. Lehr L, Rupp N, Siewert JR. Assessment of resectability of esophageal cancer by computed tomography and magnetic resonance imaging. *Surgery* 1987;**103**:344-50.
35. Quint, LE, Glazer GMN, Orringer MB. Esophageal imaging by MR and CT: Study of normal anatomy and neoplasms. *Radiology* 1985;**156**:727-31.
36. Petrillo R, Balzarini L, Bidoli P, Ceglia E, D'Ippolito G, Tess JDT, Musumeci R. Esophageal squamous cell carcinoma: MRI evaluation of mediastinum. *Gastrointest Radiol* 1990;**15**:275-8.
37. Halvorsen RA, Thompson WM. Computed tomography evaluation of esophageal carcinoma. *Semin Oncol* 1984;**11**:113-26.
38. Balzarini L, Ceglia E, D'Ippolito G, Petrillo R, Tess JDT, Musumeci R. Local recurrence of rectosigmoid cancer: What about the choice of MRI for diagnosis? *Gastrointest Radiol* 1990;**15**:338-42.

39. Torp-Pedersen S, Gronvall S, Holm HH. Ultrasonically guided fine-needle aspiration biopsy of gastrointestinal mass lesions. *J Ultrasound Med* 1984;**3**:65-68.
40. Fleischer AC, Muhletaler CA, James AE Jr. Detection of bowel lesions during abdominal and pelvic sonography. *JAMA* 1980;**244**:2096-9.
41. Fakhry JR, Berk RN. The 'target' pattern: Characteristic sonographic feature of stomach and bowel abnormalities. *AJR* 1981;**137**:969-72.
42. Kremer H, Grobner W. Sonography of polypoid gastric lesions by the fluid-filled stomach method. *J Clin Ultrasound* 1981;**9**:51-4.
43. Weighall SL, Wolfman NT, Watson N. The fluid-filled stomach: A new sonic window. *JCU* 1979;**7**:353-6.
44. Rubin C, Kurtz AB, Goldberg BB. Water enema: A new ultrasound technique in defining pelvic anatomy. *J Clin Ultrasound* 1978;**6**:28-33.
45. Mittelstaedt CA. The gastrointestinal tract. In CA Mittelstaedt (ed). *Abdominal Ultrasound*, pp 605-56. New York: Churchill Livingstone Inc, 1987.
46. Fleischer AC, Muhletaler CA, James AE Jr. Sonographic assessment of the bowel wall. *AJR* 1981;**136**:887-91.
47. Bluth EI, Merritt CRB, Sullivan MA. Ultrasonic evaluation of the stomach, small bowel and colon. *Radiology*;**133**:677-680.
48. Fleischer AC, Dowling AD, Weinstein ML, James AE Jr. Sonographic patterns of distended, fluid filled bowel. *Radiology* 1979;**133**:681-5.
49. Rifkin MD, Gordon SJ, Goldberg BB. Sonographic examination of the mediastinum and upper abdomen by fiberoptic gastroscope. *Radiology* 1984;**151**:175-180.
50. Tio TL, Tytgat GNJ. Evaluation of resectability of gastrointestinal tumors. In: Kawai K (ed). *Endoscopic Ultrasonography in Gastroenterology*. New York: Igaku-Shoin, 1988.
51. Drugsted J, Gammelgaard J. Endoluminal ultrasonic scanning in the evaluation of rectal cancer. A preliminary report of 13 cases. *Gastrointest Radiol* 1983;**8**:367-9.
52. Tio TL. *Endosonography in Gastroenterology*, Berlin. Heidelberg and New York: Springer-Verlag, 1988.
53. Yasuda K, Nakajima M, Kawai K. Malignant lesions of the gastrointestinal tract. In K Kawai (ed). *Endoscopic Ultrasonography in Gastroenterology*, pp 56. Tokyo and New York: Igaku-Shoin, 1988.
54. Caletti G, Bolondi L, Barbara L. Instrumentation and scanning techniques. In K Kawai (ed). *Endoscopic Ultrasonography in Gastroenterology*, pp 1. Tokyo and New York: Igaku-Shoin, 1988.
55. Rosenberg JC, Schwade JG, Vaitkevicius VK. Cancer of the oesophagus. In VT Devita, S Hellman, SA Roenberg (eds). *Cancer: Principles and Practice of Oncology*, pp 499-533. Philadelphia: JB Lippincott, 1982.
56. Akiyama H, Tsurumaru M, Kawamura T, Ono Y. Principles of surgical treatment for carcinoma of the esophagus. Analysis of lymph node involvement. *Ann Surg* 1981;**194**:438-46.
57. Itai Y, Kogure T, Okuyama Y, Akiyama H. Superficial esophageal carcinoma: Radiological findings in double-contrast studies. *Radiology* 1978;**126**:597-601.
58. Koehler RE, Moss AA, Margulis AR. Early radiographic manifestations of carcinoma of the esophagus. *Radiology* 1976;**119**:1-5.
59. Dodds WJ. Radiology. In AR Margulis, HJ Burhenne (eds). *Alimentary Tract Radiology*, 4th Ed. St Louis: CV Mosby Co., 1989.
60. Agha FP. Secondary neoplasms of the esophagus. *Gastrointest Radiol* 1987;**12**:187-93.
61. Gelfand DW. Abnormalities of the esophagus and esophagogastric junction. In DW Gelfand (ed). *Gastrointestinal Radiology*. Edinburgh: Churchill Livingstone, 1984.
62. Halvorsen RA, Thompson WM. CT of esophageal neoplasms. In RM Gore (ed). CT of the Gastrointestinal Tract. *Radiol Clin North Am* 1989;**27**(**4**):667-85.

63. Picus D, Balfe DM, Koehler RE, Roper CL, Owen JW. Computed tomography in the staging of esophageal carcinoma. *Radiology* 1983;**146:**433-8.
64. Balfe DM, Mauro MA, Koehler RE, Lee JKT, Weyman PJ, Picus D, Peterson RR. Gastrohepatic ligament: Normal and pathologic CT anatomy. *Radiology* 1984;**150:**485-90.
65. Inculet RI, Keller SM Dwyer A, Roth JA. Evaluation of noninvasive tests for the preoperative staging of carcinoma of the esophagus: A prospective study. *Ann Thorac Surg* 1985;**40:**561-5.
66. Lea JW, Prager RL, Bender HW Jr. The questionable role of computed tomography in preoperative staging of esophageal cancer. *Ann Thorac Surg* 1984;**38:**479-81.
67. Halvorsen RA, Magruder-Habib K, Foster W, Roberts L, Postlethwait RW, Thompson WM. Esophageal cancer: Long-term follow-up of staging by computed tomography. *Radiology* 1986;**161:**147-51.
68. Tio TL. The role of endoscopic ultrasonography in assessing local resectability of oesophagogastric malignancies. In TN Tio (ed). *Endosonography in Gastroenterology*, pp 23-32. Heidelberg: Springer-Verlag, 1988.
69. Tio TL, Cohen P, Coene PP, Udding J, Jager FCADH, Tytgat GNJ. Endosonography and computed tomography of esophageal carcinoma. Preoperative classification compared to the new (1987) TNM system. *Gastroenterology* 1989;**96:**1478-86.
70. Shirakabe H. *Atlas of X-ray Diagnosis of Early Gastric Cancer.* Philadelphia: JB Lippincott, 1966.
71. Laufer I. A simple method for routine double-contrast study of the upper gastrointestinal tract. *Radiology* 1975;**117:**513-8.
72. Shirakabe H, Ichikawa H. Early gastric cancer. In: Hodess PJ (ed). *Atlas of Tumor Radiology. Radiology of the Esophagus and Stomach.* Chicago: Year Book Medical Publ, 1973.
73. Maruyama M. Early gastric cancer. In I Laufer (ed). *Double Contrast Gastrointestinal Radiology with Endoscopic Correlation.* Philadelphia: WB Saunders 1979.
74. Hada M, Hihara T, Kakishita M. Computed tomography in gastric carcinoma: Thickness of gastric wall and infiltration to serosa surface. *Radiat Med* 1984;**2:**27-30.
75. Kleinhaus U, Militianu D. Computed tomography in the preoperative evaluation of gastric carcinoma. *Gastrointest Radiol* 1988;**13:**97-101.
76. Sussman SK, Halvorsen RA, Illescas FF, Cohan RH, Saeed M, Silverman PM, Thompson WM, Meyers WC. Gastric adenocarcinoma: CT versus surgical staging. *Radiology* 1988;**167:**335-40.
77. Mullin D, Shirkhoda A. Computed tomography after gastrectomy in primary gastric carcinoma. *J Comput Assist Tomogr* 1985;**9:**30-3.
78. Morgan CL, Trought WS, Oddson TA, Clark WM, Rice RP. Ultrasound patterns of disorders affecting the gastrointestinal tract. *Radiology* 1980;**135:**129-135.
79. Yeh H-C, Rabinowitz JG. Ultrasonography and computed tomography of gastric wall lesions. *Radiology* 1981;**141:**147-55.
80. Komaiko MS. Gastric neoplasms: Ultrasound and CT evaluation. *Gastrointest Radiol* 1979;**4:**131-7.
81. Derchi LE, Biggi E, Rollandi GA, Cicio GR, Neumaier CE. Sonographic staging of gastric cancer. *AJR* 1983;**140:**273-6.
82. Loehr WJ, Mujahed Z, Zahn FD, Gray GF, Thorbjarnarson B. Primary lymphoma of the gastrointestinal tract. A review of 100 cases. *Ann Surg* 1969;**170:**232-8.
83. Brady LW. Malignant lymphoma of the gastrointestinal tract. *Radiology* 1980;**137:**291-8.
84. Thorbjarnarson B, Pearce JM, Beal JM. Sarcoma of the stomach. *Am J Surg* 1959;**97:**36-42.

85. Solidoro A, Salazar F, De la Flor, J, Sanchez J, Otero J. Endoscopic tissue diagnosis of gastric involvement in the staging of non-Hodgkin's lymphoma. *Cancer* 1981;**48:**1053-7.
86. Nelson RS. The endoscopic diagnosis of gastric lymphoma. Gross characteristics and histology. *Gastrointest Endosc* 1974;**21:**66-8.
87. Rosch W, Hartwich G, Elster K, Ottenjann R. Gastric lymphoma. *Endoscopy* 1971;**3:**28-33.
88. Sugiyama N. Macroscopic observation and radiological diagnosis of malignant lymphoma of the stomach with special reference to the early stage. *Jpn J Gastroenterol* 1974;**71:**1118-30.
89. Sato T, Sakai Y, Ishiguro S, Furukawa H. Radiologic manifestations of early gastric lymphoma. *AJR* 1986;**146:**513-17.
90. Privett TJ, Davies ER, Roylance J. The radiological features of gastric lymphoma. *Clin Radiol* 1977;**28:**457-63.
91. Fork F-T, Ekberg O, Haglund U. Radiology in primary gastric lymphoma. *Acta Radiol* 1984;**25:**481-8.
92. Redd BL. Lymphosarcoma of the stomach. *AJR* 1959;**82:**634-50.
93. Buy J, Moss AA. Computed tomography of gastric lymphoma. *AJR* 1982;**138:**859-65.
94. Derchi LE, Banderai A, Bossi MC, De Paolis M, Musante F, Solbiati L, Subelli M. The sonographic appearance of gastric lymphoma. *J Ultrasound Med* 1984;**3:**251-6.
95. Kaftori JK, Aharon M, Kleinhaus U. Sonographic features of gastrointestinal leiomyosarcoma. *JCU* 1981;**9:**11-15.
96. Scatarige JC, Fishman EK, Jones B, Cameron JL, Sanders RC, Siegelman SS. Gastric leiomyosarcoma: CT observations. *J Comput Assist Tomogr* 1985;**9:**320-7.
97. Subramanyam BR, Balthazar EJ, Raghavendra BN, Madamba MR. Sonography of exophytic gastrointestinal leiomyosarcoma. *Gastrointest Radiol* 1982;**7:**47-51.
98. Bruneton JN, Caramella E, Cazenave P, Birtwisle Y, Hericord P, Drouillard J. Gastric leiomyosarcoma: comparative value of barium examinations, ultrasonography and CT scans. *Eur J Radiol* 1987;**7:**160-2.
99. Godwin JD. Carcinoid tumors - an analysis of 2837 cases. *Cancer* 1975;**36:**560-9.
100. Modlin IM. Carcinoid syndrome. *J Clin Gastroenterol* 1980;**2:**349.
101. Thompson GB, van Heerden JA, Martin JK, Schutt AJ, Ilstrup DM, Carney JA. Carcinoid tumors of GI Tract: Presentation, management and prognosis. *Surgery* 1985;**98:**1054-63.
102. Kothari T, Mangla JC. Malignant tumors associated with carcinoid tumors of the gastrointestinal tract. *J Clin Gastroenterol* 1981;**3(suppl 1):**43-6.
103. Cockey BM, Fishman EK, Jones B, Siegelman SS. Computed tomography of abdominal carcinoid tumour of the gastrointestinal tract. *J Comput Assist Tomogr* 1985;**9:**38-42.
104. Barloon TJ, Lu CH, Honda H, Walker WP. Primary adenocarcinoma of the duodenal bulb: Radiographic and pathologic findings in two cases. *Gastrointest Radiol* 1989;**14:**223-5.
105. Kerber GW, Frank PH. Carcinoma of the small intestine and colon as a complication of Crohn's disease: Radiologic manifestations. *Radiology* 1984;**150:**639-45.
106. Miller TL, Skucas J, Gudex D, Listinsky C. Bowel cancer characteristics in patients with regional enteritis. *Gastrointest Radiol* 1987;**12:**45-52.
107. Sellink JL. Tumors. In JL Sellink (ed). *Radiological atlas of common diseases of the small bowel.* Leiden, The Netherlands: HE Stenfert Kroese BV, 1976.
108. Ekberg O, Ekholm S. Radiology in primary small bowel adenocarcinoma. *Gastrointest Radiol* 1980;**5:**49-53.
109. Mauro MA, Koehler RE. Alimentary tract. In JK Lee, SS Sagel, RJ Stanley (eds). *Computed Body Tomography*, pp 307-40 New York: Raven Press, 1983.

110. Marshak RH, Lindner AR, Maklansky D. Lymphoreticular disorders of the gastrointestinal tract: Roentgenographic features. *Gastrointest Radiol* 1979;**4:**103-20.
111. Dodd GD. Lymphoma of the hollow abdominal viscera. In HI Libshitz (ed). Imaging the lymphomas. *Radiol Clin North Am* 1990;**28:**771-83.
112. Mueller PR, Ferrucci JT, Harbin WP, Kirkpatrick RH, Simeone JF, Wittenberg J. Appearance of lymphomatous involvement of mesentery by ultrasonography and body computed tomography: the 'sandwich sign'. *Radiology* 1980;**134:**467-73.
113. Miller JH, Hindman BW, Lam AHK. Ultrasound in the evaluation of small bowel lymphoma in children. *Radiology* 1980;**135:**409-14.
114. Starr GF, Dockerty MB. Leiomyomas and leiomyosarcomas of the small intestine. *Cancer* 1955;**8:**101-11.
115. Levine MS, Drooz AT, Herlinger H. Annular malignancies of the small bowel. *Gastrointest Radiol* 1987;**12:**53-8.
116. Koehler RE. Neoplasms. In AR Margulis and HJ Burhenne (eds). *Alimentary Tract Radiology*, pp 817-38. 4th Ed. St Louis: CV Mosby Co., 1989.
117. Heald RJ, Bussey HJR. Clinical experiences at St Mark's Hospital with multiple synchronous cancers of the colon and rectum. *Dis Colon Rectum* 1975;**18:**6-10.
118. Rhodes JB, Holmes FF, Clark GM. Changing distribution of primary cancers in the large bowel. *JAMA* 1977;**238:**1641-3.
119. Fork F-T. The diagnostic value of large bowel radiography in contemporary medicine 1982. Thesis, University Library, University of Lund, pp 28-34.
120. Silverberg E, Lubera JA. Cancer statistics 1989. *CA* 39. pp 3-20.
121. Lynch HT. Frequency of hereditary non-polyposis colorectal cancer. *Gastroenterology* 1986;**90:**486-92.
122. Mecklin JP. Frequency of hereditary colorectal cancer. *Gastroenterology* 1987;**93:**1021-5.
123. Lanspa SJ, Lynch HT, Smyrk TC, Strayhorn P, Watson P, Lynch J, Appelman H. Initial results of a colonoscopy screening program in the Lynch syndromes. *Gastrointest Endosc* 1989;**35:**173.
124. Lanspa SJ, Smyrk TC, Lynch HT. The colonoscopist and the Lynch Syndromes. *Gastrointest Endosc* 1990;**36:**156-8.
125. Dodd GD. Malignancies. In AR Margulis, HJ Burhenne (eds). *Alimentary Tract Radiology*, pp 1051-82. 4th Ed. St Louis: CV Mosby Co., 1989.
126. Fork F-T. Radiographic findings in overlooked colon carcinomas - a retrospective analysis. *Acta Radiol* 1988;**29:**331-6.
127. Stryker SJ, Wolff BG, Culp CE, Libbe SD, Ilstrup DM. MacCarty RL. Natural history of untreated colonic polyps. *Gastroenterology* 1987;**93:**1009-13.
128. Morson BC. The polyp-cancer sequence in the large bowel. *Proc R Soc Med* 1974;**67:**451-7.
129. Johnson CD, Carlson HC, Taylor WF, Weiland LP. Barium enemas of carcinoma of the colon: Sensitivity of double- and single-contrast studies. *AJR* 1983;**40:**1143-9.
130. Margulis AR, Thoeni RF. The present status of the radiologic examination of the colon. *Radiology* 1988;**167:**1-5.
131. Enterline HT. Significance of adenomatous polyps in colon carcinogenesis. In: Grundtmann E (ed). *Colon Cancer: Cancer Campaign*. Vol. 2. Stuttgart: Gustav Fischer, 1978.
132. Delamarre J, Descombres P, Marti R, Remond A, Trinez G. Villous tumors of the colon and rectum: double-contrast study of 47 cases. *Gastrointest Radiol* 1980;**5:**69-73.
133. Kaye JJ, Bragg DG. Unusual roentgenologic and clinicopathologic features of villous adenomas of the colon. *Radiology* 1968;**91:**799-806.
134. Youker JE, Welin S, Main G. Computer analysis in the differentiation of benign and malignant polypoid lesions of the colon. *Radiology* 1968;**90:**794-6.

135. Muto T, Bussey HJR, Morson BC. The evolution of cancer of the colon and rectum. *Cancer* 1975;**36:**2251-70.
136. Rappaport LB, Sperling HV, Stavrides A. Colon cancer in the Cronkhite-Canada syndrome. *J Clin Gastroenterol* 1986;**8:**199-202.
137. Drachman AH, Buck JL, Burke AP, Sobin LH. Cronkhite-Canada syndrome. Radiologic features. *Gastrointest Radiol* 1990;**14:**285-90.
138. Cripps H. Two cases of disseminated polyps of the colon. *Trans Pathol Soc London* 1882;**33:**165.
139. Stewart ET, Dodds WJ. Polyps. In: Margulis AR, Burhenne HJ (eds). *Alimentary Tract Radiology*, pp 1017-49. St Louis: CV Mosby Co, 1989.
140. Watne AL, Johnson JG, Chang CH. The challenge of Gardner's syndrome. *Cancer* 1969;**19:**266-75.
141. Dodds WJ. Clinical and roentgen features of the intestinal polyposis syndromes. *Gastrointest Radiol* 1976;**1:**127-142.
142. Seaman WB. Unusual roentgen manifestations of large bowel cancer. *Semin Roentgenol* 1976;**11:**89-99.
143. Zalev AH, Baker JP, Gardiner GW. Linitis plastica of the alimentary tract and scrotum. *Gastrointest Radiol* 1990;**15:**72-5.
144. Hodgson JR, Sauer WG. The roentgenologic features of carcinoma in chronic ulcerative colitis. *AJR* 1961;**86:**91-6.
145. Phalke IM, Smallwood CJ, Wright FW. Linitis plastica of the colon. *Clin Radiol* 1969;**20:**224-7.
146. Balthazar EJ, Rosenberg HD, Davidian MM. Primary and metastatic scirrhous carcinoma of the rectum. *AJR* 1979;**132:**711-5.
147. Luchtefeld MA, Ross DS, Zander JD, Folse JR. Late development of metachronous colorectal cancer. *Dis Colon Rectum* 1987;**30:**180-4.
148. Kremer H, Lohmoeller G, Zollner N. Primary ultrasonic detection of a double carcinoma of the colon. *Radiology* 1977;**124:**481-2.
149. Schabel SI, Rittenberg GM, Johnson EG. III. Carcinoma of the colon demonstrated by ultrasound. *JCU* 1978;**6:**436-7.
150. Gooding GAW. Ultrasonography of the cecum. *Gastrointest Radiol* 1981;**6:**243-6.
151. Howell, EJ, de Lnage EE, Frierson HF Jr. Linitis plastica of the colon: Computed tomographic findings. *Gastrointest Radiol* 1990;**15:**69-71.
152. Solomon A, Bar-Ziv J, Stern D. Staging of cecal and ascending colon carcinoma with computed tomography. *Gastrointest Radiol* 1988;**13:**152-4.
153. Grabbe E, Winkler R. Local recurrence after sphincter saving resection for rectal and rectosigmoid carcinoma. *Radiology* 1985;**155:**305-10.
154. Freeny PC, Marks WM, Ryan JA, Bolen JW. Colorectal carcinoma evaluation with CT, preoperative staging and detection of postoperative recurrence. *Radiology* 1986;**158:**347-53.
155. van Waes PFG, Koehler PR, Feldberg MAM. CT of rectal cancer: its accuracy and effect on patient management. *Radiographics* 1984;**4:**801-19.
156. Grabbe E, Lierse W, Winkler R. The perirectal fascia: Morphology and use in staging of rectal carcinoma. *Radiology* 1983;**149:**241-6.
157. Moss AA, Margulis AR, Schnyder P, Thoeni RF. A uniform, CT based staging system for malignant neoplasms of the alimentary tube, editorial. *AJR* 1981;**136:**1251-2.
158. Balthazar EJ, Megibow AJ, Hulnick D, Naidich DP. Carcinoma of the colon: Detection and preoperative staging by CT. *AJR* 1988;**150:**301-6.
159. Thoeni RF. CT evaluation of carcinoma of the colon and rectum. In RM Gore. CT of the gastrointestinal tract. *Radiol Clin North Am* 1989;**27:**731-41.

160. Malt RA. Current concepts: Surgery for hepatic neoplasms. *N Engl J Med* 1985;**313:**1591-6.
161. Devine RM, Bearet RW, Wolff BG. Malignant lymphoma of the rectum. *Dis Colon Rectum* 1986;**29:**821-3.
162. Fry DE, Amin M, Harbrecht PJ. Rectal obstruction secondary to carcinoma of the prostage. *Ann Surg* 1979;**189:**488-92.
163. Meyers MA, McSweeney J. Secondary neoplasms of the bowel. *Radiology* 1972;**105:**1-11.
164. Dixon AK, Kelsey Fry I, Morson BC, Nicholls RJ, York Mason A. Pre-operative computed tomography of carcinoma of the rectum. *Br J Radiol* 1981;**54:**655-9.
165. Pahlman L, Adalsteinsson B, Glimelius B, Lindgren PG, Scheipenpflug L. Ultrasound in preoperative staging of rectal tumours. *Acta Radiol Diagn* 1984;**25:**489-94.
166. Rifkin MD, Marks GJ. Transrectal US as an adjunct in the diagnosis of rectal and extrarectal tumours. *Radiology* 1985;**157:**499-502.
167. Rotte KH, Kluhs L, Kleinau H, Kriedermann E. Computed tomography and endosonography in the preoperative staging of rectal carcinoma. *Eur J Radiol* 1989;**9:**187-90.
168. Bryan PJ, Butler HE, Lipuma JP. Magnetic resonance imaging of the pelvis. *Radiol Clin North Am* 1984;**22:**897-915.
169. Hricak A, Alpers C, Crooks LE, Sheldon PE. Magnetic resonance imaging of the female pelvis: Inital experience. *AJR* 1983;**141:**1119-28.
170. Hricak A, Williams RD, Spring DB, Moon KL Jr, Hedgcock MW, Watson RA, Crooks LE. Anatomy and pathology of the male pelvis by magnetic resonance imaging. *AJR* 1983;**141:**1101-10.
171. Butch RJ, Stark DD, Wittenberg J, Tepper JE, Saini S, Simeone JF, Mueller PR, Ferrucci JT Jr. Staging rectal cancer by MR and CT. *AJR* 1986;**146:**1155-60.
172. Engelholm L, Segebarth C, de Toeuf J, Zalcman M, Jean-Mart J. Gastrointestinal tract. In Vanel D. and McNamara MT (eds). *MRI of the Body*, pp 179-87. Paris: Springer Verlag, 1989.
173. Kuper K, Bautz W, Gnann H. Wertigkeit der MR-Tomographie fur die Diagnostik des Rektumkarzinoms und dessen Rezidiv in Vergleich zur CT. *RöFo* 1985;**143:**301-6.
174. Lee JKT, Heiken JP, Ling D, Glazer HS, Balfe DM, Levitt RG, Dixon WT, Murphy WA Jr. Magnetic resonance imaging of abdominal and pelvic lymphadenopathy. *Radiology* 1984;**153:**181-188.
175. Butch RJ, Wittenberg J, Mueller PR, Simeone JF, Meyer JE, Ferrucci JT Jr. Presacral masses after abdominoperineal resection for colorectal carcinoma: The need for needle biopsy. *AJR* 1985;**144:**309-12.

Fibre-endoscopy versus radiology in the diagnosis of gastrointestinal cancer

Frans-Thomas Fork
Department of Diagnostic Radiology, University of Lund, Malmö, Sweden

Introduction

During the last two decades, the number of fibre-endoscopic procedures has increased in preference to radiographic barium studies. However, the total number of all gastrointestinal diagnostic procedures has decreased in the author's institution. This decline is mainly explained by the reduced number of follow-up cases but probably also by the increased number of patients with an endoscopic diagnosis of minimal inflammatory mucosal change, formerly diagnosed by chance only. In many hospitals fibre-endoscopy is today the technique of choice for detecting mucosal lesions in the upper and lower gastrointestinal tract. The reasons for its popularity are manifold:

- The combination of a rather simple performance together with high diagnostic accuracy and yield.
- Its facilities for obtaining tissue specimens.
- A number of advanced therapeutic procedures can be performed through the endoscope, but not least
- The clinician may look for himself without relying on the interpretation of a radiologist who may or may not have special interest in the gastrointestinal field.

Why Barium Examinations?

Parallel to endoscopic evolution barium studies have gone through an improvement in quality. A correctly performed double-contrast barium study covers the entire gastrointestinal tract and is highly accurate when correctly interpreted. This technique is now routine worldwide. Experience has shown that a second look increases the diagnostic yield, is a necessary quality control, and ensures continuing education [1].

The standardized imaging techniques of radiology meet any demands in this matter, whereas fibre-endoscopy does not.

Although mucosal details on the radiogram cannot compete with direct vision through an endoscope, the radiogram also shows the topography of the intestinal surroundings (Fig. 1) which can only exceptionally be predicted endoscopically, viz. duodenal ulcer and gas in the bile duct in an emergency admission with right upper quadrant pain, or the dislocation of a sigmoid loop in a female patient with ovarian tumour.

Further reasons for continuing barium studies are as follows:

- The endoscopist overlooks lesions and misinterprets findings. Follow-up studies have shown a 10-30% false negative rate for endoscopists unaware of the radiological findings [2-5].
- The intubation may be difficult due to twisted and long loops.
- Incomplete intubation due to stenosis or deformities (Fig. 2).
- Some fibre-endoscopic procedures are hazardous to the patient and this necessitates strict patient selection.
- Follow-up examination after endoscopic therapy for documentation, viz. barium enema after colonoscopic polypectomy to document absence of neoplasms, viz. a 'clean colon'.
- Barium follow-up after surgery for anastomotic control and upper GI motility studies (Fig. 3).
- Consecutive radiograms are unchallenged in describing the evolution of the disease over time (Fig. 4).
- Unchallenged demonstration of strictures, hernias and extrinsic lesions (Fig. 5) [6].

The number of examinations per hour varies greatly but in most hospitals an upper GI study with fibre-endoscopy is faster than a corresponding barium examination, while a colonoscopy takes twice

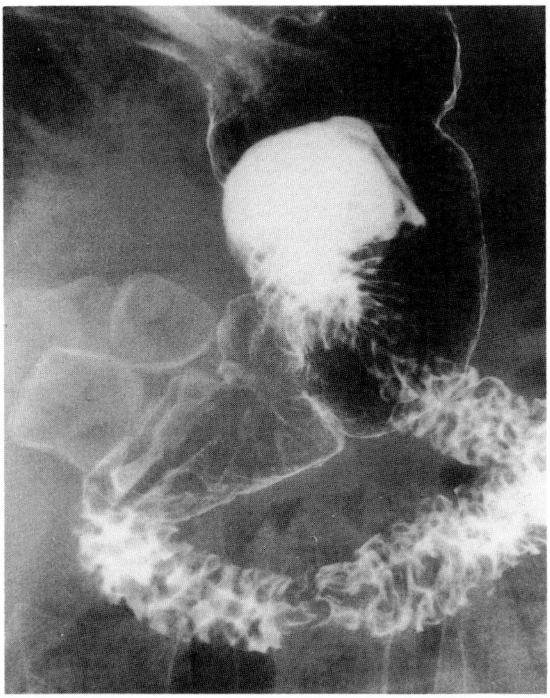

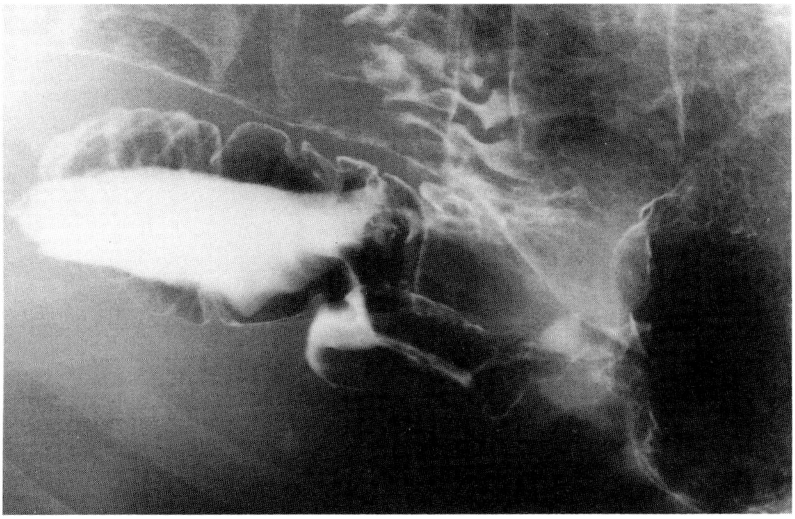

Figure 1. *Duodenal ulcer with converging mucosal folds. The four gas-containing gallstones are not possible to diagnose endoscopically.*

Figure 2. *Barium meal in an elderly lady with weight loss, anaemia and nausea. Gastric retention and a stenotic pyloric ring were found at gastroscopy. The radiogram clearly demonstrates the stricturing carcinoma.*

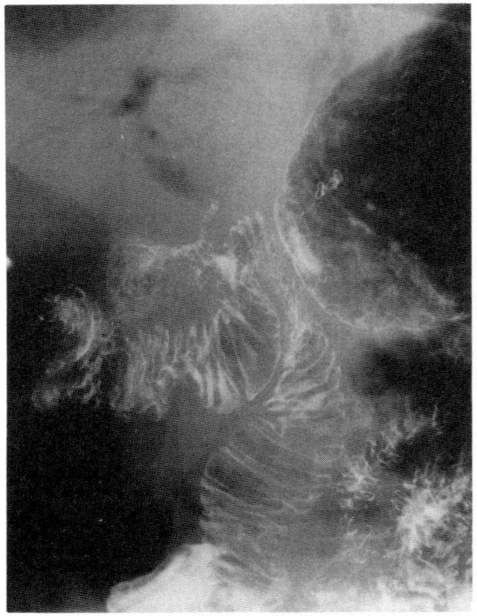

Figure 3. *Upper GI series showing a B-II stomach with a stomal stricture. Radiographic examination also shows a patent bilio-digestive shunt with air-filled bile ducts, and two sub-mucosal metastases in afferent loop - impossible to detect endoscopically.*

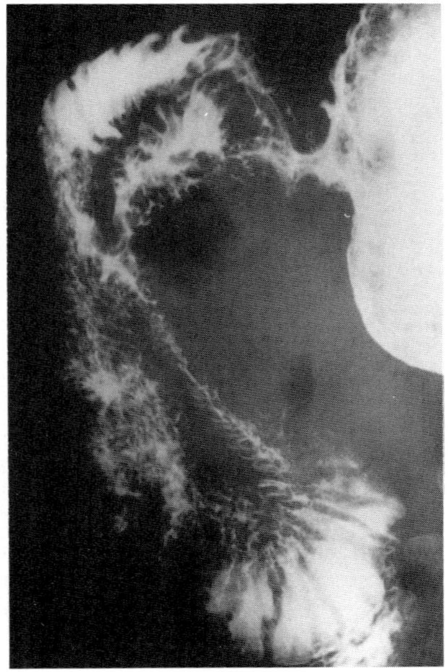

Figure 4. *Barium meal clearly demonstrating a recurrent gastric carcinoma which causes displacement and compression of adjacent bowel loops - not possible to detect endoscopically because of the stenotic stoma.*

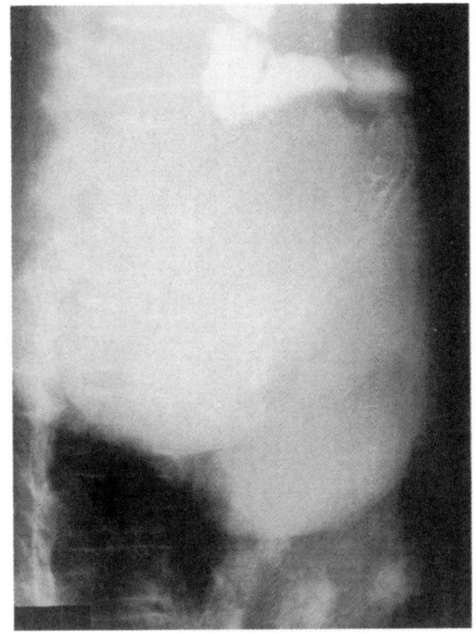

Figure 5. *Upper abdominal survey in a patient with metastatic colon cancer disease. The enlarged liver, the cranial displacement of the right hemi-diaphragm and the pulmonary metastases are radiographically evident but endoscopically hidden. Only the ventral dislocation of the gastric body might be diagnosed by endoscopy.*

the time compared to a double-contrast barium enema. However the author knows experts in both fields who would state the contrary. The literature is full of figures supporting as well as rejecting opinions in this matter. The difficulty is in finding unbiased series large enough to guarantee impeccable bio-statistics, written by colleagues in collaboration, all equally experienced in their techniques [3].

The efficacy of a procedure is usually presented in terms of sensitivity. The sensitivity of a diagnostic procedure describes the number of detected lesions to known ones in an unselected population, often given as a percentage. Unfortunately the interpretation of this percentage is affected by the prevalence of the disease, i.e. in spite of very high figures for sensitivity, the positive predictive value of a test's statement might be very low indeed if the disease is rare [8,9]. In southern Sweden early gastric carcinoma (EGC) (Fig. 6) is such a rare entity. Only a very large patient study would indicate a difference in diagnostic sensitivity of barium meals compared to gastroscopy in the diagnosis of EGC.

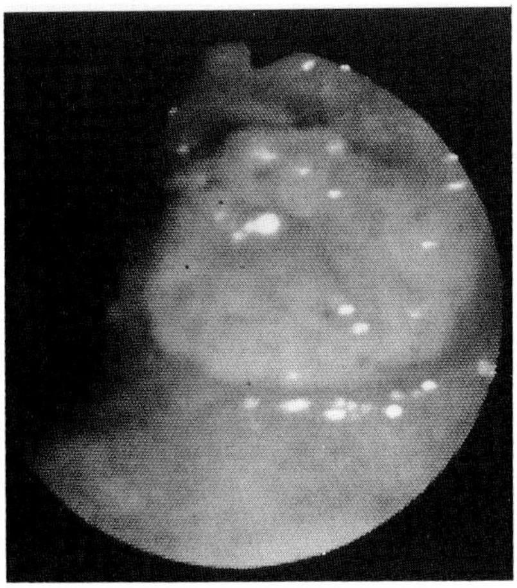

Figure 6. *Early gastric carcinoma of elevated type IIa. These lesions are more readily detected endoscopically because of the colour shift.*

It is known that microscopic lesions cannot be detected radiographically. On the other hand small malignant lesions may be equally hard to describe endoscopically [10].

Upper GI Cancer

Oesophageal cancer may be detected in up to 90% of patients with barium radiology as compared to endoscopy [11]. Mean sensitivity for barium studies of the whole upper GI tract is equally high, with no significant lesion being overlooked radiographically, as proven in follow-up series [12,13]. Although endoscopy in most series is documented as being the more accurate procedure in diagnosing gastric carcinoma [14], the sensitivity for radiographic detection of such lesions may indeed be greater compared to upper GI endoscopy, as shown in a series of 243 patients from 1978 [15].

Today upper GI endoscopy is the first-line method in the author's department. The total number of upper GI examinations in Malmö has decreased by 80% in the 10-year period from 1976 to 1986 and the mean age of patients sent for barium meals has decreased from 52 to 41.9 years during the same period. This shift can only partly be attributed to the greater accuracy of fibre-endoscopy - for example the detection rate of early gastric carcinoma in Malmö (1/100,000 annually) has not increased since gastroscopy has become the routine method. Interestingly enough, the slightly greater overall sensitivity for upper fibre-endoscopy is not mirrored in the survival rate for gastric cancer in Europe [16].

Another interesting observation by the author is that the proportion of examinations with abnormal findings at the end of the 10-year period had increased from 0.44 to 0.54, which is highly significant and cannot be explained by the overall reduction in number of patients studied. The main reason is probably the fact that of patients primarily endoscoped only 5% require a barium study, as opposed to almost 30% of patients who required follow-up gastroscopy after an initial barium meal [17].

It might be concluded that although upper GI radiology is accurate [18,19], and sometimes very much so (Fig. 7), endoscopy is still more so, is tolerable for the patient (although some demand premedication), is easily performed and offers means for treatment and for obtaining biopsies at the same time. Whether endoscopy should primarily be performed in every patient or in selected patients with clinical signs of ulcer or malignant disease, is still a matter of debate [6]. The barium meal is non-invasive and safe, whereas mortality from endoscopy is 1 in 12,000 [20]. In Sweden the price per procedure is equal. If you want to invest your money into a diagnostic

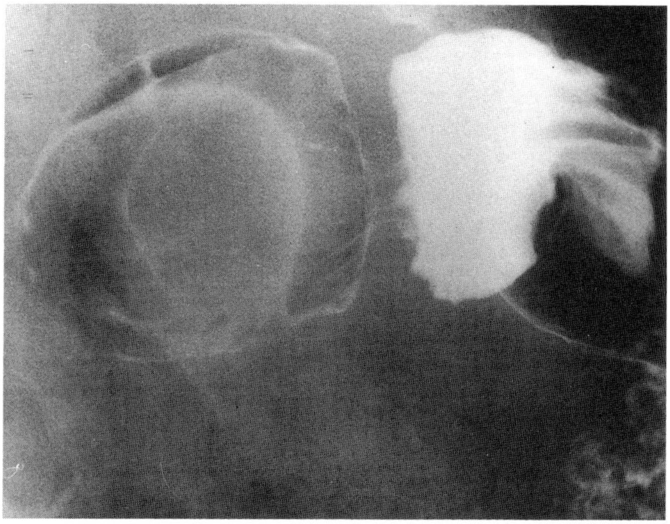

(a)

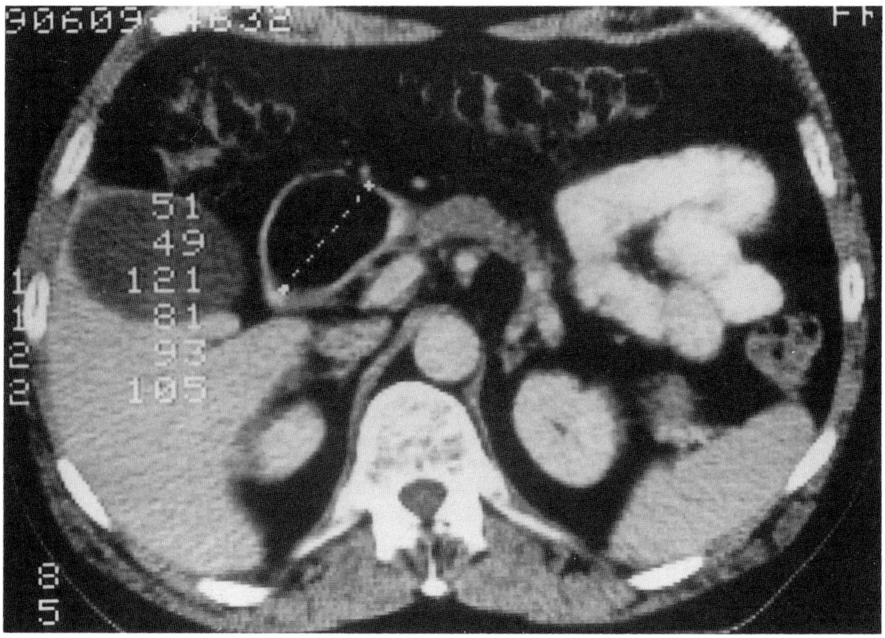

(b)

Figure 7. *A lumen-sized soft mass lesion of the duodenal cup (a), proved on CT to be a lipoma (b).*

facility today, you will have 5 to 8 fully equipped endoscopy stations for the price of just one fluoroscopy room!

Enteroscopy

Fibre-enteroscopes are available for direct visualization of enteric mucosa [21]. However, this technique is time consuming and rather uncomfortable for the patient. Combined techniques with jejunoscopy and enteroclysis have been described recently which may increase the detectability of small bowel neoplasms [22].

Lower GI Neoplasia

Sensitivities for both barium enema at its best and for total colonoscopy in diagnosing colon carcinoma are up to 95% as stated by various researchers [23-25]. It is also evident from other series that there is no significant difference in detecting polyps 7 mm or larger in diameter with either procedure [26,27], although radiology produces a higher number of false positive diagnoses [28].

Whereas colonoscopy is more sensitive in detecting lesions less than 6 mm across it also has a greater potential for perforation. As the risk for malignancy in 5-mm polyps is much less than the complication rate for polypectomy, i.e. 0.5-1% risk for perforation [29,30], the difference in detection rate for small polyps may not be clinically important [31]!

Which technique should then be used as the method of first choice? Some physicians state fibre-endoscopy to be sufficiently superior to barium enema in diagnostic accuracy, safety and patient compliance to justify colonoscopy to be their first choice [32,33], while others recommend colonoscopy in selected patients because of missed lesions and false-negative biopsy specimens [29,34]. Unfortunately many of the series comparing colonoscopy and barium enemas are written by experts without radiological experience, are retrospective and based on selected populations [35]. These works are thus wide open to the influence of bias, and the results presented difficult to interpret [36-38].

Colonoscopic tumour localization may be problematic, as reliance on distance measurements is insecure due to anatomical variants and loops. Barium enema is still recommended for localization prior to surgery [39]. Also, series with endoscopically undetected neoplasms are currently presented, including lesions ranging from small benign to large carcinomas, later depicted on radiograms of the colon [40-42].

Series on large tumours missed on endoscopy are also published. These works are usually built up by case reports from different departments and thus not based on consecutive patient material, which makes the result difficult to evaluate [43]. On the whole, reports like these are outnumbered by series showing lesions overlooked by radiology [44,45] in which failures are ascribed to inferior radiographic technique [46] or, more likely, attributable to perception errors: The lesions are depicted but overlooked or not understood [23].

In order to meet the diagnostic problems in the sigmoid colon, authors have suggested that routine flexible sigmoidoscopy to precede a double-contrast barium enema [47-49]. By this means the greater lesion detectability shown by flexible endoscopy is combined with the superior documentation of barium enema. The advantage of this combination is reflected in increased sensitivity and positive prediction value of a spectrum of colonic diseases [48].

Double-contrast barium enema performed directly after collecting colonoscopic biopsies bears no risk, whereas the larger mucosal defects produced by biopsies through a rectoscope call for some days rest.

In summary both colonoscopy and barium enema have their pros and cons. The merit of colon radiography is the outstanding documentation which allows double reading, retrospect analysis and continuing education. The weaknesses are in the sigmoid colon and right hemicolon [1,26,45]. The main merit of colonoscopy is the means it provides for therapy, the drawbacks are incomplete intubation [50] and the risk of serious complications.

In general, one could probably justify the statement that the procedures are complementary [51,52], but a skilled colonoscopist is very hard to beat. The author is usually more correct as a colonoscopist: For every small lesion missed colonoscopically there are five to eight times as many overlooked radiographically. On the other hand, very few lesions 10 mm across or larger are missed by either technique [34].

In countries where the procedures compete on equal terms without the influence of money, as in Scandinavia, enemas still precede fibre-endoscopy in most non-colitic patients [53]. This is justified by the sufficiently high sensitivity, the accurate documentation of any mucosal lesion and the unchallenged ability to unveil extracolonic disorders otherwise hidden: endometriosis, pelvic and gynaecological tumours, organ dislocations, skeletal metastases, kidney and gallbladder stones, aneurysms, fistulas etc.

On the other hand colonoscopy should be performed on every patient with [29]:

- occult bleeding [48]
- significant clinical signs and symptoms irrespective of a negative barium enema or sigmoidoscopy [54]
- patients with polypoid lesions 5 mm across or larger, i.e. 8-mm lesions as measured on radiograms
- post-operative examination after partial colectomy for carcinoma (when all metachronous lesions are removed, the 'clean colon' is then documented by a double-contrast enema)
- 10 and more years duration of ulcerative colitis.

Quoting Simpkins, it may be concluded that there is no clinical, scientific or economic justification for the wholesale replacement of barium radiology by endoscopy [55].

References

1. Ott DJ, Gelfand DW, Ramquist NA. Causes of error in gastrointestinal radiology II. Barium enema examination. *Gastrointest Radiol* 1980;**5**:99-105.
2. Cotton PB, Rosenberg MT, Axon ATR, Davis M, Pierce JW, Price AB, Stevenson GW, Waldrum R. Diagnostic yeald of fibre-optic endoscopy in the operated stomach. *Br J Surg* 1973;**60**:629-32.
3. Martin TR, Vennes JA, Silvis SE, Ansel HJ. A comparison of upper gastrointestinal endoscopy and radiography. *J Clin Gastroenterol* 1980;**2**:21-5.
4. Fraser GM, Earnshaw PM. The double-contrast barium meal: A correlation with endoscopy. *Clin Radiol* 1983;**34**:1-000.
5. Gjörup T, Agner E, Bording-Jensen L, Nörup-Jensen A, Möllmann K. The endoscopic diagnosis of gastric ulcer. A randomized clinical trial of interobserver variation and bias induced by knowledge of the radiographical diagnosis. *Scand J Gastroenterol* 1985;**20**:554-8
6. Colin-Jones DG. Endoscopy or radiology for upper gastrointestinal symptoms.? *Lancet* 1986;**1**:1022-3.
7. Kim U, Rudick J, Aufses AH. Surgical management of acute upper gastrointestinal bleeding. *Arch Surg* 1978;**113**:1444-47.

8. Galen RS, Gambino SR. *Beyond normality: The predictive value and efficiency of medical diagnoses*. New York: John Wiley & Sons, 1975.
9. Kundel HL. Disease prevalence and radiological decision making. *Invest Radiol* 1982;**17**:107-9.
10. Graham DY, Schwartz JT, Cain GD, Gyorkey F. Prospective evaluation of biopsy number in the diagnosis of esophageal and gastric carcinoma. *Gastroenterology* 1982;**82**:228-31.
11. Ott, DJ, Gelfand DW, Wu WC. Sensitivity of single-contrast radiology in esophageal disease: A study of 240 patients with endoscopically verified abnormality. *Gastrointest Radiol* 1983;**8**:105-10.
12. Munitz HA, Gelfand DW, Ott DJ. Upper gastrointestinal series: Patient management and a study of 199 cases. *Gastrointest Radiol* 1985;**10**:277-81.
13. Gjörup T, Agner E, Bording-Jensen L, Mörup-Jensen A, Möllmann KM. Accuracy of radiologic and endoscopic diagnosis of gastric ulcer. *Acta Radiol* 1987;**28**:421-3.
14. Olearchyk AS. Gastric carcinoma. A critical review of 243 cases. *Am J Gastroenterol* 1978;**70**:24-45.
15. Dooley CP, Larson AW, Stace NH, Renner IG, Valenzuela JE, Eliasoph J, Colletti PM, Halls JM, Weiner JM. Double-constrast meal and upper gastrointestinal endoscopy. *Ann Int Med* 1984;**101**:538-45.
16. Holdstock G, Bruce S. Endoscopy and gastric cancer. *Gut* 1981;**22**:673-6.
17. Editorial. Upper gastrointestinal endoscopy - is it a first-line diagnostic service? *Gastrointest Endosc* 1982;**28**:213-4.
18. Hedeman N, Kruse A, Madsen EH, Mathiasen MS. X-ray examination or endoscopy? *Gastrointest Radiol* 1977;**1**:331-4.
19. Clark ML. Upper intestinal endoscopy. *Lancet* 1985;**1**:629.
20. Dawson J, Cockel R. Oesophageal perforation at fibreoptic gastroscopy. *Br Med J* 1981;**283**:533.
21. Lewis BS, Waye JD. Small bowel enteroscopy in 1988: Pros and cons. *Am J Gastroenterol* 1988;**84**:1413-5.
22. McGovern R, Barkin JS. Enteroscopy and enteroclysis: An improved method for combined procedure. *Gastrointest Radiol* 1990;**15**:327-8.
23. Kelvin FM, Gardiner R, Vas W, Stevenson GW. Colorectal carcinoma missed on double contrast barium enema study: a problem in perception. *AJR{* 1981;**137**:307-13.
24. Gelfand DW, Ott DJ, Munitz HA, et al. Radiology and endoscopy: A radiologic viewpoint. *Ann Intern Med* 1984;**101**:550.
25. Bolin S, Franzén L, Nilsson E, Sjödahl R. Carcinoma of the colon and rectum. Tumors missed by radiologic examination in 61 patients. *Cancer* 1988;**61**:1999-2008.
26. Fork F-T. Double contrast enema and colonoscopy in polyp detection. *Gut* 1981;**22**:971-7.
27. Williams CB, Macrae FA, Bartram CI. A prospective study of diagnostic methods in adenoma follow-up. *Endoscopy* 1982;**143**:74-8.
28. Ott, DJ, Ablin DS, Gelfand DW, Meschan I. Predictive value of a diagnosis of colonic polyp on the double-contrast barium enema. *Gastrointest Radiol* 1983;**8**:75-80.
29. Abrams JS. A second look at colonoscopy. *Arch Surg* 1982;**117**:913-7.
30. Gilbert DA, Shaneyfelt SL, Mahler AK, et al. The national ASGE colonoscopy survey: Preliminary analysis of complications of colonoscopy. *Gastrointest Endosc* 1983;**29**:176.
31. Whalen E. Colon cancer: Diagnosis in an era of cost containment. ACR conference, Nov 8, 1989. *AJR* 1990;**154**:875-881.
32. Reilly JC, Rusin LC, Theuerkauf FJ. Colonoscopy, Its role in cancer of the colon and rectum. *Dis Colon Rectum* 1982;**25**:532-8.
33. Durdey P, Weston PMT, Williams NS. Colonoscopy or barium enema as initial investigation of colonic disease. *Lancet* 1987;**2**:549-51.

34. Fork F-T. Diagnostic procedures in colo-rectal cancer; barium enema or colonoscopy? or both? *Europ J Surg Oncol* 1987;**13:**147-9.
35. Shinya H, Cwern M, Wolf G. Colonoscopic diagnosis and management of rectal bleeding. *Surg Clin North Am* 1982;**62:**897-903.
36. Lindsay DC, Freeman JG, Cobden I, Record CO. Should colonoscopy be the first investigation for colonic diseases? *Brit Med J* 1988;**296:**167-9.
37. Martin D. Letter: Should colonoscopy be the first investigation for colonic disease? *Br Med J* 000;**296:**571-2.
38. Gelfand DW, Ott DJ. Methodologic considerations in comparing imaging methods. *AJR* 1985;**144:**1117-21.
39. Frager DH, Frager JD, Wolf EL, Beneventano TC. Problems in the colonoscopic localization of tumours. Continued value of the barium enema. *Gastrointest Radiol* 1987;**12,**343-6.
40. Laufer I, Smith NCW, Mullens JE. The radiological demonstration of colorectal polyps undetected by endoscopy. *Gastroenterology* 1976;**70:**167-70.
41. Miller RE, Lehman G. Polypoid colonic lesions undetected by endoscopy. *Radiology* 1978;**139:**295-7.
42. Kelvin FM, Maglinte DDT. Colorectal carcinoma: a radiologic and clinical review. *Radiology* 1987;**164:**1-8.
43. Glick SN, Teplick SK, Balfe DM, Levine MS, Gasparaitis, AE, Maglinte, DDT, Shortsleeve MJ, Brandon JC. Large colonic neoplasms missed by endoscopy. *AJR* 1989;**152:**513-7.
44. Bartram CI. Radiology in investigation of rectal bleeding. *Dis Colon Rectum* 1980;**23:**318-9.
45. Aldridge MC, Sim AJW. Colonoscopy findings in symptomatic patients without X-ray evidence of colonic neoplasms. *Lancet* 1986;**2:**833-4.
46. Holloway R, Goulston K, Schieb M. The barium enema as a diagnostic procedure. *Austral Radiol* 1982;**26:**144-8.
47. Thoeni RF, Petras A. Detection of rectal and rectosigmoid lesions by double-contrast barium enema examination and sigmoidoscopy. *Radiology* 1982;**142:**59-62.
48. Irvine EJ, O'Connor J, Frost RA, Shorvon P, Somers S, Stevenson GW, Hunt RH. Prospective comparison of double contrast barium enema plus flexible sigmoidoscopy versus colonoscopy in rectal bleeding: barium enema versus colonoscopy in rectal bleeding. *Gut* 1988;**29:**1188-93.
49. Saito Y, Slezak P, Rubio C. The diagnostic value of combining flexible sigmoidoscopy and double-contrast barium enema as a one-stage procedure. *Gastrointest Endosc* 1989;**14,**357-9.
50. Gelfand DW, Wu WC, Ott DJ. The extent of successful colonoscopy: Its implication for the radiologist. *Gastrointest Radiol* 1979;**4:**75-78.
51. Thoeni RF, Menuck L. Comparison of barium enema and colonoscopy in the detection of small colonic polyps. *Radiology* 1977;**124:**631-5.
52. Thoeni RF, Petras A. Double-contrast barium-enema examination and endoscopy in the detection of polypoid lesions in the cecum and ascending colon. *Radiology* 1982;**144:**257-60.
53. Bloomfield JA. Reliability of barium enema in detecting colonic neoplasia. *Med J Aust* 1981;**1:**631-3.
54. Hixson LJ, Sampliner RE, Chernin M, Amberg J, Kogan F. Limitations of combined flexible sigmoidoscopy and double contrast barium enema in patients with rectal bleeding. *Eur J Radiol* 1989;**9:**254-7.
55. Simpkins KC. Bring out your barium. *J Can Assoc Radiol* 1989;**40:**5-11.

Angiography in diagnosis and treatment of lower gastrointestinal bleeding

J. Rösch
Charles Dotter Institute of Interventional Therapy, Oregon Health Sciences University, Portland, Oregon, USA and

K. Ivancev
Charles Dotter Institute of Interventional Therapy, Oregon Health Sciences University and University Hospital, Lund, Sweden

Introduction

Lower gastrointestinal bleeding (LGIB) originates, in the majority of patients, from lesions in the large bowel or small intestine. Up to 10% of patients with LGIB, however, have the bleeding source proximally to the ligament of Treitz, in the duodenum, stomach, or even in the oesophagus [1]. LGIB may be chronic and present with intermittent melanotic stools and cause chronic anaemia. Acute LGIB often presents as single or recurrent episodes of massive haemorrhage. Occasionally, the massive LGIB is continuous or explosive and results in significant hypovolaemia and even exsanguination. LGIB can be caused by various bowel lesions. Diverticula, congenital arteriovenous malformation (AVM), acquired angiodyplasias, ischaemia, inflammation, ulcerations, benign or malignant tumors, and iatrogenic injury such as polypectomy are among its more common causes [1,2]. Aorto-enteric fistula, visceral artery aneurysm, small or large bowel varices, faecal disimpaction, haemobilia, or bleeding from the pancreas are some of its less common causes [1,2].

Since the first use of operative mesenteric arteriography in 1960 [3], angiography has become an important method in the diagnosis of chronic and acute LGIB. In the 1970s angiographic interventional techniques were also introduced into the treatment of LGIB [1].

Diagnosis

Techniques

In older patients the authors often select the left femoral approach for catheter introduction because it facilitates catheterization of the inferior mesenteric artery. Occasionally, the authors use a left axillary approach, particularly when super-selective catheterization for embolization treatment is not possible from the femoral approach. In patients where an aortoenteric fistula is suspected, particularly in patients with a history of aortic bypass surgery or aortic aneurysm, the authors start with abdominal aortography using a 5 Fr pigtail catheter [1] (Fig. 1). Aortograms are obtained in frontal and lateral projections the latter demonstrating bleeding better, particularly if done in a prone position [4].

In patients, with aorto-iliac grafts or an iliac aneurysm, aortography is complemented by pelvic angiography to exclude a leak at the distal anastomosis or aneurysmal rupture [5]. Pelvic angiography is also an essential part of the study in patients after colectomy with residual rectal pouch and in pelvic malignancies, particularly those treated by radiation; their vascular bowel anatomy is usually grossly distorted, and they can bleed from the hypogastric arteries and their branches [6] (Fig. 2).

The majority of our patients with LGIB, however, have only selective visceral angiographic studies with use of 6 Fr Torcon visceral catheters (Cook Inc.) preshaped according to the anatomy of the individual vessels [1]. We usually perform the inferior mesenteric angiography first (Fig. 3). If the study is negative, superior mesenteric angiography follows (Fig. 4). In the case of a suspicious finding, super-selective angiography of the area in question is performed, usually with a magnification technique to facilitate diagnosis of small lesions. For super-selective catheterization, we use a long tapered tip (6 cm to 10 cm) 6 Fr Torcon catheter, or a 3 Fr catheter coaxially introduced via the 6 Fr catheter [1].

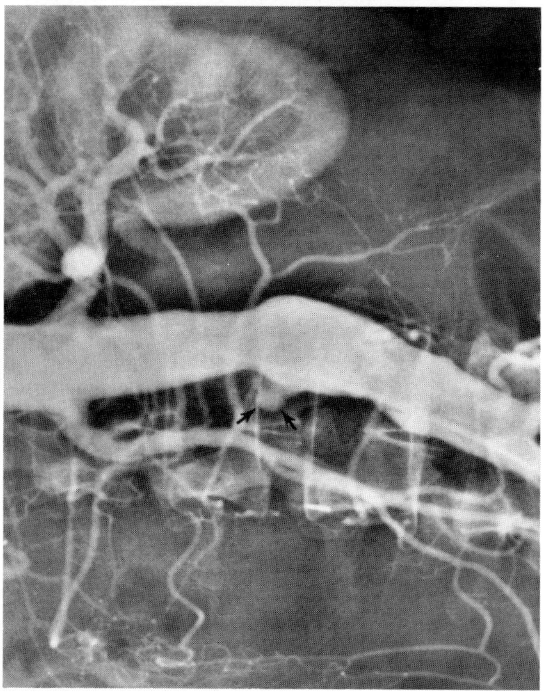

Figure 1. *Abdominal aortogram in a patient with history of multiple aorto-right renal bypass grafts and recurrent lower GI bleeding reveals a pseudoaneurysm of the aorta in the area of an aortoduodenal fistula (arrows).*

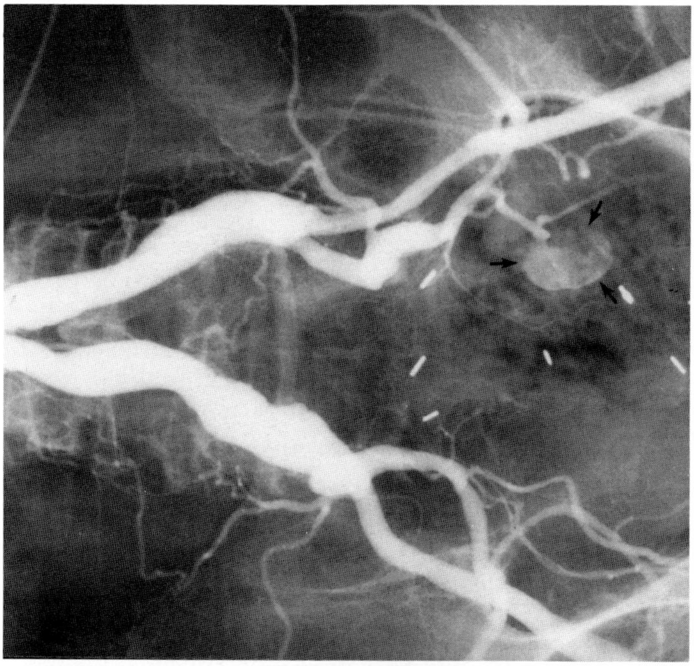

Figure 2. *Pelvic angiogram in a patient with recto-sigmoid carcinoma resection and acute bleeding from rectal pouch shows extravasation into the pouch from a branch of the left hypogastric artery (arrows).*

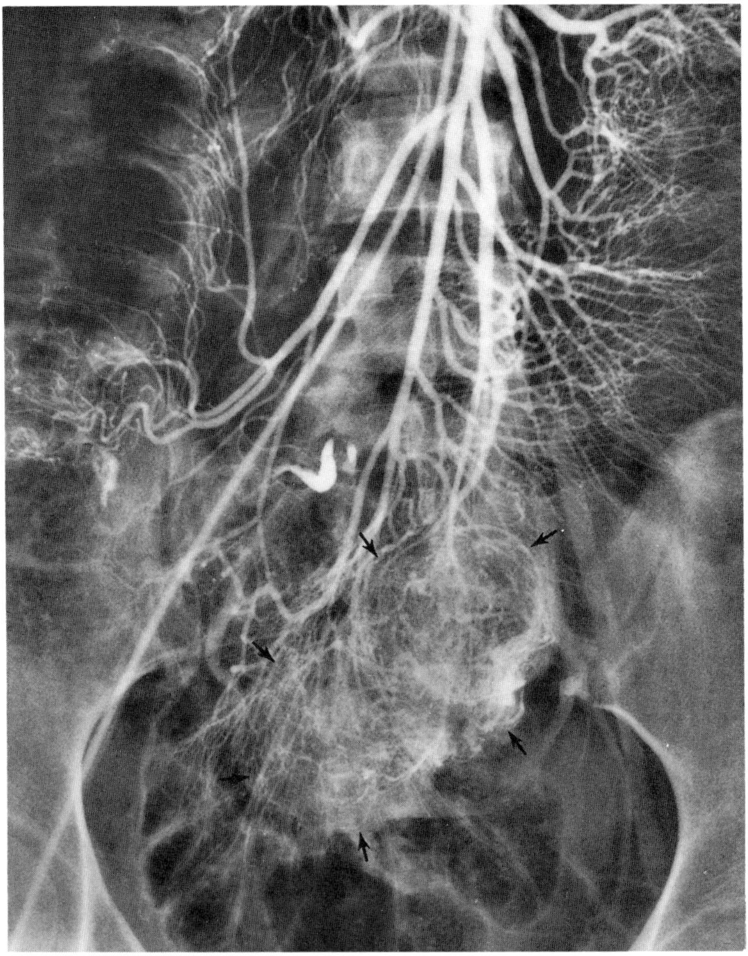

Figure 3. *Inferior mesenteric angiogram in a patient with recent renal transplant and massive hemotochezia reveals extensive extravasation in the distal rectum from large ulcer (arrows).*

When mesenteric angiograms are negative, coeliac angiography is performed. This not only helps to exclude bleeding from the stomach, duodenum, liver, and pancreas manifesting as LGIB, but also may visualize an accessory middle colic artery occasionally originating from the coeliac artery, which may supply a bleeding site in the transverse colon [2]. The authors perform 5-second contrast medium injections at a rate of 2-4 ml/s for inferior mesenteric arteriography and 7-9 ml/s for superior mesenteric and celiac arteriography.

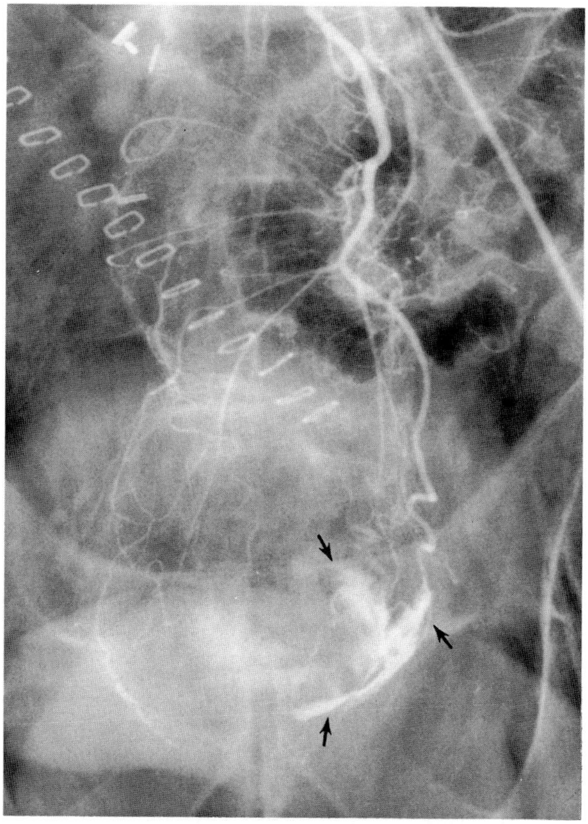

Figure 4. *Superior mesenteric angiogram in a patient with recurrent lower GI bleeding demonstrates a large hypervascular tumour - leiomyosarcoma - in the distal ileum (arrows).*

When pharmaco-angiography with the use of vasodilators is performed for better visualization of small vascular lesions, the injection rate is increased. The authors use tolazoline, usually 25 mg for the inferior mesenteric artery and 37.5-50 mg for the superior mesenteric artery injection. Tolazoline is diluted in 10 ml of normal saline and injected over 20 seconds. Angiography is performed 30 seconds later. The injection rate of contrast medium is 4-5 ml/s for the inferior mesenteric and 9-12 ml/s for the superior mesenteric. The first seven films are taken at a rate of one per second and are followed by seven films exposed every other second. In patients with portal hypertension, the filming is extended to 25-30 seconds.

The authors use conventional large film angiography in the diagnosis of LGIB. Satisfactory result were also reported with digital subtraction angiography. However, peristalsis can cause artifacts and confuse diagnosis. Digital subtraction angiography, however, is very useful during embolization to evaluate efficacy of the treatment.

The angiographer can also help the surgeon by facilitating exact localization of a bleeding site or vascular lesion at surgery by selective intraoperative mesenteric methylene blue injection [2]. This is important mainly in lesions of the small intestine where exact intraoperative localization may be difficult. When a vascular lesion or active bleeding is found on a superior mesenteric angiogram, the 6 Fr catheter is advanced into the branch of the superior mesenteric artery supplying the segment of bowel containing the lesion. A 3 Fr catheter is then coaxially introduced through the 6 Fr catheter and advanced deep into the supplying artery close to the bowel wall (Fig. 5). After super-selective angiography confirms the position, both catheters are

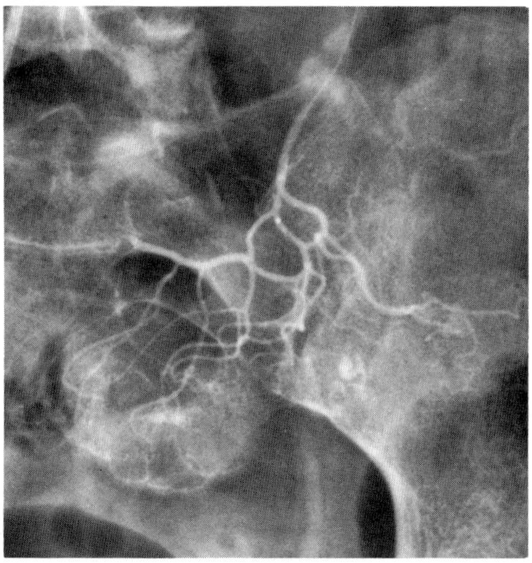

Figure 5. *Super-selective angiogram of a small ileal branch in a patient with lower GI bleeding reveals two foci of vascular ectasias (arrows). Catheter was left in place for visualization of the affected ileal loop at surgery.*

securely taped to the skin to prevent their dislodgement and are perfused with heparinized saline. At surgery, 1 ml of methylene blue is injected through the small catheter and the segmental bluish colouration of the small intestine exactly delineates the area of the lesion. This technique enables the surgeon to perform a selective, short-segment bowel resection [2].

Chronic Bleeding

In recurrent, low-grade rectal bleeding, angiography is indicated in patients in whom other investigations, particularly barium studies and endoscopic examinations, failed to define the source of haemorrhage. Done on an elective basis, angiography is obtained to demonstrate a structural, vascular lesion in the bowel as a potential bleeding source. There is about a 45% chance of finding such a lesion, but the incidence of false-negative findings is high, about 13% [1]. Use of pharmaco-angiography with vasodilators enhancing visualization of vascular lesions may decrease this high false-negative rate. Angiography is particularly important in the diagnosis of lesions located in the small intestine, where they easily escape detection by other techniques. Acquired angiodysplasias, congenital AVMs, and benign or malignant tumours are the most frequently found lesions. Visceral artery aneurysm, Meckel's diverticulum, or regional enteritis are among other causes of chronic LGIB.

Acquired angiodysplasias or vascular ectasias are seen in the elderly, with a higher incidence in patients with aortic valvular disease [7,8]. They are often located in the caecum and ascending colon, but they may also occur in other parts of the colon or small intestine. Angiodysplasias appear as small localized clusters of tangled arteries or vascular tufts with focal opacification of the bowel wall, 5 mm to 2 cm in size. They are often multiple and occasionally diffusely involve the caecum or a portion of the ascending colon. Angiodysplasias are supplied by slightly dilated arteries and show early drainage through dilated veins [7,9] (Fig. 6). Angiographic findings of angiodysplasias are often difficult to document at surgery or examination of the resected specimen unless a special injection technique is used [2,7].

Congenital AVMs can be localized in any portion of the bowel. They can be solitary lesions or part of a generalized vascular disorder such as Rendu-Osler-Weber syndrome [2,10] (Fig. 7). Depending on the prevalence of their vascular structures, they have various angiographic appearances. They sometimes appear as multiple telangiectasia consisting of closely packed networks of minute vessels or small

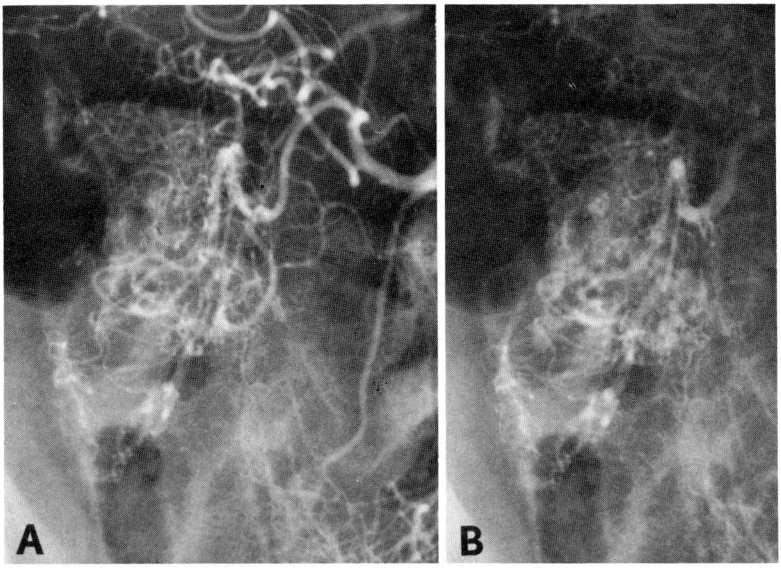

Figure 6. *Large angiodysplasia of the cecum and ascending colon causing recurrent low-grade rectal bleeding. A. Close-up of the arterial phase of superior mesenteric angiogram shows increased vascularity and multiple areas of tangled vessels in the cecum and ascending colon. B. Parenchymal phase shows increased blush of the angiodysplastic area and dense filling of the draining veins.*

focal densities in the bowel wall. They are usually supplied by normal-sized vasa recta and do not exhibit early venous filling. Magnification angiography is helpful in their visualization.

Arteriovenous fistulas occasionally occur in the bowel as clusters of vascular lakes supplied by an enlarged artery and exhibiting early and dense venous drainage via an enlarged vein. Localized phlebectasias, which may present in the form of a few ectatic veins but more often as nets of enlarged veins, usually present a challenge to angiographic diagnosis. They show no arterial changes or only minimal arterial dilation, and may not be obvious on a conventional study because of dilution of contrast medium in the enlarged venous structures. Tolazoline pharmaco-angiography enhances their visualization and facilitates their diagnosis. Occasionally, diffuse venous angiomatosis is found involving a major portion of the bowel, such as the rectum of sigmoid colon. It consists of multiple vascular lakes, appearing in the late parenchymal and venous phase of the study.

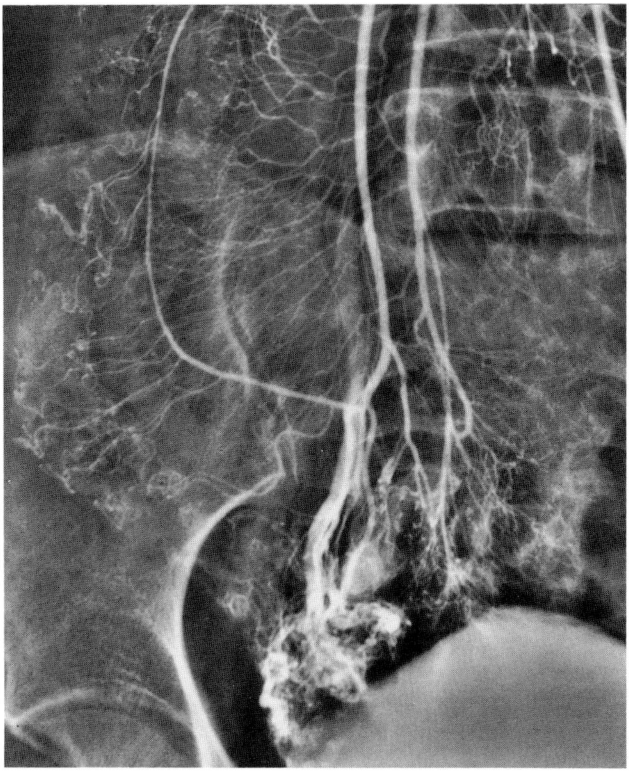

Figure 7. *Large arteriovenous malformation of the terminal ileum and cecum and multiple telangiectasias of the ascending colon in a patient with Rendu-Osler-Weber syndrome and recurrent LGIB. The patient also had multiple lung AVMs.*

Aneurysms of the visceral arteries may occasionally be the cause of chronic bleeding, particularly when localized close to the bowel lumen or inside the liver (haemobilia) or pancreas. However, even ruptured aneurysm of the splenic artery may cause LGIB. In patients with portal hypertension, varices are often seen in the mesentery close to the bowel wall, particularly at the sites of post-surgical adhesions. Their relationship to LGIB, however, is uncertain.

Tumours of the small intestine, particularly leiomyoma and leiomyosarcoma, present angiographically as hypervascular masses containing nets of irregular tumour vessels, tumour blush in the capillary phase, and early dense venous filling (Fig. 4). Other tumours, such as carcinoid or melanoma, are less obvious. Carcinoid is usually diagnosed by its desmoplastic reaction in the mesentery causing irregularity and retraction of surrounding vessels. Melanoma of the small bowel may be hypervascular or present only by irregular encasement of surrounding vessels.

Acute Bleeding

In patients with acute LGIB, angiography should be performed on an emergency basis when the patient is actively bleeding. Extravasation of contrast medium into the bowel lumen is the main finding to look for on angiograms (Figs. 3 and 8). Finding of a hypervascular lesion, as described in chronic bleeding, is also important but is only suggestive of a potential bleeding source. Before angiography, patients should have digital rectal and proctosigmoidoscopic examinations to exclude an anal or rectal source of haemorrhage. Many gastroenterologists also perform colonoscopy, but in massive bleeding it may be difficult to evaluate the study because of the presence of large amounts of blood in the entire colon. Bleeding from a source in the upper gastrointestinal tract must always be excluded before angiography; aspiration of gastric content is helpful but endoscopy may be required to exclude a duodenal ulcer [8].

Success of angiography in visualization of the site of haemorrhage by contrast medium extravasation depends on proper timing of the examination; it has to be done during active bleeding at a rate greater than 0.5 ml/min. Patients with continuous massive rectal bleeding who are haemodynamically unstable are usually actively bleeding and should have angiography as the first study. In these patients angiography has shown an efficacy of visualization of extravasation in the range of 67-92% [2]. In haemodynamically stable patients, activity of LGIB is much more difficult to assess, particularly when it originates from the small bowel or proximal colon. It is often intermittent in nature, from minute to minute, and a bloody rectal discharge can continue for several hours after bleeding has actually stopped [11]. Angiography performed solely on the basis of clinical criteria in haemodynamically stable patients has often been unrevealing, with an efficacy of 30-40% [2,12].

These patients should first be evaluated by radionuclide scanning for activity of bleeding.

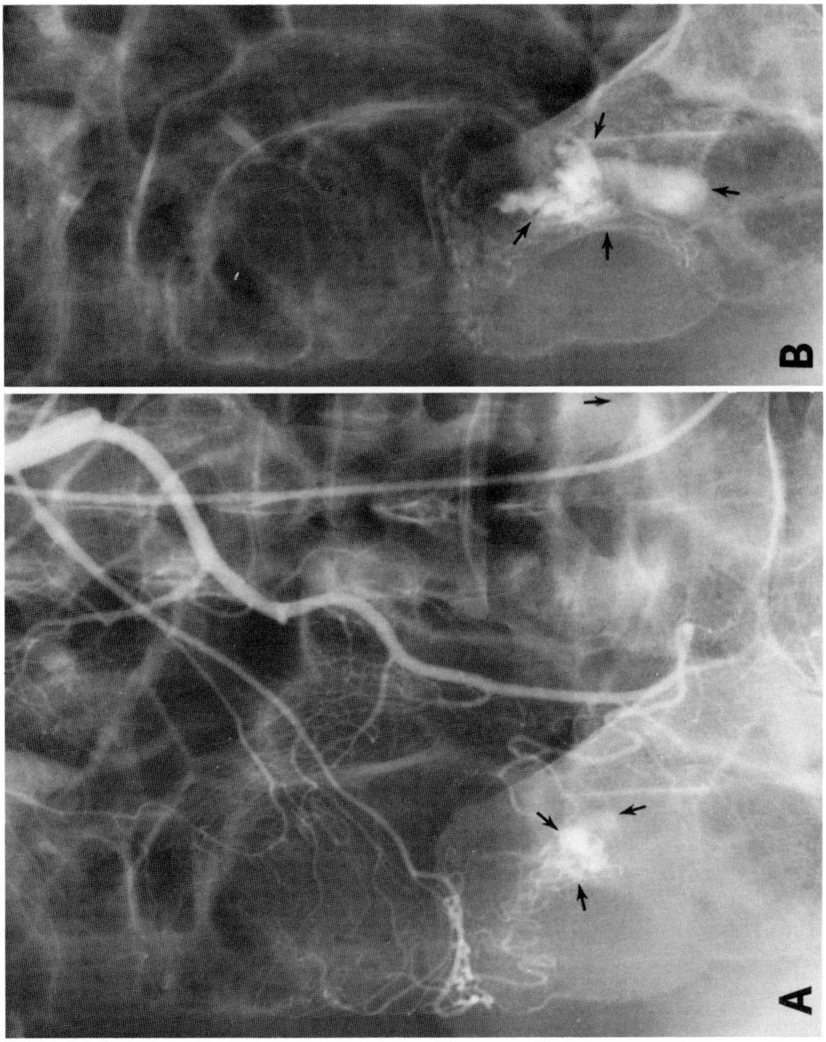

Figure 8. *A: Acutely bleeding angiodysplasia in the cecum in a patient with massive lower GI bleeding. Arterial phase of superior mesenteric angiogram reveals increase vascularity of the cecum with contrast medium extravasation (arrows). B. Late parenchymal phase shows persistent pooling of contrast medium in the cecal lumen (arrows).*

Technetium-labeled sulphur colloid or technetium-labeled red blood cells help to determine the state of haemorrhagic activity with higher sensitivity than angiography and can detect bleeding of as little as 0.1 ml/min [13]. If the radionuclide study is negative, the patient should be followed by sequential images to detect a temporarily ceased, intermittent bleeding. If the radionuclide scan is positive for active bleeding on either early or delayed images, angiography should be performed without delay.

Efficacy of angiography in visualization of active bleeding in haemodynamically stable patients can be enhanced by several interventions that help to prolong, augment, or reactivate bleeding [1,14]. In the authors' experience, these interventions increased the diagnostic yield of angiography for demonstration of extravasation from 32 to 65%; moreover, they decreased the percentage of negative studies from 27 to 16%, and the percentage of angiograms revealing only a vascular lesion as a possible bleeding source from 41 to 19% [15]. Diagnostic interventions, however, should be used only in patients who constitute diagnostic and therapeutic dilemmas, and in whom risk of prolonging or reactivating bleeding is outweighed by the potential diagnostic gains.

Anticoagulants, in particular heparin, are used first, with the objective of prolonging the existing bleeding until angiography can be performed. It is administered intravenously at the time of angiography scheduling when the radionuclide scan indicates active bleeding - 1000 U of heparin per 10 kg body weight (Fig. 9). After the study successfully demonstrates extravasation, protamine sulphate is given to neutralize the effects of heparin - 10 mg of protamine sulphate being sufficient to neutralize each 1000 U of heparin. The dose of protamine sulphate, however, should be decreased in proportion to the duration of the procedure, since heparin has a half-life of about 2 hours.

When angiography after heparin does not reveal extravasation or an obvious vascular lesion as the potential bleeding site, the authors proceed to a further interventional measure, use of the vasodilator tolazoline (Fig. 10). This used to augment low volume bleeding or reactivate a recently-ceased haemorrhage to a greater rate then 0.5 ml/min. Induced vasodilation opens constricted vessels at the bleeding site and, together with increased blood flow, can dislodge a soft fibrin plug in the bleeding vessel. Selection of the site of tolazoline injection reflects the suspected level of bleeding. The superior

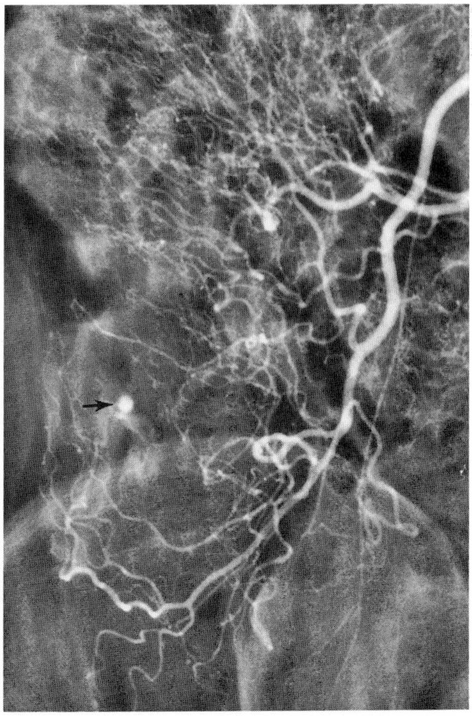

Figure 9. *Recurrent, massive bleeding from a diverticulum in the ascending colon diagnosed with the help of systemic heparinization. The patient had a negative angiographic study during his previous episode of active bleeding. When acute rectal haemorrhage recurred, he was given 6000 U of heparin intravenously. Follow-up superior mesenteric angiography showed active extravasation of contrast medium into a diverticular sack (arrow) with some spilling into the bowel lumen.*

mesenteric artery is most often used because haemorrhage of the small intestine and right colon is difficult to diagnose without angiography. The dose of tolazoline depends on the size of the catheterized vessel and the weight of the patient, and ranges from 25 to 50 mg. Tolazoline is injected over 20 seconds. Angiography follows 60 seconds later with increased volume and injection rate of contrast material (Fig. 11).

Further interventional measures in the case of negative tolazoline angiography depend on the urgency of need for diagnosis. In most cases the catheter is left in the artery supplying the presumed

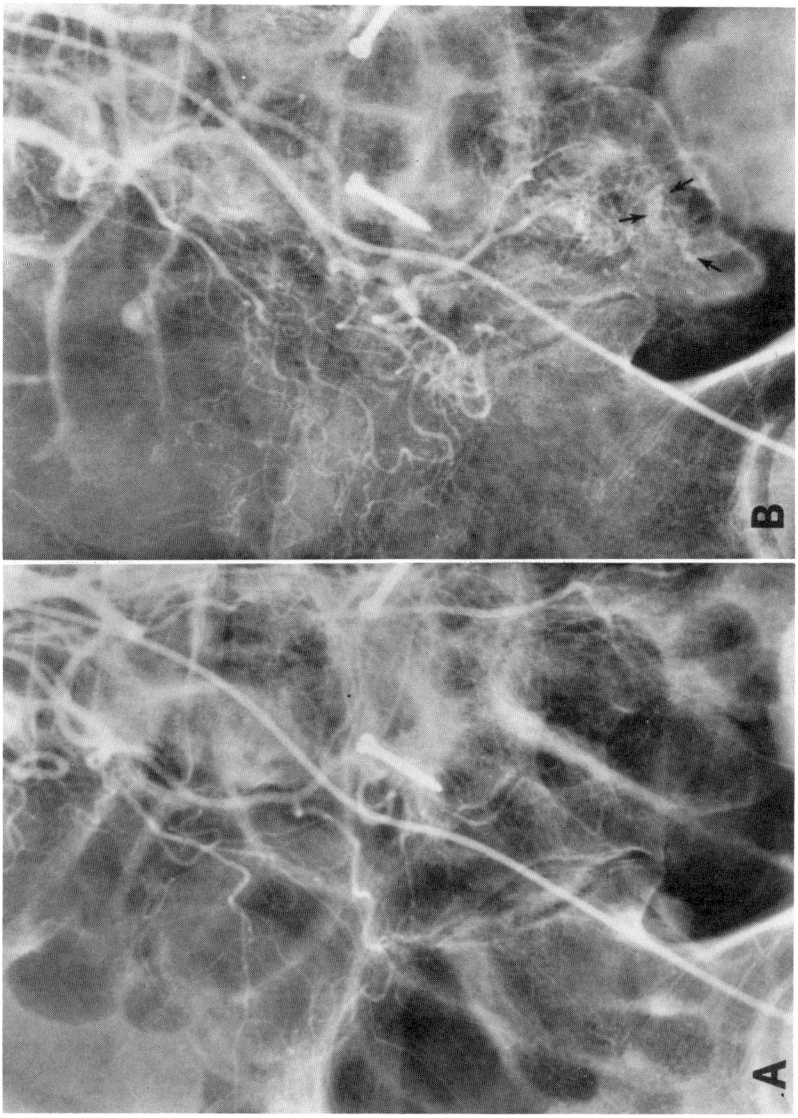

Figure 10. *Recurrent massive rectal haemorrhage from an angiodysplasia in the terminal ileum and cecum diagnosed with use of heparin and tolazoline. A. Superior mesenteric angiogram after heparin shows extensive vasoconstriction of the ileocolic artery braches and no angiodysplasia or extravasation B. Tolazoline pharmaco-angiogram, which was done after the patient had a large bowel movement of bloody stool, reveals enlarged ileocolic branches feeding several angiodysplastic areas in the terminal ileum and cecum and extravasation of contrast medium (arrows).*

Figure 11. *Acute bleeding from an ulcerated carcinoid tumour in the distal ileum diagnosed with the use of heparin and tolazoline. Superior mesenteric angiography after intravenous administration of 7500 U heparin was negative for active bleeding. Pharmaco-angiography performed after 50 mg of tolazoline revealed small extravasation of contrast medium (arrows). A. Arterial phase. B. Parenchymal phase.*

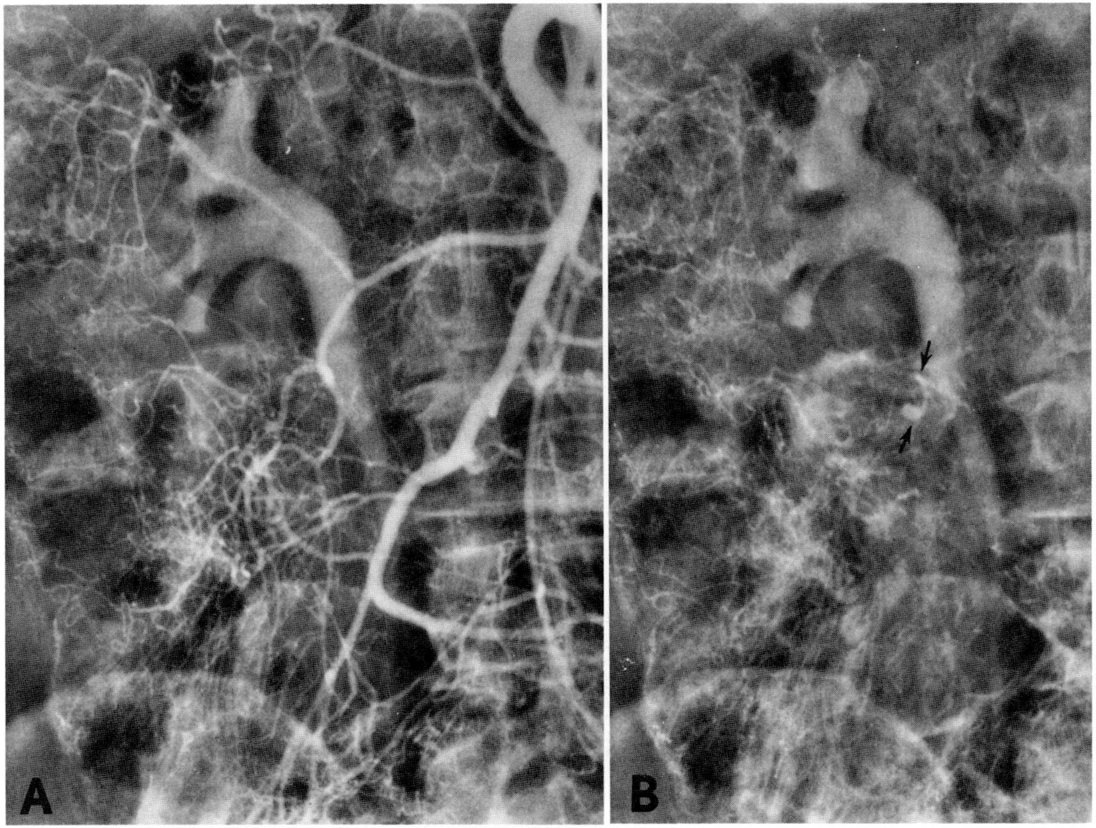

bleeding area and the patient is returned to the ward. The indwelling catheter allows prompt repeat angiography when clinical evidence of active bleeding recurs (Fig. 12). The indwelling catheter is some times the only intervention in patients with severe underlying disease in whom use of heparin and tolazoline is contraindicated [15]. The catheter is left in the artery for 1-3 days, depending on the patient's clinical condition.

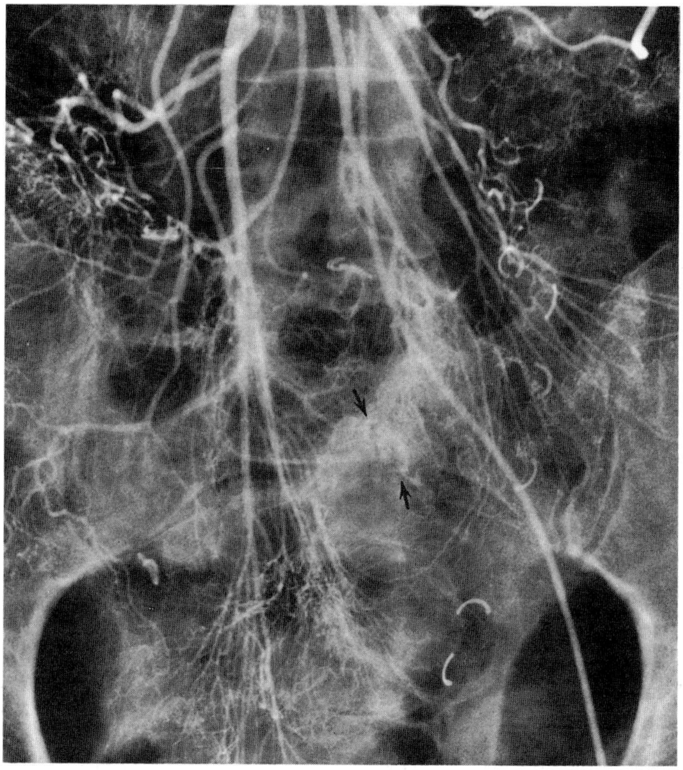

Figure 12. *Acute bleeding from a lymphoma in the mid-ileum diagnosed with the use of an indwelling catheter. After a superior mesenteric angiographic study was negative for active bleeding, the catheter was left in place for 3 days. When the patient started to pass bloody stools again, a repeat study was done. It showed extravasation of contrast medium (arrows).*

When the need for diagnosis is desperate, particularly when a patient continues to bleed despite previous resective surgery for LGIB, use of fibrinolytic agents - streptokinase or preferably urokinase - is indicated to reactivate the bleeding. They are likely to reactivate bleeding that has recently ceased, no more than a few hours before the procedure. Their effectiveness decreases with the age of the haemostatic plug, and a short-term infusion will probably have no effect on an established, well-organized, haemostatic thrombus [14,15]. Tolazoline angiography is performed after infusion of fibrinolytic agents because the induced vasodilation and increased flow may help to break up and dislodge the partially lysed thrombus and reactivate the bleeding. All decisions about the use of fibrinolytic agents, however, have to be reached in conjunction with the referring gastroenterologist and surgeon, and blood for transfusion must be at hand for emergency needs. The fibrinolytic agent is infused selectively into the artery supplying the presumed bleeding site, usually the superior mesenteric, for 30-60 minutes. With streptokinase, the authors have used an initial bolus of 20,000 to 40,000 U which was followed by infusion of 2000 to 4000 U/min, depending on the patient's weight (Fig. 13). With urokinase the dose is 20,000 to 30,000 U/min (Fig. 14). These low-dose, short-term selective infusions usually do not produce a systemic thrombolytic effect with undesired remote bleeding; however, the induced bleeding may require corrective fluid replacement.

The diagnostic interventional measures have their contraindications and carry certain risks. Use of heparin, tolazoline, and fibrinolytic agents is contraindicated in patients with severe underlying disease combined with coagulopathy or impaired cardiac function. These measures are also contraindicated in patients with potential aorto-enteric fistulas because they can result in explosive, uncontrollable haemorrhage. Tolazoline also should not be used in patients with hypotension. In patients with compromised renal function, the amount of contrast material has to be limited and the approach altered [15].

Contrast medium extravasation in LGIB is practically always at the arterial or arteriolo-capillary level and appears early or later in the arterial phase of angiography and persists in the parenchymal and venous phases. With a large amount of blood or fluid in the involved bowel, it may become diluted and decrease in density or even disappear on later venous films. Its amount varies, depending on severity of bleeding, from barely visible extravasation to a massive pooling outlining or filling the lumen of the involved bowel, particularly in a brisk haemorrhage in the small intestine.

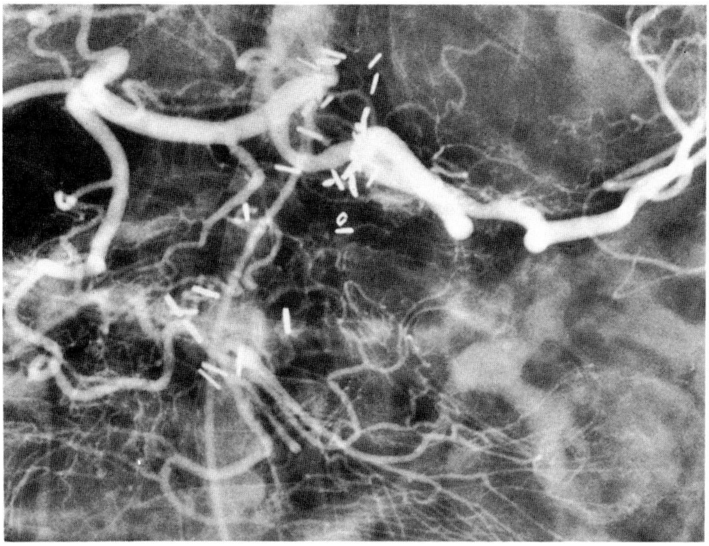

Figure 13. *Recurrent LGIB from small venous ectasias in the upper jejunum diagnosed with the use of heparin, streptokinase, and tolazoline. After the celiac and superior mesenteric angiographic studies with the use of heparin and tolazoline were negative, 60 000 U of streptokinase was infused over a period of 30 minutes in the superior mesenteric artery followed by 50 mg of tolazoline. Massive haematemesis immediately ensued, and celiac angiogram revealed extravasation of contrast medium (arrows) into the upper jejunum, which was filled by pancreaticoduodenal collaterals.*

Extravasation provoked by vasodilators and fibrinolytic agents are usually small and in a diagnostically borderline range. High-quality angiograms and careful evaluation are necessary if they are not to be overlooked. The majority of extravasations occur in a normal bowel and are easily diagnosed. Extravasation occurring in a pathologically changed bowel, as in a hypervascular wall due to inflammation or ischaemia, angiodysplasia, AVM, or tumour may be difficult to differentiate from the underlying lesion. Late angiographic phases may help; extravasation persists, while filling of the underlying lesion disappears. Location of the extravasation is usually easy to establish by tracing the arterial branch feeding the bleeding point. With overlapping vessels of different portions of the bowel, it may be more difficult. It may happen in the hepatic flexure and low-positioned transverse colon where the right and middle colic arteries are superimposed over the inferior pancreaticoduodenal and jejunal arteries feeding the duodenum and the jejunum. In case of doubt, superselective angiography helps to find the exact site of haemorrhage.

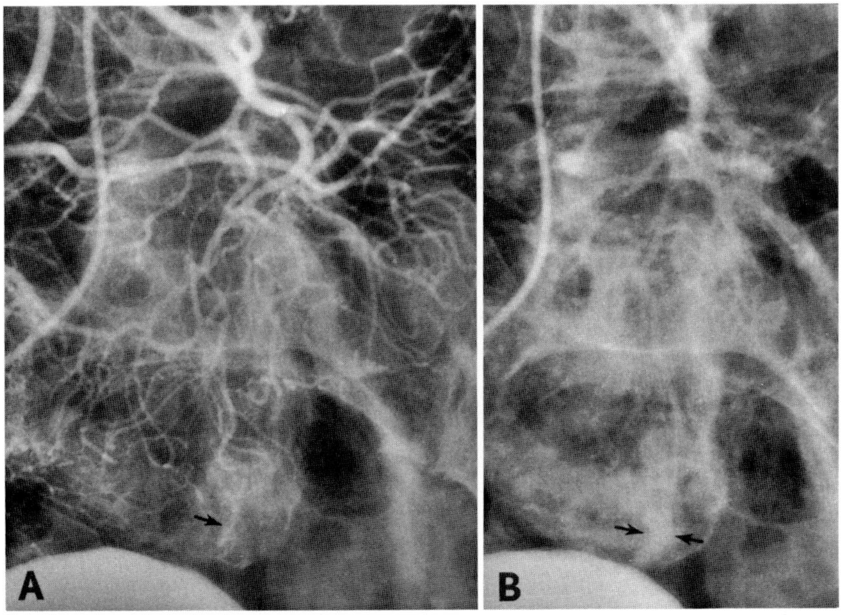

Figure 14. *Recurrent LGIB from vascular ectasia in the ileum in a patient with previous right hemicolectomy. Bleeding was diagnosed with the use of heparin, urokinase and tolazoline. After angiograms with the use of heparin and tolazoline were negative one million units of urokinase was infused at a rate of 30 000 units per minute into the superior mesenteric artery followed by 25 milligrams of tolazoline and superior mesenteric angiogram. A. Close-up view of superior mesenteric angiogram in arterial phase reveals vascular ectasia in ileum (arrow). B. Early venous phase demonstrates extravasation of contrast medium at the area of vascular ectasia (arrows).*

The source of haemorrhage can be diagnosed only occasionally when bleeding originates from a hypervascular, well-defined lesion. Occasionally, a small rate diverticular bleeding also gives a characteristic picture of a well localized, rounded density by contrast medium filling of a diverticular sack. With major diverticular haemorrhage, contrast medium usually spills freely into the bowel lumen. In colonic diverticula, bleeding is more frequent and more severe from those localized in the right colon, even when more diverticula occur in the left colon and sigmoid [2]. Post-operative bleeding is usually at the area of an anastomosis, particularly if metallic clips were used, and the area must be well evaluated. With an aortoenteric fistula, which most often occurs in the duodenum, the extravasation is seen only rarely and mainly on a lateral aortogram in the prone position [4,16]. More often, however, only a pseudo-aneurysm at the area of the graft anastomosis or a bulging aneurysm is seen [16,17].

Haemobilia, which has recently been occurring with increased incidence because of interventional percutaneous treatment of obstructive jaundice, often is manifested by haematemesis; with slow rate or intermittent haemorrhage, however, LGIB may be its only sign. A slow rate haemorrhage into the biliary tract may not be visualized directly by angiography. However, indirect but diagnostically important findings such as intrahepatic pseudoaneurysm and arteriovenous or arterioportal fistula are indicative of the bleeding source [18]. In bleeding from the pancreas, extravasation into the pancreatic duct is occasionally seen, but finding of a pseudoaneurysm or aneurysm of pancreatic vessels is also important for diagnosis and suggestive of a bleeding source.

Vasoconstrictive Therapy

Selective infusion of a vasoconstrictive agent into the artery supplying the bleeding site is the primary angiographic therapy for control of LGIB [1]. Vasopressin, an aqueous solution of the pressor component of the posterior pituitary gland, is presently the choice of a vasoconstrictive agent. It causes contraction of the vascular bed of the perfused intestine - especially of its capillaries, small arterioles and venules - and produces a significant and sustained reduction in splanchnic blood flow. Vasopressin infusion is best in controlling capillary, arteriolar, and small vessel bleeding in patients with normal haemocoagulation (Fig. 15). Prolonged vasoconstriction enables formation of a stable clot at the area of haemorrhage and control of the bleeding. In patients with a coagulopathy, usually temporary control only is achieved during infusion, and bleeding recurs after cessation of infusion. Vasopressin is also less effective in bleeding from larger arteries particularly those changed by tumour, inflammation, or abscess [19].

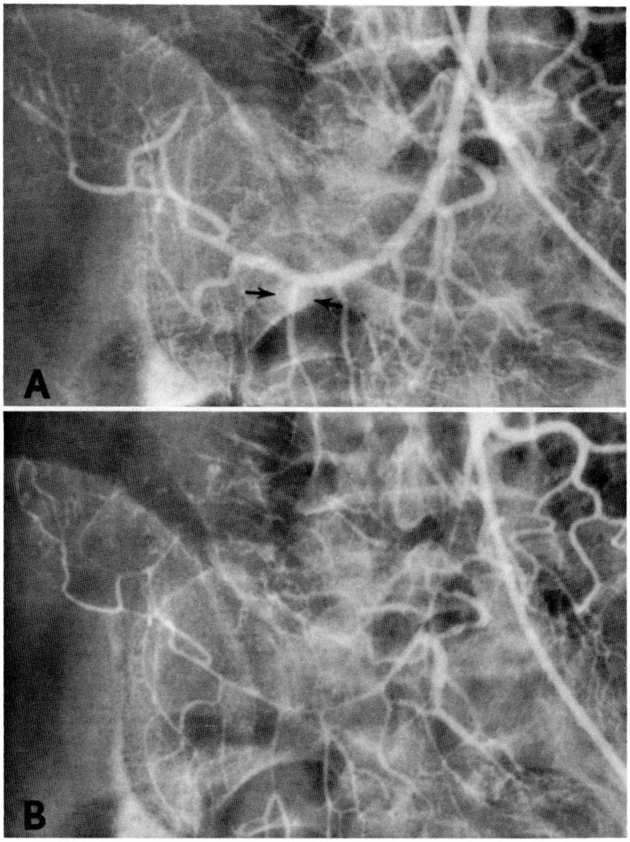

Figure 15. *Acute bleeding from an ileal ulcer in a patient with total colectomy successfully treated with selective vasopressin infusion. A. Close-up view of mesenteric angiogram shows early extravasation in the ileum (arrows). B. Close-up view of angiogram done after 20-minute infusion of vasopressin at a rate of 0.3 U/min shows extensive vasoconstriction and no extravasation. Infusion was continued for 24 hours at a rate of 0.2 U/min. No bleeding recurred, no surgery was necessary.*

In patients with colonic diverticula, which represent the majority of LGIB in the elderly, vasopressin infusion can control haemorrhage in about 90% [2,20]. Bleeding recurs in only about 30% of patients, from hours to months after initial control [2], thus surgery can be prevented in more than half of patients with diverticular haemorrhage. Patients with lesions that have higher recurrence rates of rebleeding after infusion, such as major angiodysplasias, or with lesions that have to be treated surgically, such as large AMVs, can also profit from vasopressin infusions. The temporary control of bleeding during infusion gives time to stabilize the patient so that surgery can be performed on an elective basis. If effective control of bleeding cannot be achieved by vasopressin infusion and the patient is not a candidate for surgery, selective embolization of the bleeding artery should be considered. Clinically significant coronary artery disease, particularly recent myocardial infarction, advanced peripheral and cerebral vascular disease, congestive heart failure, and renal failure with fluid retention, are among the main contraindications to vasopressin use.

Vasopressin is selectively infused into the artery supplying the bleeding point, usually the main trunk of the inferior or superior mesenteric artery [19]. In patients with a replaced hepatic artery originating from the superior mesenteric, the infusion catheter has to be positioned beyond the origin of the replaced artery to prevent loss of vasopressin to the liver. When a large ileocolic artery causes bleeding in the distal ileum or cecum, the catheter can be advanced into a super-selective position to achieve more localized effect. Direct jejunal artery infusion is preferable for bleeding control of a jejunal ulcer, particularly if it is at the site of a surgical anastomosis. In bleeding from an aberrant middle colic artery originating from the coeliac artery, direct catheterization has to be achieved. In catheterization of these smaller vessels, the catheter has to be in a free position to allow adequate blood flow around it, otherwise infarction of the infused bowel can occur.

Vasopressin is diluted in normal saline or 5% dextrose into a 0.2 U/ml concentration and is delivered with an arterial infusion pump. Infusion dose rate depends on the size of the catheterized artery [1]. For the inferior mesenteric artery, the initial rate is 0.1-0.2 U/min and for the superior mesenteric artery 0.2-0.3 U/min. An initial 20-minute test infusion is performed in the angiography room and is followed by a repeat angiogram to assess the efficacy of the infusion (Fig. 16). If no further bleeding is demonstrated and no excessive vasoconstriction is seen, the catheter is secured at the groin, and the infusion is continued in the intensive care unit. If bleeding persists after a 20-minute vasoconstrictive infusion, the vasopressin dose is increased, but no more than 0.3 U/min for the inferior mesenteric and 0.4 U/min for the superior mesenteric artery for a further 20-minute test infusion. Failure to control the bleeding using these high doses or

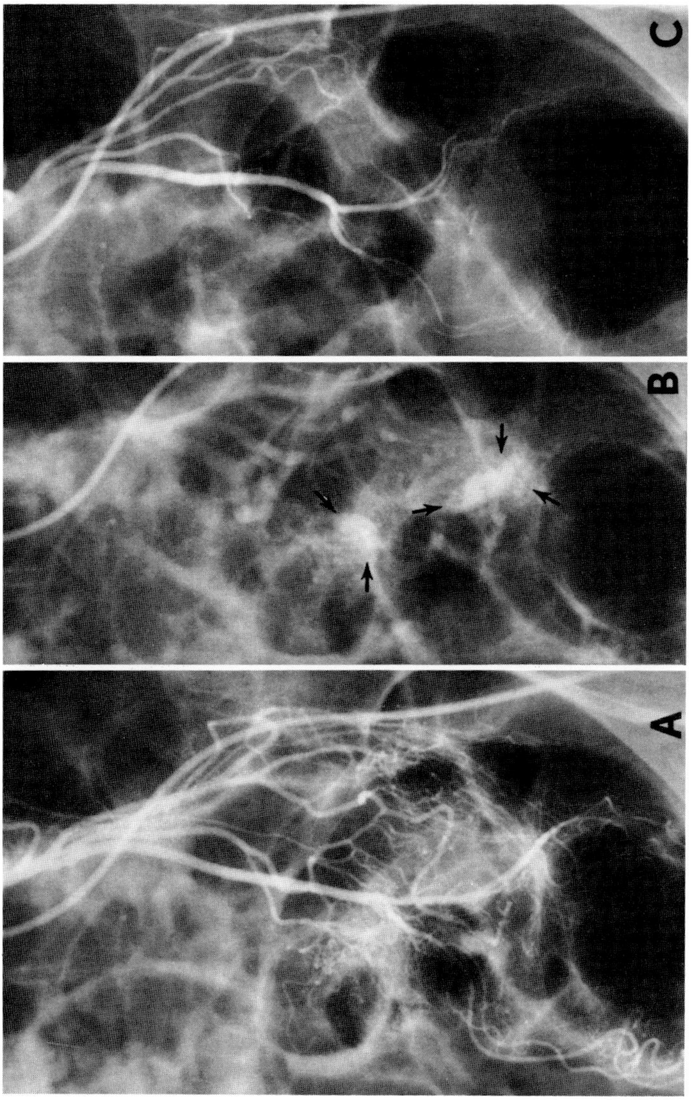

Figure 16. *Acute massive bleeding after endoscopical removal of a sigmoid colon polyp controlled by selective vasopressin infusion. A and B. Inferior mesenteric arteriogram reveals hypervascularity of sigmoid in the arterial phase and extensive contrast medium extravasation in the venous phase (arrows). C. Angiogram after 20 minutes infusion of vasopressin at a rate of 0.2 U/min shows extensive vasoconstriction and no more bleeding.*

absence of significant vasoconstrictive effect on follow-up angiogram indicates that safe vasoconstrictive control cannot be expected, and alternative therapeutic methods should be used. With a good vasoconstrictive response on follow-up angiograms, infusion is continued at full dose rate for 12-24 hours, depending on the patient's condition and clinical response. The initial rate is then halved for the ensuing 24 hours and the infusion is discontinued if there is no clinical evidence of further bleeding. The catheter may be kept in place with a low volume 5% dextrose infusion for another 12 to 24 hours to be ready for repeat vasopressin infusion should the bleeding clinically recur.

During the first 20 minutes of vasopressin infusion, some patients may experience abdominal cramps or abdominal pain because of vasopressin-induced bowel contractions, which may result in a beneficial emptying of the bowel of the accumulated blood clots. The cramps and pain should subside in 30 minutes, and their persistence or later occurrence is indicative either of too high a dose rate or of dislodgement of the catheter tip and selective infusion into a small branch. A decreased infusion rate and check of the catheter position will help to define the cause of patient discomfort.

Selective mesenteric vasoconstrictive treatment is not without risk, and complications may result from the prolonged presence of an intravascular catheter or from the vasopressin infusion rate [2,20,21]. Vascular spasm and thrombosis may occur at the puncture site of the femoral artery and result in leg ischaemia; spasm and thrombosis of the infused artery or arteries may cause bowel infarction. Chest pain, cardiac arrhythmias, in particular bradycardia, and even myocardial infarction may occur. The antidiuretic effect of vasopressin may lead to decreased diuresis, oedema, and hyponatraemia. The incidence of complications can be expected to be in the range of 3-5% and can be kept at a minimum by strict observance of contraindications, limiting the time of intravascular catheter placement and keeping the dose rate of vasopressin at the lowest effective level.

Embolization therapy

Embolization of the bleeding artery of the small intestine and large bowel has to be approached with much greater caution than that of the stomach and duodenum, where a multiple-vessel blood supply minimizes the risk of significant ischaemic injury [1]. The sections of the small intestine and large bowel, with the exception of the splenic flexure and distal rectum, are supplied by only one artery and have less large vessel collateral capacity than the stomach and duodenum. Small bowel collaterals consist of small vessel arcades in the mesentery close to the bowel wall; large bowel arteries are interconnected by a marginal artery in the mesentery. Vasa recta of both the small intestine and large colon arise predominantly as single, non-communicating arteries. In the bowel wall their branches anastomose and form rich intermural vascular networks at the level of submucosal arterioles. Because of the paucity of larger collaterals, embolization therapy of LGIB involves a risk of ischaemic injury. Review of the reported cases indicates that risk may range between 15 and 25% for embolization in the small intestine and 10 and 15% for the large bowel [21-25]. Ischaemic injury may be acute and manifested by transmural necrosis and bowel infarction. Ischaemic necrosis involving only mucosa may cause bowel stricture after healing [26]. Risk of bowel injury, however, can be kept at a minimum by careful performance of the embolization procedure.

Embolization is usually used as a secondary angiographic intervention for control of massive LGIB after vasoconstrictive infusion failure and when the patient is not a good candidate for emergency surgery (Fig. 17). Embolization, however, can easily be justified as a primary procedure for fast haemostasis when the patient is bleeding profusely, his clinical condition is rapidly deteriorating, and large amounts of blood are necessary for stabilization [1]. It should be considered particularly in lesions that respond poorly to vasoconstrictive treatment, such as bleeding from major AVMs or large vessels. In this situation, embolization may be a life-saving procedure replacing emergency surgery, which has high morbidity and mortality - particularly in elderly and debilitated patients. It allows stabilization of the patient, and with lesions requiring surgical removal, an elective operation can be performed with much less risk. In lesions amenable to medical treatment, embolization may be the definitive therapy. If bowel ischaemia requiring surgery occurs, the operation is usually done on an improved, stabilized patient, and usually no more bowel has to be removed than would ordinarily be resected if surgery had been performed for the initial control of bleeding. Embolization may also be the only effective palliative treatment for control of bleeding

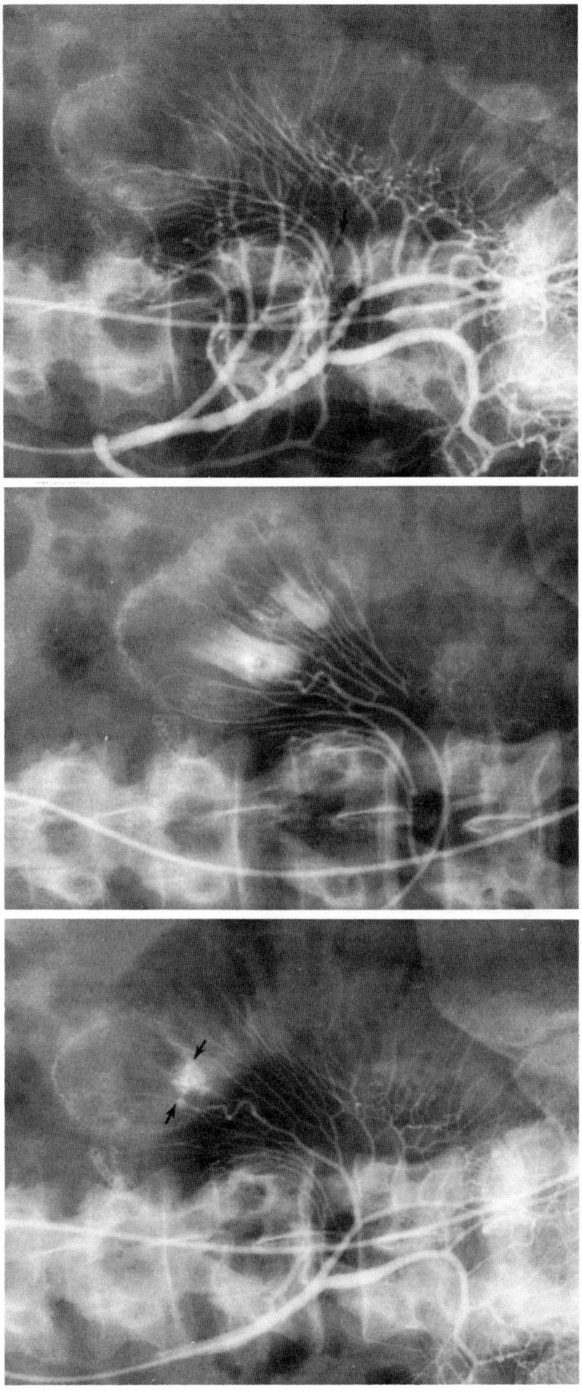

Figure 17. *Massive bleeding from a recent surgical anastomosis in the jejunum in a patient with hepatitis and coagulopathy. Bleeding was controlled for 2 days by selective infusion of vasopressin but recurred immediately after discontinuation of infusion. It was successfully treated by selective embolization. No complications developed. A. Selective angiogram of jejunoileal branch shows extravasation of contrast medium (arrows) at the area of metallic clips. B. Selective angiogram of the bleeding artery using a long tapered 6 Fr Torcon catheter shows increased extravasation. The catheterized artery was occluded with one Gelfoam strip. C. Follow-up angiogram shows occlusion of the embolized artery (arrow), absence of extravasation, and collateral filling of the embolized area. Post-catheterization spasm of the larger arteries is also present.*

from inoperable tumours, particularly when located in the rectum [6] (Fig. 18).

Safety of bowel embolization is closely related to the techniques used, and to decrease its risks, several rules should be followed [1].

(1) The embolization has to be super-selective and only the bleeding artery or its small feeder should be occluded. Direct catheterization and embolization of the bleeding artery is often possible in hypervascular lesions such as larger AVMs or angiodysplasias that have enlarged feeding arteries. Occasionally a nidus of this lesion may be directly catheterized and occluded. Embolization of lesions supplied by a normal-sized artery is technically more demanding, but with use of long tapered 6 F Torcon catheters or 3 F coaxial catheters, a high degree of selective catheterization can usually be achieved. During catheterization, care has to be taken to minimise major spasm and avoid intimal dissection of vessels not supplying the bleeding site. Decreased flow to the non-embolized bowel diminishes chances of development of collaterals and increases the risks of significant bowel ischaemia. If major spasm develops during catheterization, selective intra-arterial administration of small doses of nitroglycerin and a few minutes of waiting help to decrease or resolve it. Pre-medication with calcium antagonists may also be useful for prevention of the catheter-induced spasm.

(2) Except in cases in which direct occlusion of a nidus of a hypervascular lesion is possible, embolization should not be peripheral. It should spare distal communicating arcades in the small intestine, the marginal artery in the large bowel, and intramural vascular networks. Only the distal intestinal branches and proximal communicating arcades should be occluded. The goal of embolization is to decrease the pulse pressure at the bleeding site and thus allow for spontaneous haemostasis. Such embolization is safe and usually effective in patients with normal coagulation. In patients with coagulation defects, however, it may not be sufficient and bleeding may continue from collaterals. A decision about more distal and thus less safe embolization has to be made on the basis of the patient's condition. Sometimes it is necessary to take a higher risk and manage complications late. In patients with bleeding from rectal lesions, particularly malignant tumours, embolization can be more aggressive [6] (Fig. 18). Because of dual supply of the rectum from the inferior mesenteric and hypogastric arteries, the superior haemorrhoidal artery can be occluded with low risk of ischaemic consequences.

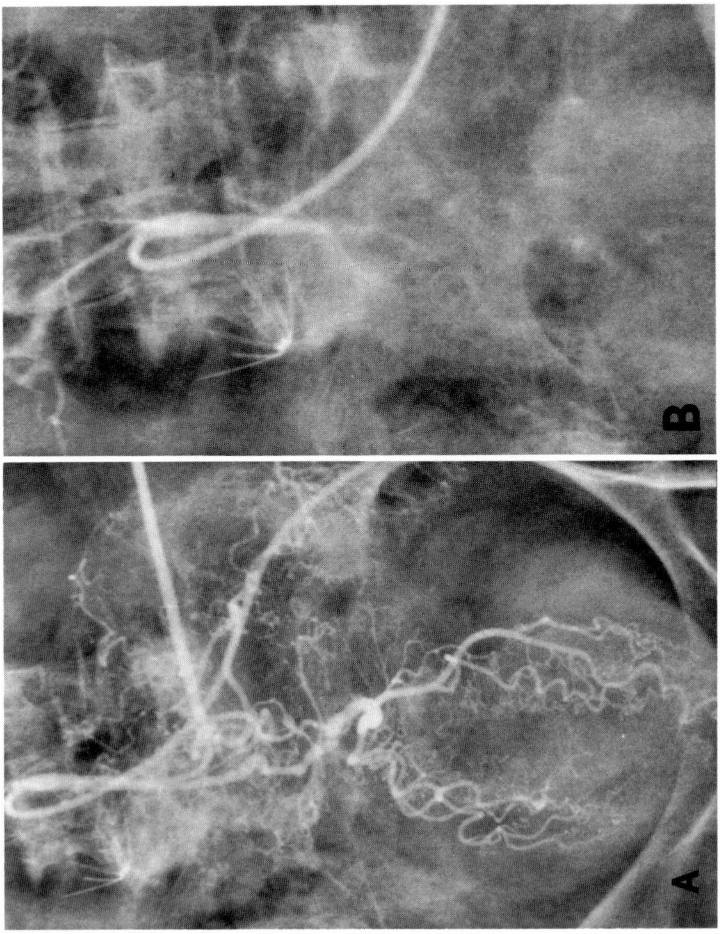

Figure 18. *Recurrent massive rectal bleeding from uterine carcinoma invading the rectum and sigmoid colon. Diffuse bleeding in rectum was seen at proctoscopy, and the patient, who was not a surgical candidate, was referred for angiographic treatment. Bleeding was controlled by embolization of the superior haemorrhoidal artery with Ivalon particles. No complications developed. The patient has a Mobin-Uddin filter in the right common iliac vein. A. Inferior mesenteric angiogram reveals encasement of the superior hemorrhoidal artery and diffuse hypervascularity of the rectum and sigmoid colon. Catheter for embolization was placed below the origin of the large sigmoid branch. B. Follow-up angiogram after embolization shows occlusion of the superior hemorrhoidal artery. The large sigmoidal branch went into spasm during catheterization.*

(3) The number of occluded vessels has to be kept to a minimum, and optimally only the bleeding artery should be occluded. After embolization of the catheterized vessel, the catheter is pulled back proximally and an angiogram obtained to document the distal vessel occlusion and absence or persistence of bleeding. With ongoing extravasation, another branch feeding the bleeding site should be catheterized and occluded, and a follow-up angiogram obtained. Embolization of more than one branch, however, increases the risk of ischaemia and bowel infarction, and decisions about the number of branches to be occluded when bleeding persists on follow-up angiograms has to be made again, depending on the patient's condition and location of the bleeding lesion.

(4) No vasopressin infusion should be performed after embolization as it would impair chances of development of collateral circulation [1]. Vasoconstrictive effect would add to the vascular compromise and increase the risk of bowel infarction. When embolization follows ineffective vasopressin infusion it should be done after the vasopressin effect disappears or substantially diminishes, when the catheterized vessels are not constricted and over sensitive to catheter and wire manipulation.

(5) Choice of the proper occlusive material is important for the safety of embolization. For the majority of patients with LGIB, the material of choice is surgical gelatin (Gelfoam) in particulate form. Particles of Gelfoam are easily delivered through the 6 Fr catheters, achieve a rapid and temporary vessel occlusion that persists from a few days to a few weeks, and is satisfactory for control of LGIB. The authors use small strips (torpedoes) 2-3 mm in diameter and 3-5 mm in length, and inject one strip at a time. It is rolled, compressed and inserted into the nozzle of a tuberculin syringe containing contrast medium. We inject the strip directly into the catheter without a stopcock using a 5 ml syringe filled with contrast medium to control the embolization [1]. Carefully injected contrast medium helps to check the degree of obstruction and the need for injection of more strips. Strict attention to aseptic technique is necessary as wetted Gelfoam shows rapid contamination.

With use of 3 Fr catheters and peripheral catheterization of vessels 1-2 mm in diameter where Gelfoam particles are difficult to inject, the authors use occlusive Gianturco mini-coilsprings (Cook Inc.) 2 mm in size [1]. They can be easily and safely introduced through these small catheters and stay at the point of placement in a small artery (Fig. 19). They result in an instantaneous, localized, permanent occlusion and favour development of peripheral collateral circulation.

Tissue adhesive isobutyl-2-cyanoacrylate (IBC) is another possible occlusive material; it causes an immediate, permanent, and - mixed with iophendylate and tantalum - controlled vessel occlusion. In our opinion, however, it should be used only as a last resort in patients with malignant diseases, particularly tumours, when other occlusive materials or devices are not suitable or have failed to occlude the lesion (Fig. 20).

A long-term occlusive agent, polyvinyl alcohol (Ivalon) also has its place in embolization treatment of LGIB. It is suitable mainly for embolization of hypervascular lesions supplied by enlarged arteries when a catheter can be advanced close to or directly into the lesion. Delivered through 6 Fr catheters as small (0.5-1 mm) particles or as larger (1-2 mm) plugs, it can directly occlude the vascular nidus of the lesion and result in long-term bleeding control [27,28].

With bleeding from medium-sized vessels larger than 2-3 mm in diameter, which may happen in haemobilia and pancreatic bleeding, a 3 mm coilspring can be used for occlusion, if the bleeding vessel can be directly catheterized [1]. When direct catheterization is impossible, a small detachable balloon can be a useful occlusive device. Its location can be checked with contrast medium injection after being positioned, and it is not detached until it is lodged properly in the bleeding vessel [29].

Bleeding from a larger vessel, particularly from a hypogastric artery aneurysm perforating into the rectum, is best managed by combination of occlusive devices and materials. Depending on the size of the aneurysm, various sizes of occlusive coilsprings (5, 8, 12 mm) are placed directly into the aneurysmal sac or its feeding vessel. With a large aneurysm, multiple coilsprings often have to be used. Thrombin, particulate occlusive material (Gelfoam or Ivalon), or liquid polymer (IBC), can then be injected and interspersed between the coil springs to accelerate thrombus formation and thrombosis of the entire aneurysm or its feeder (Fig. 20).

(6) Bowel embolizations should be done with antibiotic coverage because of easy contamination of Gelfoam and presence of bowel bacteria, which can easily migrate across the ischaemic bowel wall [21].

Successful occlusion of the bleeding vessel(s) results in immediate

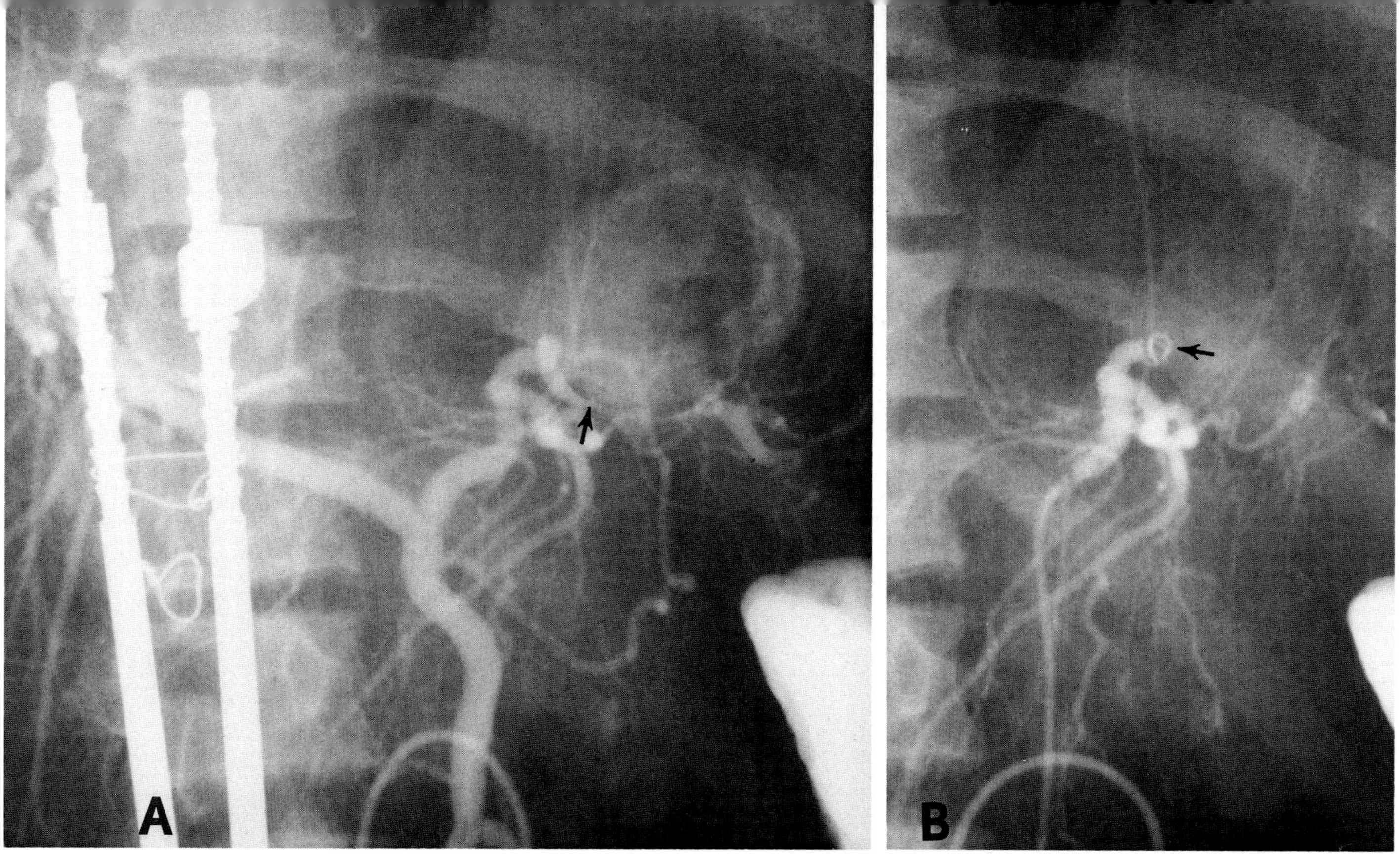

Figure 19. *Post-traumatic haemobilia presenting by recurrent melena successfully treated by selective embolization; no complication developed. A. Close-up view of selective hepatic angiogram in a slight oblique projection reveals a large (6 by 5 cm) pseudo-aneurysm in the left liver lobe originating from a third order branch (arrow). B. Selective left hepatic angiogram after occlusion of the involved branch with a 3 mm Gianturco coil-spring (arrow) placed through a long tapered-tip 6 F Torcon catheter shows absence of aneurysm filling.*

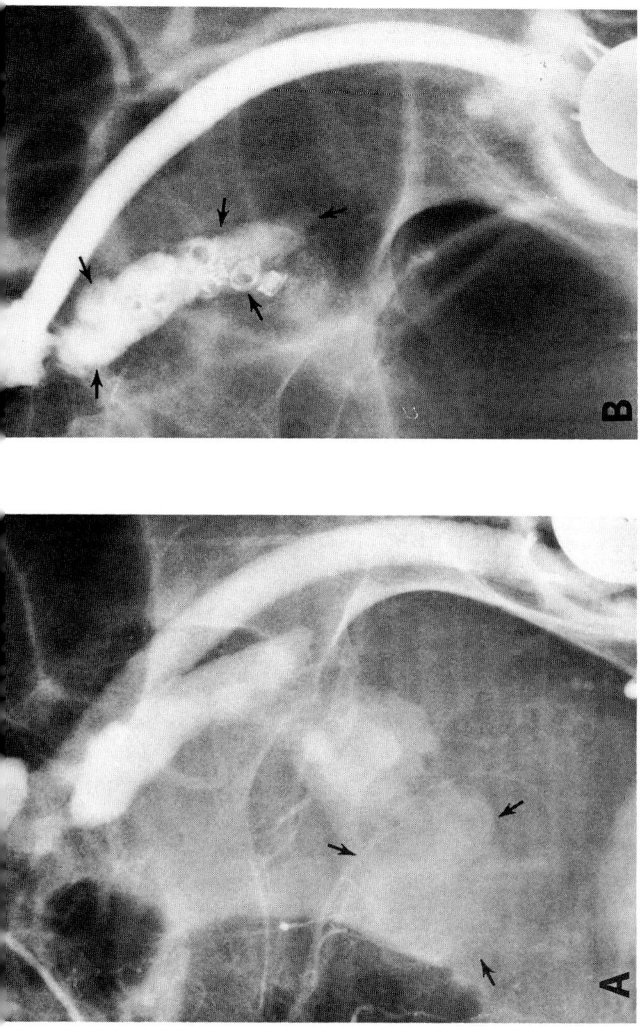

Figure 20. *Recurrent massive rectal haemorrhage from a large aneurysm of the left hypogastric artery eroding into the rectum in patient with recent left common iliac-femoral graft. Ligation of the hypogastric artery was attempted at surgery with only partial success. Placement of multiple occlusive coilsprings and large Gelfoam particles decreased bleeding, which was finally controlled by cast occlusion by tissue adhesive -IBC. A. Late phase of pelvic angiogram reveals diffusely dilated left hypogastric artery entering into a large aneurysm from which contrast medium extravasates into the rectum (arrows). B. Follow-up common iliac angiogram shows a cast occlusion of the hypogastric artery with coilsprings and tissue adhesive opacified by tantalum (arrow) and no filling of aneurysm.*

cessation of bleeding and the patient's rapid stabilization. Bloody stools usually continue for a few hours because of the large amount of blood retained in the bowel from previous bleeding. With occlusion of a small-sized vessel, the patient usually does not have any significant discomfort or has only minor abdominal pain persisting for a few hours. With occlusion of a larger mesenteric branch or several branches supplying larger segments of bowel, discomfort and abdominal pain are usually significant, persist for a few days, and require narcotic medication. Localized ileus may sometimes be present with abdominal distention. A febrile reaction and mild leukocytosis often occur, even with small vessel embolization; however, they need not be signs of bowel infarction. They can be caused by migration of bowel bacteria across the wall due to transient loss of integrity of ischaemic bowel [21]. All these symptoms should resolve in 2-4 days. If they persist, and particularly if they increase in intensity, the major complication of embolization, significant bowel ischaemia and infarction, has to be considered. All decisions about embolization therapy of LGIB have to be made together with clinicians and surgeons. Surgeons should follow-up the patient after embolization as primary physicians and make decisions about the need for surgical intervention if complications of embolization develop.

Summary

Diagnosis and catheter therapy of LGIB has been and will continue to be an important part of the work of the interventional angiographers. Even with refinement and wider use of endoscopic techniques, there will be need for angiographic diagnosis for chronic, recurrent, and acute, massive bleeding. Angiography is particularly important for diagnosis of haemorrhage from lesions of the small intestine. Interventional diagnostic measures significantly improve the diagnostic efficacy of emergency angiography in patients who constitute diagnostic dilemmas. Interventional therapeutic techniques have much to offer for the control of LGIB. Selective infusion of vasopressin is the primary technique for treatment of active haemorrhage and should be considered in all patients except where the use of vasopressin is contraindicated. Embolization techniques are gaining in popularity even when they carry risk of complications. Careful selection of patients and performance of the procedure, however, can decrease risks of embolization to an acceptable minimum, with the gains outweighing the risks of the treatments.

References

1. Rösch J. Lower gastrointestinal bleeding. In: Dondelinger RF, Rossi P. Kirdziel JC, Wallace S eds. *Interventional Radiology*. Stuttgart: George Thieme Verlag, 1990:349-367.
2. Athanasoulis CA. Lower gastroinestinal bleeding. In: Athanasoulis CA, Pfister RC, Greene RE, Roberson GH eds. *Interventional radiology*. Philadelphia: Saunders, 1982:115-148.
3. Margulis AR, Heinbecker P, Bernard HR. Operative mesenteric arteriography in the search for the site in unexplained gastrointestinal hemorrhage. *Surgery* 1960;**48:**534.
4. Pingoud EG, Pais SI. Usefulness of the prone position for aortography of aortic graft-intestinal fistulae. *AJR* 1979;**132:**836.
5. Husted J, Dempsey D. Angiographic management of arteriocolic fistulae. *Cardiovasc Intervent Radiol* 1986;**9:**158.
6. Chuang VP, Charnsangavej C, Carrasco H, Wallace S, Soo CS, Bechtel W, Strohlein J. Transcatheter treatment of gastrointestinal hemorrhage in cancer patients. *J Intervent Radiol* 1986;**1:**43.
7. Baum S, Athanasoulis CA, Waltman AC, Galdabini J, Schapiro RH, Warshaw AL, Ottinger LW. Angiodysplasia of the right colon: a cause of gastrointestinal bleeding. *AJR* 1977;**129:**789.
8. Boley SJ, Brandt LJ, Frank MS. Severe lower intestinal bleeding: diagnosis and treatment. *Clin Gastroenterol* 1981;**10:**65.
9. Vallee C, Legmann P, Favriel JM, Garnier T, Levesque M. Colonic angiodysplasia: clinical, endoscopic, arteriographic signs and histopathological correlations. *Eur J Radiol* 1984;**4:**258.
10. Nyman U, Boijsen UN, Lindstrom C, Rosengren JE. Angiography in angiomatous lesions of the gastrointestinal tract. *Acta Radiol Diagn* 1980;**21:**21.
11. Sos TA, Lee JG, Wixson D, Sniderman KW. Intermittent bleeding from minute to minute in acute massive gastrointestinal hemorrhage: arteriographic demonstration. *AJR* 1978;**131:**1015.
12. Rahn NH, Tishler JM, Han SY, Russinovich NA. Diagnostic and interventional angiography in acute gastrointestinal hemorrhage. *Radiology* 1982;**143:**361.
13. Foelich JW, Winzelberg GG. Radionuclide detection of gastrointestinal hemorrhage. In: Athanasoulis CA, Pfister RC, Greene RE, Roberson GH eds. *Interventional radiology*. Philadelphia: Saunders, 1982:149-156.
14. Rösch J, Keller FS, Wawrukiewicz AS, Krippaehne WW, Dotter CT. Pharmacoangiography in the diagnosis of recurrent massive lower gastrointestinal bleeding. *Radiology* 1982;**145:**615.
15. Rösch J, Kozak BE, Keller FS. Interventional diagnostic in acute-lower-gastrointestinal bleeding. *Semin Intervent Radiol* 1988;**5:**10.
16. Pelz DM, Rankin RN. Alternate bleeding sites in suspected graft-enteric fistula. *AJR* 1981;**136:**707.
17. Thompson WM, Jackson DC, Johnsrude IS. Aortoenteric and paraprosthetic-enteric fistulas: radiologic findings. *AJR* 1976;**127:**235.
18. Rösch J, Putnam JS, Keller FS. Diagnosis and management of hemobilia. *Semin Intervent Radiol* 1988;**5:**49.

19. Rösch J, Dotter CT, Rose RW. Selective arterial infusions of vasoconstrictors in acute gastrointestinal bleeding. *Radiology* 1971;**99**:27.
20. Waltman AC. Transcatheter embolization versus vasopressin infusion for the control of arteriocapillary gastrointestinal bleeding. *Cardiovasc Intervent Radiol* 1980;**3**:289.
21. Gomes AS, Lois JF, McCoy RD. Angiographic treatment of gastrointestinal hemorrhage: comparison of vasopressin infusion and embolization. *AJR* 1986;**146**:1031.
22. Gerlock AJ, Muhletaler CA, Berger JL. Halter SA, O'Leary JP, Avant GR. Infarction after embolization of the ileocolic artery. *Cardiovasc Intervent Radiol* 1981;**4**:202.
23. Palmaz JC, Walter JF, Cho KJ. Therapeutic embolization of the small-bowel arteries. *Radiology* 1984;**152**:377.
24. Rosenkrantz H, Bookstein JJ, Rosen RJ, Goff WB, Healy JR. Postembolic colonic infarction. *Radiology* 1982;**142**:47.
25. Walker WJ, Goldin AR, Shaff MI, Allibone GW. Per catheter control of haemorrhage from the superior and inferior mesenteric arteries. *Clin Radiol* 1980;**31**:71.
26. Mitty HA, Efremićis S, Keller RJ, Colonic stricture after transcatheter embolization for diverticular bleeding. *AJR* 1979;**133**:519.
27. Tadavarthy AM, Castaneda-Zuniga W, Zollikofer C, Nemer F, Barron J, Amplatz K. Angiodysplasia of the right colon treated by embolization with ivalon (polyvinyl alcohol). *Cardiovasc Intervent Radiol* 1981;**4**:39.
28. Tisnado J, Cho SR, Beachley MC, Margolius DA. Transcatheter embolization of angiodysplasia of the rectum. *Acta Radiol Diagn* 1985;**26**:677.
29. Mitchell SE, Shuman LS, Kaufman SL, Chang R, Kadir S, Kinnison ML, White RI. Biliary catheter drainage complicated by hemobilia; treatment by balloon embolotherapy. *Radiology* 1985;**157**:645.

Current trends in the management of obstructive jaundice

Aksel Kruse
Department of Surgical Gastroenterology, Aarhus Municipal Hospital, Aarhus, Denmark

Introduction

Management of the jaundiced patient includes careful history recording and physical examination, supplemented by biochemical analysis of blood samples. Additional information is obtained by ultrasound investigation of the liver, biliary duct and upper abdomen. By this means a differential diagnosis between so-called surgical and medical jaundice can be obtained with very high accuracy.

Analysis of the final diagnosis of more than 1,000 consecutive patients with jaundice in Copenhagen, where almost all jaundiced patients are hospitalized, showed that 60% had 'medical' jaundice, primarily related to hepatitis or liver cirrhosis. Among the 40% of patients with 'surgical' jaundice, i.e. large duct obstruction, there were slightly more malignant than benign cases, 22% with respect to 18%.

Improvements in non-invasive as well as invasive diagnostic procedures have paralleled the introduction of new modalities for non-surgical treatment for cure as well as palliation for a large number of patients with benign and malignant biliary diseases.

This chapter discusses present trends in management of patients with obstructive jaundice.

Benign Obstructive Jaundice

Application of a decision 'tree' based upon clinical and bio-chemical parameters for differentiation between benign and malignant cases in patients presenting with obstructive jaundice produces a correct diagnosis in three out of four cases [1]. Ultrasound scanning will improve these figures, and may even be diagnostic for stones in the common bile duct (Fig. 1). Direct cholangiography, either percutaneous transhepatic cholangiography (PTC) or endoscopic retrograde cholangiopancreatography (ERCP) will differentiate between gallstone obstruction and obstructions due to other benign diseases or malignancy [2]. The concomitant mapping of the biliary tree obtained by PTC or ERCP gives valuable information about the therapeutic strategy which should be chosen in each individual case.

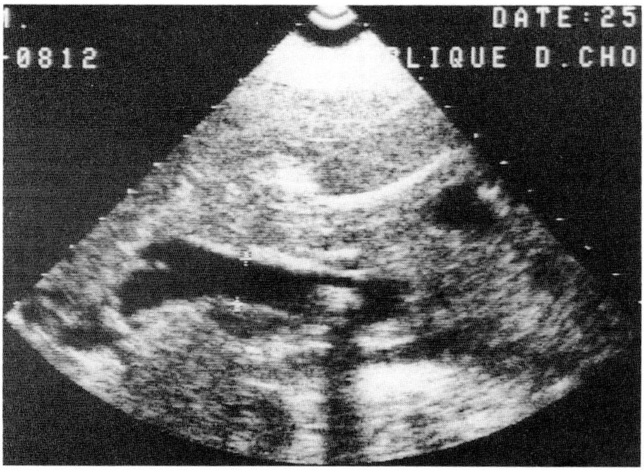

Figure 1. *Ultrasound scan of the liver and biliary duct in a jaundiced patient with a stone in the dilated common bile duct*

Common Bile Duct Stones

Since the introduction of endoscopic sphincterotomy with stone extraction in 1974, this non-surgical treatment has become the treatment of first choice in an increasing proportion of patients presenting with symptomatic common bile duct stones.

The low morbidity and mortality of this method in patients considered unfit for surgical treatment contributed to the rapid spread of this technique worldwide. The original spectrum of indications for endoscopic sphincterotomy and stone removal were cases with previous cholecystectomy and patients with common bile duct stones and intact gall-bladders where old age or complicating diseases contra-indicated surgical treatment.

Endoscopic sphincterotomy and stone removal can be performed in 90-95% of patients and the common bile duct can be cleared in about 90% of cases leaving a few with unextractable, usually large, gallstones in the common bile duct [3,4].

If these patients are left with their stones untreated, they run a 50% risk of cholangitis and a high mortality risk [3,4].

If an endoprosthesis or a nasobiliary drain is placed above the obstructing large stone (Fig. 2) in the common bile duct the cholangitis can be prevented. Later attempts can then be made to remove the stones non-operatively, for example by mechanical or shock-wave lithotripsy (Fig. 3) or lithotripsy performed cholangioscopically by intraductal electrohydraulic or pulsed laser technique [5].

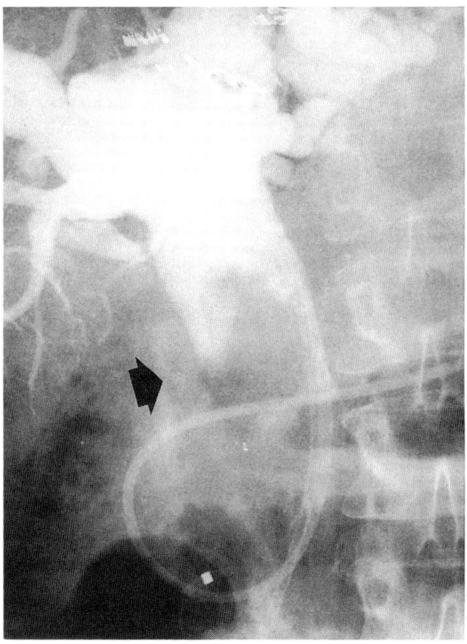

Figure 2. *Giant stone in severely dilated biliary tree in a patient with recurrent jaundice and cholangitis after previous complicated biliary surgery. An endoprosthesis and nasobiliary drain are seen.*

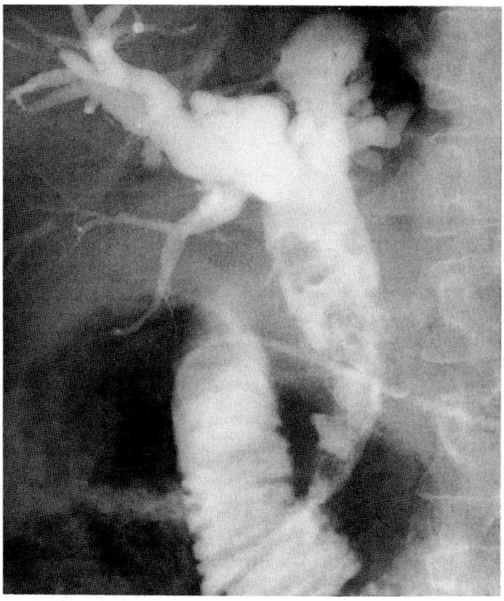

Figure 3. *The same patient as in Fig. 2 after shock-wave lithotripsy.*

If the patients are considered unfit for surgery or if they refuse an operation, they may be referred to highly specialised centres, where cholangioscopic evaluation and treatment can be undertaken either perorally - introducing a slender endoscope through a so-called mother-endoscope in the duodenum into the common bile duct and then advancing it under direct vision, or by previous percutaneous transhepatic puncture of the dilated biliary tree above the stones. The PTC-tract in the liver is dilated over several days to a size sufficient to allow insertion of a cholangioscope into the biliary tree which allows removal of stones or fragments of stones after lithotripsy [5].

Emergency Cases

Recurrent jaundice associated with fever and upper epigastric pain - the so-called Charcot's triad - is highly suggestive of common bile duct stones with cholangitis. Such patients are in danger of progression into a condition characterized by shock, renal insuffiency and mental confusion. Decompression of the biliary tree in such cases is mandatory and should be under-taken as soon as possible. Performed surgically the decompression has a high morbidity and mortality but endoscopic decompression with sphincterotomy and stone removal

(Fig. 4) or sphincterotomy with drainage of the obstructed biliary tree can be performed with a reported much lower morbidity and mortality [6]. The endoscopic treatment should be undertaken as soon as possible after admission of the severely ill patient. If the obstructing common bile duct stone cannot be easily removed, the patient is better treated by decompression either with internal stents or nasobiliary catheters.

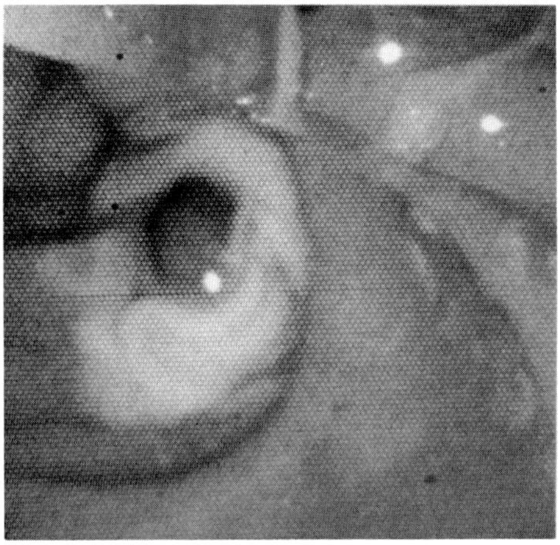

Figure 4. *Endoscopic view of the descending duodenum after urgent sphincterotomy in a patient with cholangitis and jaundice. A stone is seen amidst a collection of pus.*

In the author's experience with urgent biliary drainage in patients with obstructive jaundice due to stones, the jaundice subsided in 94% of cases and cholangitis was controlled in 90% [4]. Similar very favourable experience has been reported from other centres [6,7] and it has become widely accepted that obstructive jaundice with cholangitis is a condition to be treated by expert endoscopists, surgery being considered the method of second choice.

In the author's series [4] and in the experience reported from Hong Kong [6] some patients with mental confusion due to their cholangitis accidentally removed the nasobiliary drains and therefore had to undergo a new endoscopic procedure. It is the author's policy in such patients to insert an internal endoprosthesis as well as the nasobiliary drain (Fig. 2). When the cholangitis is controlled and the patient is in a stable condition attempts can be made to remove the obstructing stones either surgically, endoscopically or after attempts to reduce the size of the stones by infusion of solvent via the nasobiliary catheter or by fragmentation by extracorporeal shock-wave lithotripsy (ESWL).

However, a significant proportion of patients of very old age and poor general condition are probably better treated by internal drains only. In the author's experience [4], shared by others [3,6,7], the internal biliary drains in patients with unextractable common bile duct stones have a much longer functional life than biliary endoprostheses in patients with malignant stenoses. This is probably due to the fact that the endoprosthesis prevents the stone from impaction rather than serves as a stent. In 63 patients with permanent internal drains the median function time of the endoprostheses was 19 months and where the patient had recurrent symptoms the endoprosthesis was exchanged with excellent clinical results [4]. Similar experience is reported from London and Durham with a median patency for internal endoprosthesis of 15.9 months [3].

The rapid spread of use of interventional biliary endoscopy over the last 10 years is fully justified by the results obtained in management of biliary lithiasis.

PTC

Invasive and interventional radiological methods have become less important in the same time span, but in selected cases where endoscopic methods fail or cannot be performed, PTC should be performed as an easy and very effective way of mapping the biliary tree and for decompression of obstructed bile ducts. Close co-operation between interventional radiologists and biliary endoscopists has widened the spectrum of non-surgical treatment in selected cases where the radiologist inserts a wire-guide through a PTC catheter and advances it through the biliary duct and the papilla into the bowel, where it is then taken by the endoscopist, who can thereby advance the endoscope into an otherwise unattainable position for endoscopic treatment [8,9]. For example, patients who have previously undergone partial gastrectomy and Roux-en-Y gastroenteroanastomosis, and more frequently patients who have undergone a Whipple's pancreatico-duodenal resection of the right side of the pancreas are candidates for this combined technique. The so-called rendezvous technique is applied also as the initial step in a number of patients for palliative biliary stenting in case of malignant stenosis and will be discussed later.

Other Benign Biliary Obstructions

Benign strictures in the biliary tree are most frequently seen after biliary surgery and become symptomatic in the post-operative period (Fig. 5) or may be detected years after previous surgery because of intermittent jaundice and cholangitis (Fig. 6).

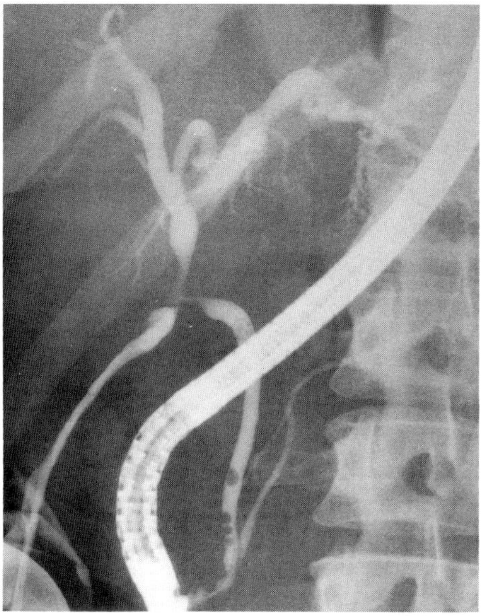

Figure 5. *Biliary leakage and stenosis of the common hepatic duct after cholecystectomy. The patient was jaundiced and had dilatation of the intrahepatic biliary tree.*

The benign strictures can be treated non-operatively by dilatation either via endoscopically introduced balloon catheters or via PTC introduced balloons. The immediate success of dilatation of benign strictures seems satisfactory but there is a high recurrence rate which increases with any increase in delay in follow-up after dilatation. Probably the best results are obtained by inserting biliary stents through the dilated benign stricture and leaving the stent in situ several months. The best results have been obtained treating patients with a stenosed bilio-enteric anastomoses. A 70% patency rate after 3 years has been reported, but life-long follow-up in these often young patients is necessary because, if symptoms or biochemical indices suggest recurrent stricture, the patient might be better treated by reconstructive biliary surgery which should be performed only in hospitals with special expertise in this field [10].

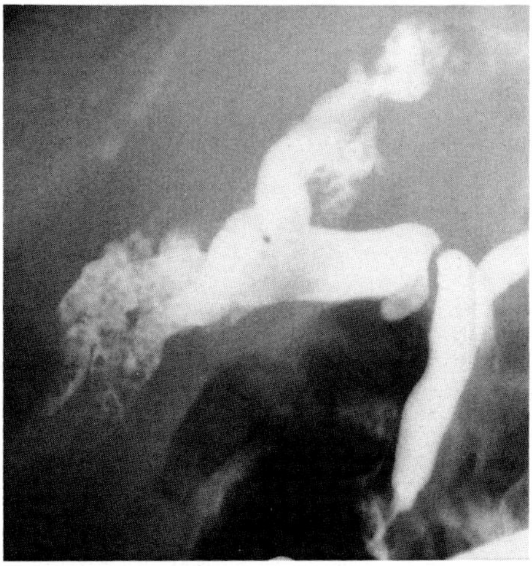

Figure 6. *Intermittent jaundice with cholangitis in a patient with multiple intrahepatic biliary calculi after benign stricture complicating previous cholecystectomy.*

If reconstructive surgery fails there is perhaps a case for considering the newly designed self-expanding biliary stent [11,12]. Initial experience with these stents in malignant as well as benign cases has been encouraging but long-term results are as yet unavailable. It is not without concern that one hears of placement of such metallic stents in patients with benign strictures because - so far - these stents cannot be removed. Multi-centre protocols for application and follow-up of these self-expanding stents have been designed and long-term experience with this technique is awaited with great interest.

Primary sclerosing cholangitis (Fig. 7), is a progressive disease with liver insufficiency or cholangiocarcinoma as the end stage, unless liver transplantation is offered to the patient. Direct cholangiography, normally by ERCP but sometimes by PTC, is necessary to confirm the diagnosis and to map the biliary tree prior to palliative dilatation of strictures or prior to liver transplantation. The effect of dilatation procedures (Fig. 8) is unpredictable and in most cases short lasting. Probably only stenoses of the extrahepatic biliary duct should be subjected to dilation.

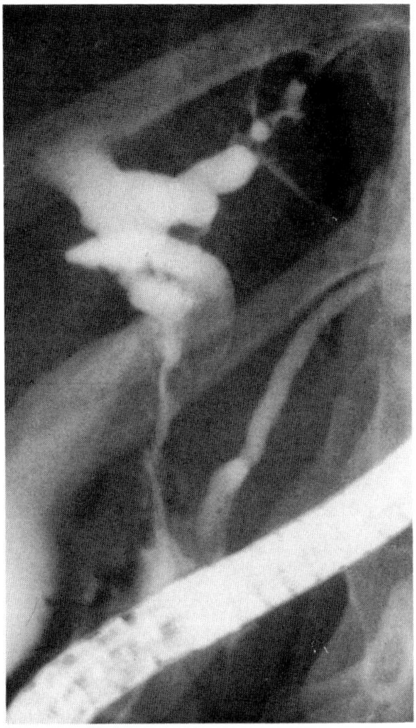

Figure 7. *Severe stenosis of the common bile duct in a young patient with sclerosing cholangitis and jaundice.*

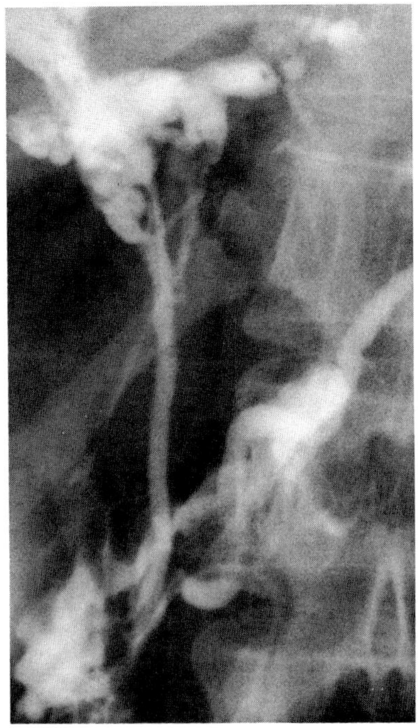

Figure 8. *Common bile duct after balloon dilatation (same patient as Fig. 7).*

Primary sclerosing cholangitis carries a 10-20% risk of cholangiocarcinoma. Early detection of cholangiocarcinoma may be very difficult and almost impossible by normal imaging techniques such as ultrasound CT scan and magnetic resonance imaging (MRI), because there is no mass lesion to be identified, but direct cholangiography in these conditions is very difficult to interpret. Suspicion of malignancy should be confirmed by intraductal biopsy. Staging of cholangiocarcinomas in the extrahepatic bile duct can be achieved by endoscopic ultrasound where the 7.5 MHz probe can be placed very close to the lesion. Impressive correlation between endoscopic ultrasound findings and histological examination of the resected specimen was reported recently [13].

Malignant Obstructive Jaundice

Transabdominal ultrasound has an undisputed role as the method of first choice for imaging of the liver and biliary duct in jaundiced patients known or thought to suffer from obstructive jaundice. In experienced hands ultrasound scanning gives as precise information as CT scan. Demonstration of mass lesion affecting the biliary tree is very suggestive of malignancy but the diagnosis should be confirmed by biopsy or fine needle aspiration cytology. The easiest way of obtaining such material is percutaneously, guided by ultrasound, but it can be obtained as precisely when guided by CT.

The accuracy of biopsies and aspiration cytology from a tumour mass in the head of the pancreas is very high but from a mass affecting the biliary tree the accuracy is lower. Metastatic nodules and primary tumours in the liver are visualized and diagnosed very reliably.

Cholangiocarcinomas, often small and fibrotic, are often not seen in ultrasound or CT-scan (Figs. 9 and 10) but they are easily detected

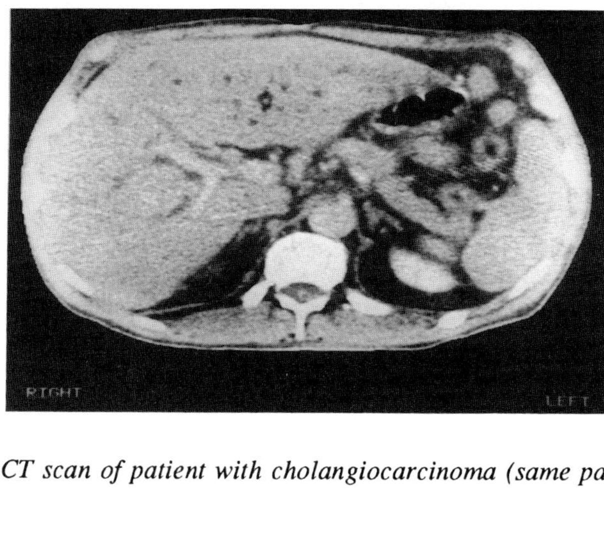

Figure 9. *CT scan of patient with cholangiocarcinoma (same patient as Fig. 12).*

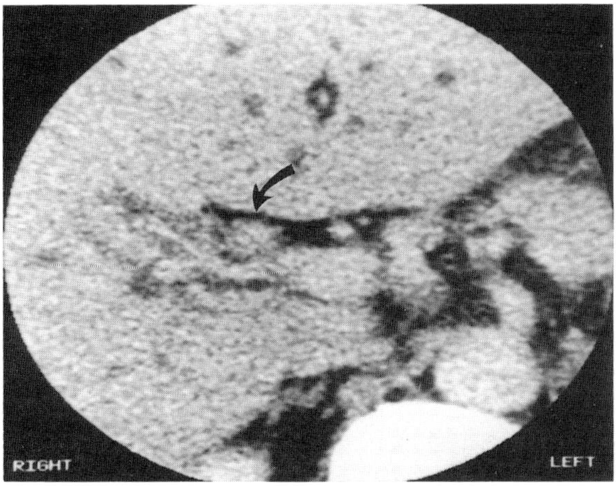

Figure 10. *CT scan after contrast in the same patient as in Fig. 12.*

on direct cholangiography, for example ERCP (Fig. 11). Although a high quality ultrasound scan (Fig. 12) may demonstrate a small cholangiocarcinoma at the bifurcation of the biliary tree, the so-called Klatskin-tumour, confirmation of the diagnosis may be very difficult.

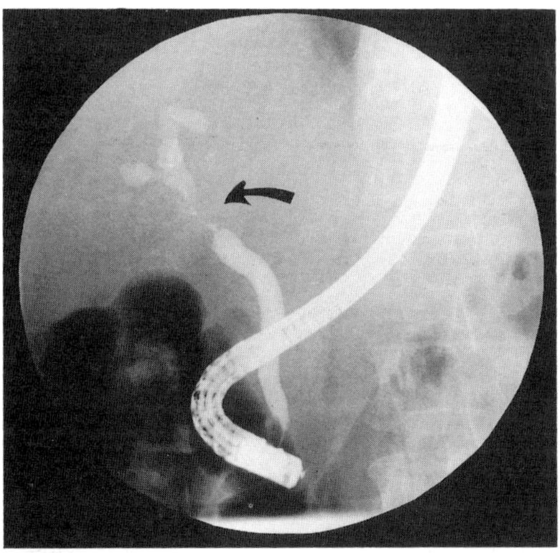

Figure 11. *Cholangiogram demonstrating cholangiocarcinoma not seen on ultrasound or CT scan.*

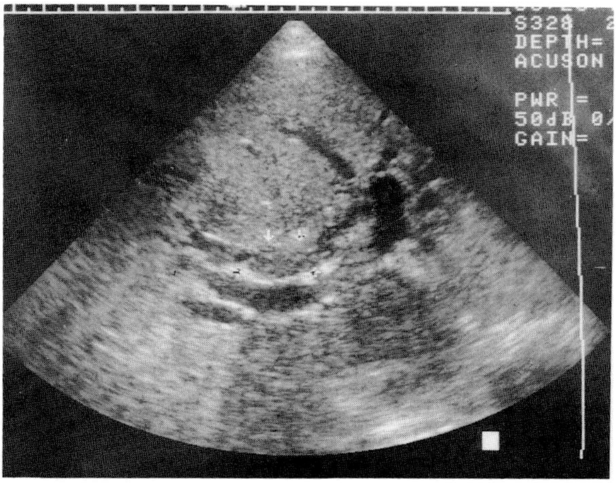

Figure 12. *Ultrasound scan of the liver in a patient with a small cholangiocarcinoma (Klatskin tumor) affecting the right and the left hepatic duct. (Courtesy of A. Haubek).*

Positive aspiration cytology is obtained in less than 50% of such small tumours. In such cases the assumed malignant diagnosis may be confirmed by obtaining cytology scraping intraductally with a device introduced via the endoscope and guided by a soft wire pushed through the stenosis (Fig. 13). Intraductal biopsies (Fig. 14)

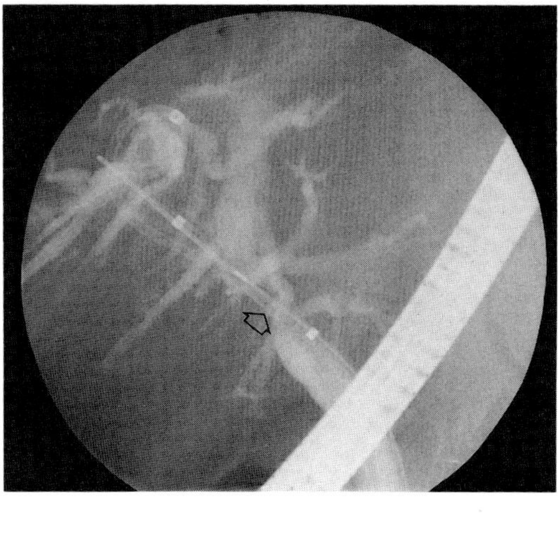

Figure 13. *Intraductal cytology brush along endoprosthesis (same patient as Fig. 11).*

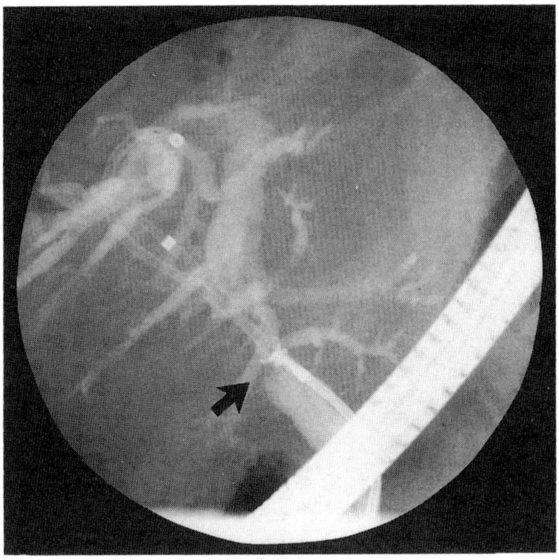

Figure 14. *Intraductal biopsy from cholangiocarcinoma (same patient as Fig. 11).*

can also be obtained but they are usually very small. False negative diagnoses are frequent.

Tumors involving the papilla of Vater are easily detected endoscopically (Fig. 15) and biopsy is easy.

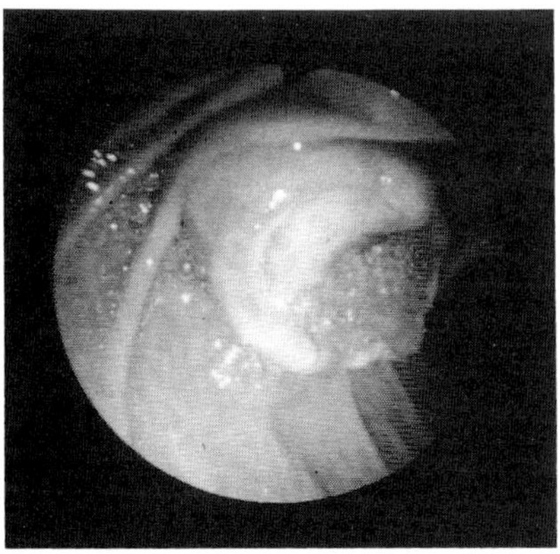

Figure 15. *Ulcerated carcinoma of the ampulla of Vater in a 66 year old patient with jaundice.*

Cholangioscopic access to a suspected malignant stenoses in the biliary tree permits biopsy under direct visual control [14]. The differentiation between benign and malignant strictures can also be made from observation of differences in mucosal vascular patterns in the malignant and benign stenosis. Percutaneous transhepatic cholangioscopy is not without risk and peroral transendoscopic cholangioscopy is troublesome and expensive, and the exact role for these techniques in a diagnostic context has not yet been defined.

Direct cholangiography, either PTC or ERC, is a valuable contribution to the diagnosis of the jaundiced patient. The anatomy and the site of a stricture or multiple strictures is valuable information when deciding therapy in individual cases. If, for example, the stenotic lesion in the lower part of the common bile duct does not involve the cystic duct and a dilation of the gall-bladder, cystic duct and common hepatic duct is documented, the therapeutic options differ from cases with high biliary duct strictures and strictures involving the intrahepatic bile ducts. Although some features of cholangiography favour malignancy over benign conditions, the discriminating power is relatively low if clinical and biochemical information is withheld.

Assessment of Operability

When a malignant obstruction of the biliary tree has been proven or is the most obvious probability, the patient should be carefully assessed for operability with the goal of selecting patients who stand a fair chance of cure by surgical resection of the tumour.

Whereas operability in this context means tumour resectability, it is of equal importance that before any decision is made the patient's general condition is assessed. Complicating diseases, mainly cardiovascular, can preclude operation on a patient who has a relatively small tumour with no evidence of metastatic spread or involvement of vital structures. A few patients do not want an operation but accept non-operative palliation.

Surgical removal of the obstructing tumour is the only potentially curative treatment at present. Unless metastatic spread of the tumour has been proven or the tumour has been demonstrated to have invaded/encased vital structures such as the inferior caval vein or the mesenteric vessels, younger and fit patients should be offered operation even when the chance of curability is small. Otherwise patients who might be cured will be offered only palliative treatment.

Patients suffering from tumours of the papilla of Vater will often undergo an attempt at curative resection. Less common is resectability in patients with cancer in the head of the pancreas (Fig. 16) and cholangiocarcinomas. Only about 10% of these patients can be offered an attempted curative resection [15].

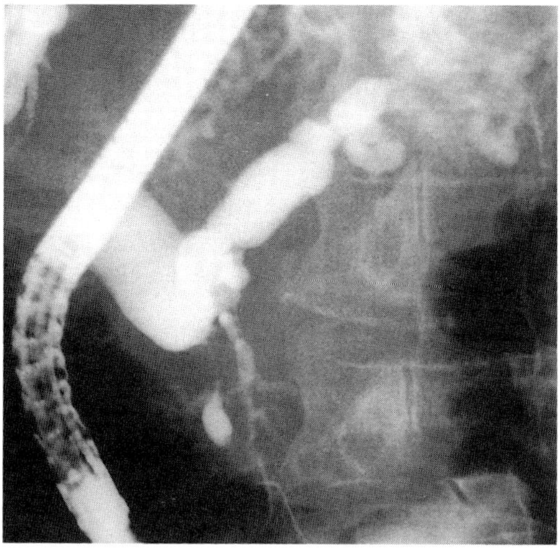

Figure 16. *ERCP demonstrating tumour stenosis of the pancreatic duct and the lower common bile duct in a patient with cancer in the head of the pancreas. Severe pre-stenotic dilatation of both ducts is seen.*

Patients who cannot be operated on with curative resection can frequently have a surgical bypass operation for palliation.

None of the imaging techniques for hepato-biliary diseases can demonstrate curability of patients with malignant biliary obstructions, but incurability can be documented by ultrasound, CT scan and angiography by demonstrating metastatic spread of the tumour or tumour involvement of adjacent vital structures.

Biliary Drainage in Malignant Obstructive Jaundice

Insertion of drains into the obstructed biliary tree can be achieved via the percutaneous transhepatic route - percutaneous transhepatic biliary drainage (PTBD), or by the endoscopic route - endoscopic biliary drainage (EBD). PTBD used to be the most frequently applied decompression of obstructed bile ducts, but the past decade has witnessed a dramatic change towards EBD as the most frequently applied technique.

PTBD is usually performed by interventional radiologists but also by a few surgeons and physicians. PTC will visualize the obstructed part of the biliary tree and permit insertion of wire-guides over which catheters can be introduced into the biliary tree and left for internal drainage, for external drainage or combined internal/external drainage.

If PTBD is meant to be of longer duration, an attempt is made to insert an internal endoprosthesis through the obstructing lesion into the duodenum or to leave a catheter for combined internal and external drainage [16]. External drainage alone leads to a loss of fluid, electrolytes and lack of bile in the bowel. The external catheters may become displaced and non-functioning, and furthermore many patients find the external catheter and bag for collection of bile repulsive. PTBD may be performed in a two-step procedure with external drainage of the dilated biliary tree for a few days when the control of a wire-guide in the dilated biliary tree is difficult and attempts to negotiate the stenosing lesion fail. New attempts can be performed with a higher success rate when the dilation of the intrahepatic tree has diminished after a few days of external biliary drainage. In the second stage, if the stricture is successfully passed with a wire-guide, an internal stent can be placed [16].

In the early days of PTBD the indication was mainly pre-operative decompression of the obstructed biliary tree because it was assumed to be beneficial for the patients. Operation was postponed for a couple of weeks, while se-bilirubin concentrations approached normal values. The initial enthusiasm disappeared over a period of a decade because careful studies demonstrated that biliary drainage either had no effect or even had a negative influence on the post-operative outcome [17].

Endoscopic Biliary Drainage

EBD was introduced only 10 years ago. It is a relatively safe technique with few early procedure-related complications and can be applied with a success rate around 90% [18]. Initially small calibre endoprostheses were introduced and provided a rapid decline in se-bilirubin and alkaline phosphatase (Figs. 17 and 18). However, after a few weeks or months most of these endoprostheses ceased to function and the patients showed recurrent jaundice and cholangitis [18].

Since the introduction of endoprostheses with larger calibres, 10-12 French, the duration of adequate biliary drainage after insertion has significantly increased and the median function of large calibre endoprostheses is now longer than the median survival of patients with unresectable malignant biliary obstructions [19].

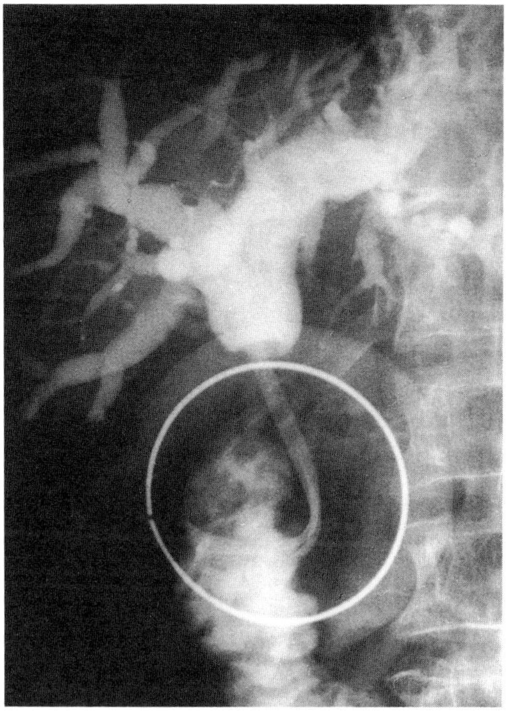

Figure 17. *Well functioning endoprosthesis in a patient with obstructive jaundice due to pancreatic cancer. Free flow of contrast into the duodenum is apparent.*

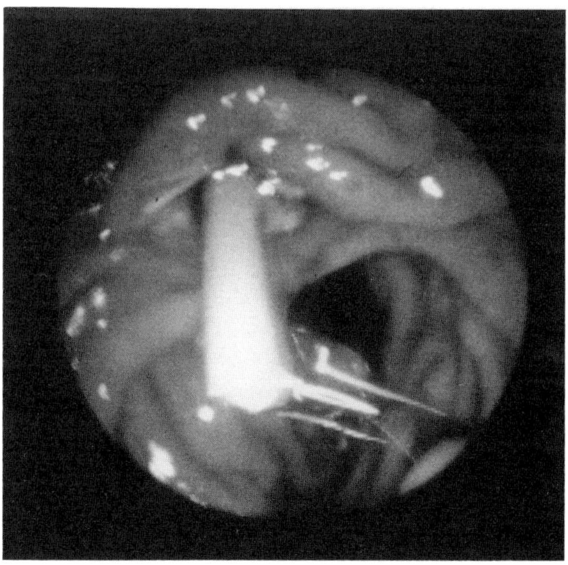

Figure 18. *Duodenal aspect of biliary stent with a stream of bile.*

Insertion of the larger stent is normally preceded by endoscopic sphincterotomy [18,19].

The most important complications after EBD are infections with cholangitis and sepsis [19,20]. In the author's initial experience the early procedure-related mortality rate was 9%. Half of the patients died from septicaemia and infectious complications were most often seen in patients with unsuccessful or only partial drainage of the obstructed biliary tree.

Since then the author has given prophylactic antibiotics to patients with assumed malignant biliary obstruction to prevent infectious complications. At present 2 g of piperacillin is given intravenously prior to ERCP. The infection rate now is only 50% of that seen previously. A more detailed analysis of the author's most recent figures shows that only when the biliary tree is sufficiently drained does prophylactic antibiotic treatment appear to be beneficial.

If EBD fails or if drainage of the biliary tree is incomplete, the patient is sent to PTBD within the first 24 hours [21].

When symptoms of malfunction of the endoprosthesis occur (cholangitis and/or jaundice) the patient is offered exchange of the biliary stent. This procedure is often easily performed endoscopically, [16], and most patients can be treated on an outpatient bases [16,19,21]. Endoprostheses inserted via PTC can be exchanged endoscopically or additional stents can be inserted.

Blocking of Biliary Endoprostheses

Endoprostheses inserted through any biliary stricture tend to become blocked as time passes after insertion [16,18-21]. This occurs whether the endoprosthesis reaches the duodenum or not. Most endoscopically-inserted biliary stents project into the duodenum and they tend to block after a few weeks to a few months. Examination of clogged endoprostheses has shown that the occluding material consists of a bacterial biofilm alternating with layers of calcium bilirubinate and the duodenal end of the endoprosthesis may contain vegetable fibres [16].

Biliary stents with larger internal diameter take a longer time to become blocked and the median function of 10 French stents exceeds that of the median survival time of patients with malignant biliary obstruction. Speer and Co-workers recommended biliary stents at least 10 French in diameter [19].

Other studies showed that straight endoprostheses, so-called

Amsterdam type stents, had a longer median function time than curved endoprostheses such as single pigtail catheters or double pigtail catheters. Therefore straight endoprostheses are recommended instead of pigtail stents [18,19].

Different materials for biliary stents have been investigated in vivo and in vitro. Teflon catheters have a very low friction coefficient and are more easily inserted through the endoscopes than, for example, polyurethane catheters, which have a very high friction coefficient. Polyethylene catheters have been found to be better than endoprostheses made from other materials [19,22].

Recently reports of preliminary experience with expandable metallic biliary stents (Fig. 19) appeared in the literature [19,12,23].

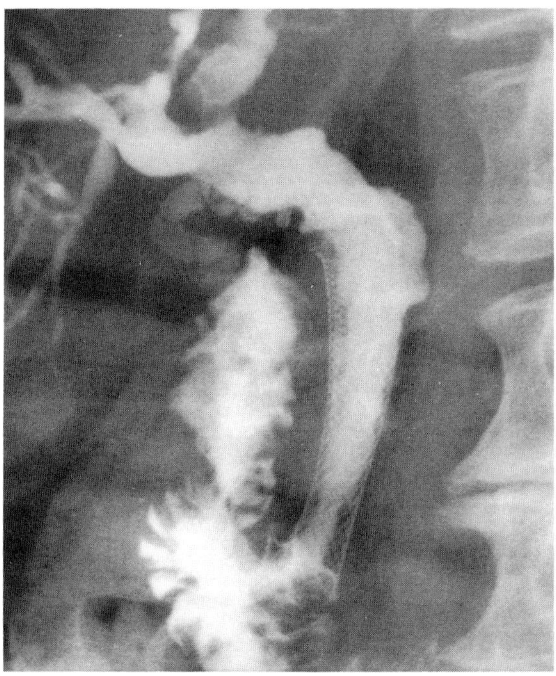

Figure 19. *Expanded wall-stent in a patient with pancreatic cancer. (Courtesy of P. Matzen).*

The results are certainly promising but long-term experience is needed before conclusions can be drawn about indications for this type of stent. Although the so-called wall stents have been able to dilate up to a diameter of 30 French, tumour growth through the meshes in the metallic stent has been reported. In such cases the usual endoprostheses can be inserted through the obstructed wall stent.

The effect of incorporating silver, copper or antibiotics into stents with a goal of retarding deposition of the bacterial film is being studied [16,22,24]. No convincing data from these studies have yet been reported. A recent paper from the very active group in Amsterdam demonstrated that the presence of side holes in the endoprosthesis seemed to precipitate deposition of sludge around the side holes [22]. However, an endoprosthesis with only an end hole can be more easily occluded when it is pressed against the wall of the duodenum or the biliary duct, although the in vivo study did not show incomplete drainage or a higher complication rate [22].

Palliation of Incurable Malignant Biliary Obstruction

Surgery of Biliary Drainage?

After confirmation of the malignant tumour affecting the biliary tree and careful assessment, a large group of patients can be identified as incurable or in fact inoperable.

A small group of patients with small well-defined tumours and no evidence of metastatic spread or involvement of neighbouring vital structures can be identified as probably curable, but there is a 'grey zone' where incurability is not demonstrated but curability/resectability remains doubtful. If fit for surgery, this group of patients should be offered the chance of cure, however small this chance may seem [15]. Many surgeons advocate resection or surgical bypass for palliation in patients found incurable at laparotomy [15]. There is, however, a significant morbidity and mortality related to surgical palliation of the incurable malignant jaundice.

The cost of the operation and the post-operative days in hospital should be taken into consideration when alternative palliative treatment is contemplated.

The expected mean survival of incurable patients is 5 or 6 months but is less in patients with widespread metastases at the time of diagnosis. In patients with cholangiocarcinomas the survival can be much longer, even several years. It is important in these cases to establish a decompression of the obstructed biliary tree as longlasting as possible because recurrent infection and jaundice experienced by the patients when the biliary endoprostheses block will necessitate many stent exchange procedures compared to a perhaps long-lasting surgical bypass.

Patients with cancer in the head of the pancreas may develop duodenal obstruction due to invading tumour and gastroenterostomy is then indicated. Few of the patients without initial duodenal obstruction live long enough to develop this complication. The proportion of patients initially treated with palliative non-surgical drainage, who developed duodenal obstruction has been reported to be around 15%.

The risk of later duodenal obstruction has lead surgeons to add a prophylactic gastroenterostomy to the surgical biliary bypass operation. The addition of such a prophylactic duodenal bypass procedure does not seem to increase post-operative morbidity or mortality.

Malignant biliary obstruction is a disease of the elderly with rapidly increasing incidence after the age of 70 years. The median age of patients in reported studies in the literature 72-77 years. In these elderly patients post-operative morbidity and mortality related to palliative treatment is significantly higher than after non-surgical palliation.

A substantial number of patients with malignant biliary obstruction are not candidates for surgical palliation at all, namely old and frail patients with complicating diseases and/or advanced malignancy. This group of patients could be offered palliative biliary drainage. In some of them even palliative drainage is hardly justified.

In the 'grey zone' of patients with incurable malignant biliary obstruction, not unfit for surgical palliation, the important question arises: Should the patient be offered operative biliary bypass or biliary drainage? In recent years randomized prospective studies have been published and in brief the conclusions of these studies have been that biliary drainage is at least as effective as surgical palliation and the resources spent are probably less [25,26]. Days spent in hospital among patients treated with biliary stenting have been less than in the surgically treated group. However, the longterm follow-up has demonstrated exactly the same survival in these two groups [26].

In a report from London, patients considered unfit for surgical palliation for their malignant biliary obstruction were randomized prospectively to biliary stenting either PTBD or EBD. The number of significant complications after PTBD was significantly higher than complications after EBD, namely 67% versus 19% and so also was 30-day mortality, 33% versus 15%. Furthermore, EBD was found to be significantly more successful for relief of jaundice than PTBD, 81% versus 61%. The authors concluded that endoscopic stenting should be the method of choice in patient considered for non-surgical palliation of malignant obstructive jaundice [27].

The experience of a lower success rate for PTBD and more complications might be attributed to the insertion of larger stents, 12 F compared to 10 F stents inserted endoscopically. The larger the stents inserted transhepatically, the higher the risk of bleeding as well as other complications, and if bleeding occurs, clots may prevent endoprosthesis from functioning.

PTBD or EBD?

It is not an easy task to answer this important question so often posed at post-graduate courses and scientific meetings. In some hospitals the endoscopic expertise is high and the capacity is there to provide high quality biliary drainage in the majority of patients with a good indication for this procedure. In such centres interventional radiology comes in as a supplementary technique to provide additional drainage in the case of incomplete drainage obtained endoscopically or as a way of obtaining biliary drainage in the case of failed endoscopic decompression.

In other hospitals the expertise lies more in the field of interventional radiology for management of biliary strictures.

PTBD should aim at inserting internal endoprostheses and to avoid external catheters for a drainage except for a few days. Most patients find it difficult to accept external catheters because of the bag for collection of bile, odor, skin infection, soiling of clothes and bed linen, etc. Patients are generally old and frail and unable to manage proper care of external catheters.

The last decade has witnessed a competition between interventional radiologists and biliary endoscopists in the nonoperative management of patients with biliary diseases. This constituted a fertile ground for technical improvements of stents, wire-guides and adjuvant therapy. Endoscopists and radiologists have recognized that they work better together than against each other. The advantages of EBD over PTBD are recognized by most interventional radiologists, especially concerning obstructions below the liver hilum.

One example of collaboration between radiologists and endoscopists is the so-called rendezvous procedure, where a wire-guide is advanced by the radiologist via PTC into the duodenum and small bowel and taken by the endoscopist, who can then use the wire-guide to lead the endoscope to the papilla or perhaps use the wire-guide to insert large stents through obstructing biliary diseases [8,9].

Endoluminal Radiotherapy

Inoperable malignant biliary obstructive lesions can be subjected to endoluminal radiotherapy after insertion of catheters/stents through the obstructive lesion. This method seems particularly indicated in patients with inoperable cholangiocarcinomas because some of these patients may live for years and the combination of stenting and radiotherapy provides a much better and longer-lasting palliation than stenting alone [28]. Placing radioactive iridium-192 in the tumour can be done via nasobiliary catheters inserted endoscopically or via PTC catheters. Endoscopic implantation of iridium-192 has been reported but this method carries an unacceptable risk of radiation to the endoscopist and his assistant [29].

Goals for Palliative Biliary Decompression

The objective should be to provide a better quality of life for the incurable patient by relieving distressing pruritus and relieving jaundice. A non-jaundiced patient finds it easier to associate with family members and other people than a patient whose shining yellowish-brown colour is a constant reminder for the patient and for other people of impending death. Furthermore, prevention of cholangitis and liver insufficiency that might be a problem in patients with a long survival should be sought.

Concluding Remarks

In the last decade the spectrum of diagnostic and therapeutic biliary interventions has expanded enormously. Some of these new techniques now have a well-established role in the management of patients, for example endoscopic treatment of common bile duct stones and insertion of biliary endoprostheses. Other techniques are still being evaluated.

In our enthusiasm for new technology we should not forget that a large number of patients can and should be treated surgically. Decision on optimal management of biliary problems in the individual patient may not always be easy and a multidisciplinary tailoring of treatment programs should be the standard in the next decade.

Introduction of new stent materials and models in a combination with endoluminal radiation or endoluminal laser therapy may improve management of the many patients with incurable malignant biliary obstruction.

References

1. Malchow-Møller A, Thomsen C, Hilden J, Matzen P, Mindeholm L, Juhl E. A decision tree for early differentiation between obstructive and non-obstructive jaundice. *Scand J Gastroenterol* 1988;**23**:391-401.
2. Matzen P. *Differentialdiagnostik ved icterus* 1985. Copenhagen: FADL's Forlag.
3. Cairns SR, Dias L, Cotton PB, Salmon PR and Russell RCG. Additional endoscopic procedures instead of urgent surgery for retained common bile duct stone. *Gut* 1989;**30**:535-40.
4. Kiil J, Kruse A, Rokkjaer M. Large bile duct stones treated by endoscopic biliary drainage. *Surgery* 1989;**105**:51-6.
5. Yasuda K, Nakajima M, Cho E, Mukai H, Kawai K. Comparison of peroral and percutaneous cholangioscopy. *Endoscopy* 1989;**21**:347-50.
6. Leung JWC, Chung SCS, Sung JJY, Banez VP, Li AKC. Urgent endoscopic drainage for acute suppurative cholangitis. *Lancet* 1989:**i**:1307-9.
7. Soomers AJ, Nagengast FM, Yap SH. Endoscopic placement of biliary endoprostheses in patients with endoscopically unextractable common bile duct stones. *Endoscopy* 1990;**22**:24-6.
8. Dowsett JF, Vaira D, Hatfield ARW, Cairns SR, Polydorou A, Frost R, Croker J, Cotton PB, Russell RCG, Mason RR. Endoscopic biliary therapy using the combined percutaneous and endoscopic technique. *Gastroenterology* 1989;**96**:1180-6.
9. Chespak LW, Ring EJ, Shapiro HA, Gordon RL, Ostroff JW. Multidisciplinary approach to complex endoscopic biliary intervention. *Radiology* 1989;**170**:995-7.
10. Pitt HA, Kaufman SL, Coleman J, White RI, Cameron JL. Benign post-operative biliary strictures: Operate or dilate? *Ann Surg* 1989;**210**:417-42.
11. Irving JD, Adam A, Dick R, Dondelinger RF, Lunderquist A, Roche A. Gianturco expandable metallic biliary stents: Results of a European clinical trial. *Radiology* 1989;**172**:321-6.
12. Coons HG. Self-expanding stainless steel biliary stents. *Radiology* 1989;**170**:979-83.
13. Dancygier H, Rosch T, Lorenz R, Gossner W, Siewert JR, Classen M. Pre-operative staging of a distal common bile duct tumor by endoscopic ultrasound. *Gastroenterology* 1989;**95**:219-22.
14. Nimura Y, Kamiya J, Hayakawa N, Shionoya S. Cholangioscopic differentiation of biliary strictures and polyps. *Endoscopy*, 1989;**21**:351-6.
15. Bismuth H, Castaing D, Traynor O. Resection or palliation: Priority of surgery in the treatment of hilar cancer. *World J Surg* 1988;**12**:39-47.

16. McLean GK, Burke DR. Role of endoprostheses in the management of malignant biliary obstruction. *Radiology* 1989;**170**:961-7.
17. McPherson GAD, Benjamin IS, Hodgson HJF, Bowley NB, Allison DJ, Blumgart LH. Pre-operative percutaneous transhepatic biliary drainage: The results of a controlled trial. *Br J Surg* 1984;**71**:371-5.
18. Huibregtse, K. *Endoscopic biliary and pancreatic drainage* 1988. Stuttgart: Georg Thieme Verlag, 1988.
19. Speer AG, Cotton PB, MacRae KD. Endoscopic management of malignant biliary obstruction: Stents of 10 French gauge are preferable to stents of 8 French Gauge. *Gastrointest Endosc* 1988;**34**:412-17.
20. Kiil J, Kruse A, Rokkjaer M. Endoscopic biliary drainage. *Br J Surg* 1987;**74**:1087-90.
21. Deviere, J, Baize M, de Toeuf J, Cremer M. Long-term followup of patients with hilar malignant stricture treated by endoscopic internal biliary drainage. *Gastrointest Endosc* 1988;**34**:95-101.
22. Coene, PPLO, Groen AK, Cheng J, Out MMJ, Tytgat GNJ, Huibregtse K. Clogging of biliary endoprostheses: A new perspective. *Gut* 1990;**31**:913-17.
23. Huibrege K, Cheng J, Coene PPLO, Fockens P, Tytgat, GNJ. Endoscopic placement of expandable metal stents for biliary strictures - A preliminary report on experience with 33 patients. *Endoscopy* 1989;**21**:280-2.
24. Alvarado R, Palmaz JC, Garcia OJ, Tio FO, Rees CR. Evaluation of polymercoated balloon expendable stents in bile ducts. *Radiology* 1989;**170**:975-8.
25. Shepherd HA, Royle G, Ross APR, Diba A, Arthur M. Colin-Jones D. Endoscopic biliary endoprosthesis in the palliation of malignant obstruction of the distal common bile duct: A randomized trial. *Br J Surg* 1988;**75**:1166-8.
26. Andersen JR, Sørensen SM, Kruse A, Rokkjaer M, Matzen P. Randomised trial of endoscopic endoprosthesis versus operative bypass in malignant obstructive jaundice. *Gut* 1989;**30**:1132-5.
27. Speer AG, Cotton PB, Russell RCG, Mason R, Hatfield ARW, Leung JWC, MacRae KD, Houghton J, Lennin CA. Randomised trial of endoscopic versus percutaneous stent insertion in malignant obstructive jaundice. *Lancet* 1987;**ii**:57-62.
28. Ede RJ, Williams SJ, Hatfield ARW, McIntyre S, Mair G. Endoscopic management of inoperable cholangiocarcinoma using iridium-192. *Br J Surg* 1988;**76**:867-9.
29. Siegel JH, Lichtenstein JL, Pullano WE, Ramsey WH, Rosenbaum A, Halpern G, Nonkin R, Jacob H (1988). Treatment of malignant biliary obstruction by endoscopic implantation of iridium-192 using a new double lumen endoprosthesis. *Gastrointest Endosc* 1988;**34**:301-6.

Percutaneous stone extraction from the biliary tract

Constantin Cope
Department of Radiology, Hospital of the University of Pennsylvania, Philadelphia, Pennsylvania, USA

Introduction

Gallstones are very prevalent in Europe and the Americas. It is estimated that there are 20 million people in the United States of America who have stones and that one million new cases develop every year. In 10-20% of the population, stones will also be found to have migrated to the bile ducts. Way and Pelligrini give a good review of gallstone disease [1].

Most subjects with gallstones have either no related detectable symptoms or only mild post-prandial discomfort. The rate of development of symptoms is 1-2% per year and they consist generally of a limited episode of colicky pain of short duration without complication. Once symptomatic with pain, 40-70% of subjects will have recurrence within 5 years. However, serious complications such as cholecystitis develop usually only in patients who have had multiple frequent attacks or attacks of longer duration.

The mortality rate of complications is approximately 1-3%. Every year, approximately half a million subjects with gallstones become sufficiently symptomatic to require cholecystectomy, and of those, 1-4% are found post-operatively to have retained stones in the bile duct that require extraction.

Depending on the age of the patient and the severity of coexisting systemic diseases, the mortality for cholecystectomy varies from 0.25-2%, and the serious morbidity from 4-10%. If additional common bile duct exploration is performed, surgical mortality rate can rise to 5-10%, and the morbidity rate to 10-20%. Mortality rate of patients over 70 is estimated at 2-3% for elective surgery and 11% for emergency surgery.

Because the average gallbladder colic is of short duration and uncomplicated and, moreover, can usually be prevented by adherence to a low fat diet, there have been increasing efforts made in the past one to two decades to develop more definite, safer methods for treating symptomatic stone disease to prevent complications without the need for cholecystectomy.

Nonsurgical or minimally invasive techniques for extracting stones include oral litholysis with chemo- or ursodesoxycholic acid, percutaneous T-tube or trans-hepatic bile duct manipulation, retrograde endoscopic sphincterotomy, ESWL, percutaneous MTBE perfusion, and mechanical extraction of gallbladder stones.

The composition of stones is generally divided into two classes: cholesterol (80%) and pigment (20%). Cholesterol stones contain over 50% cholesterol and are usually mixed with calcium salts and mucin bilirubin complex salts. These stones are generally breakable with a basket; when such stones grow to large size and become diffusely calcified, they may need, however, to be fractured with EHL or laser.

Black pigment stones, usually of polymerized bilirubin, are small, hard stones, usually under 1 cm, which can most often be extracted whole.

Brown pigment stones, commonly found in Asia, are soft, spongy, and usually associated with bile duct obstruction and chronic cholangitis. They are composed of calcium bilirubinate.

Stones can also readily form around foreign bodies such as retained suture, catheters, and metal clips (Fig. 1).

Stone Extraction Through a T-tube Tract

Despite the increasing use of operative cholangiography, bile duct calculi can be missed in over 6% of cases following cholecystectomy [2]. The surgeon will usually insert a T-tube if he suspects that there are small retained stones or if the cholangiogram is technically unsatisfactory. Surgical duct re-exploration for retained stones is no longer performed, since calculi can be safely removed through the T-tube tract if present or else by retrograde endoscopy. The trans-hepatic approach is not favoured in this situation because it is

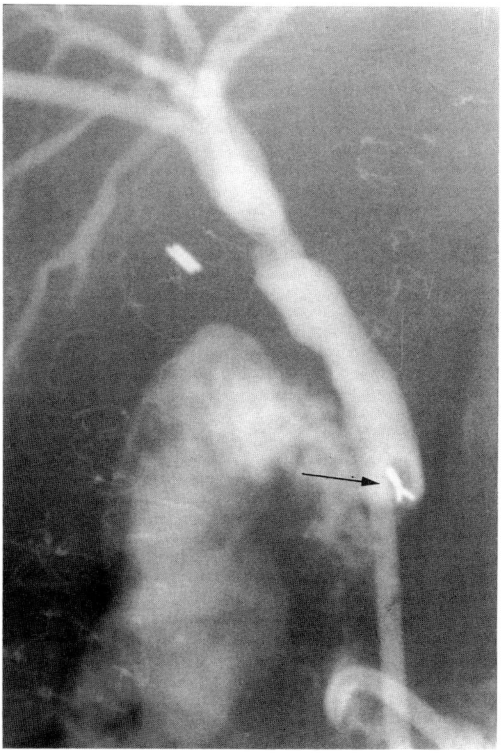

Figure 1. *Symptomatic stone formed around a metal clip expelled into the duodenum.*

unnecessarily difficult to cannulate decompressed hepatic biliary radicles.

Stone extraction through a T-tube tract should be delayed for 4-6 weeks following surgery in order to allow a good trans-peritoneal fibrous channel to form [3]. If the T-tube tract is under 14 French and the retained stones are large, the operator may decide to allow the tract to mature an extra 1-2 weeks, to ensure that it will not perforate if it needs to be dilated to over 16 to 18 French.

T-tube stone extraction is usually performed on an outpatient basis, unless the patient is old, infirm, or lives far away from the hospital. Two or more sessions are usually required to ensure that the patient is stone free. Prophylactic antibiotic coverage and pain medications are administered intravenously. The procedure is best done on a tilting fluoroscopic table to allow directional gravitational movements of stones.

Following opacification of the biliary tract, the T-tube is removed over a guidewire and replaced with either an 8 French Cobra-type angiographic catheter or a 10 French Burhenne steerable catheter. It is wise to insert a safety wire with its tip usually in a main intra-hepatic duct to ensure against accidental loss of access. If the operator anticipates a difficult extraction procedure due to the presence of large or multiple calculi or a small, tortuous tract, a 14 French or 18 French catheter sheath introducer with a side irrigation arm is inserted to protect the tract lining from the trauma of back-and-forth basketing and other painful mechanical retrieval manoeuvres, and also to simplify access to and opacification of the biliary tract, as well as suctioning of small calculi. Occasionally, a 24 French to 30 French sheath may need to be inserted when stones cannot be broken up.

Unless the stones are over 8-10 mm, it is preferable to extract them whole through the tract or push them out into the duodenum, rather than break them into small fragments, which then have to be chased and retrieved individually. With a catheter near the junction of the hepatic duct, a careful cholangiogram is performed with multiple views to assess the number, position, and size of calculi. All calculi should be herded into the common bile duct before attempting this extraction procedure. This is done by tilting the table or injecting dilute, bubble-free contrast medium from the distal right or left hepatic duct to flush the stones caudad where they can be more easily extracted. Four to 8 mm stones, if fairly hard, can usually be extracted by basketing through the tract. Flat wire Segura baskets or helical 4-wire Dormia baskets matched in diameter to the size of the common bile duct are used [4]. Once past the level of the stone, the collapsed basket is opened and gently brought back to engage the stone by a process of back-and-forth, as well as to-and-fro, rotational movements. Once the stone is trapped, the basket assembly is smoothly withdrawn through the sinus tract or the sheath. If, on the other hand, there are multiple small calculi or the larger stones break up into smaller fragments during the basketing procedure, it is then easier to drive the stones through the ampulla. Before proceeding with this approach, sphincteroplasty must be performed by threading 6-10 mm angioplasty balloon catheter over a guidewire and inflating it across the ampulla to allow free access to the duodenum [5]. Although the endoscopic literature reports a common incidence of pancreatitis following retrograde endoscopic balloon sphincteroplasty [6], this has not been the author's experience when this is performed in an antegrade manoeuvre. Multiple small stones or fragments are then directed into the distal common bile duct by irrigation, gravity, or by means of small occlusive balloon (Fig. 2a) or Fogarty catheters. The multiple stones are then pushed through the ampulla to the duodenum with a larger 11-15 mm occlusion balloon inflated to the diameter of the common duct (Fig. 2b) [7]. Alternatively, stones can

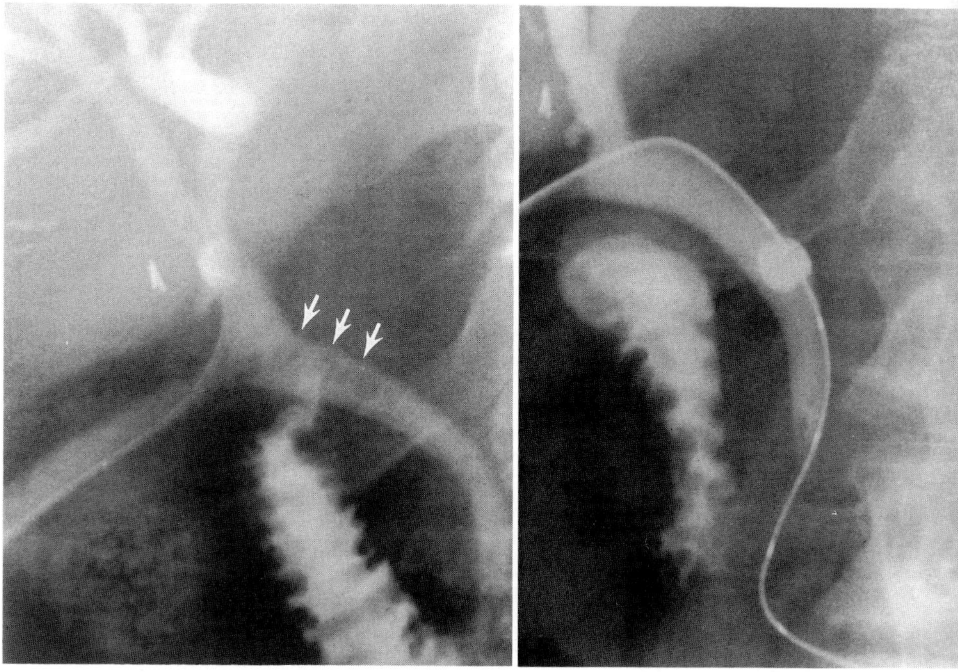

(a) **Figure 2.** *(a) Small balloon catheter used to drag multiple small stones from hepatic duct into common bile duct. (b) Larger occlusion balloon advanced over a guidewire to expel stones into duodenum.* (b)

be trapped and deposited into the duodenum with a Pfister-Schwartz type helical basket, which is equipped with a 3-5 cm floppy wire tip. Because part of this tail remains in the duodenum during manoeuvres, the basket can be smoothly and safely advanced and withdrawn across the ampulla without danger of duct perforation (Fig. 3).

The extraction procedure should be done as gently as possible and as quickly as possible (preferably within one hour). It is discontinued when all the stones have been extracted or when it is difficult to

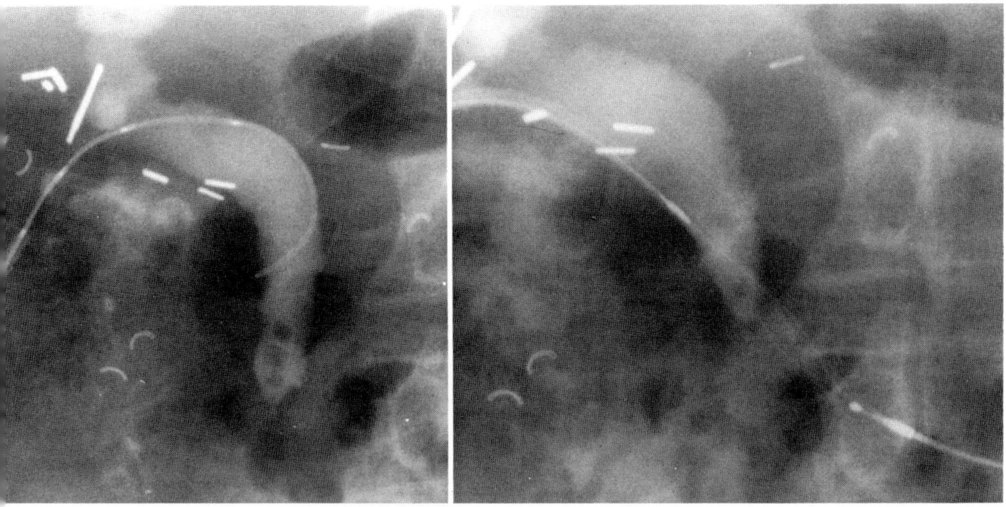

(a) **Figure 3.** *(a) Multiple small stones in common bile duct have been secured with a long tail basket and (b) expelled into duodenum.* (b)

carry on because blood clots or air bubbles are interfering with visualization of stones. A straight drain or a T-tube is left in place for external drainage to maintain patency of the tract until the next cholangiogram or extraction session. When it is difficult to reinsert a standard T-tube because of discomfort or suspected damage to the sinus tract, an articulated T-tube can be quickly fashioned from radio-opaque Silastic or red rubber or soft polymethane tubing (Fig. 4) and inserted atraumatically as follows.

The articulated T-tube crosspiece is cut to 4-5 cm length and a central side drain hole fashioned with a blade. A strong plastic 3ō suture is wrapped around the midsection of the crosspiece and its ends brought out internally through the rim of the side hole at diametrically opposite points along its long axis. The stem of the articulated tube is made of the same material and about 20 mm long. The long suture ends are then threaded through the distal end of the stem and brought out externally through the wall at about 5 cm from its proximal end or head. The cross piece and stem can then be aligned end-to-end over the guide with or without a coaxial 5 or 6 French stiffening catheter and advanced until the cross piece is completely within the common hepatic duct. The guidewire and stiffening catheter are removed. Back traction on the suture ends will

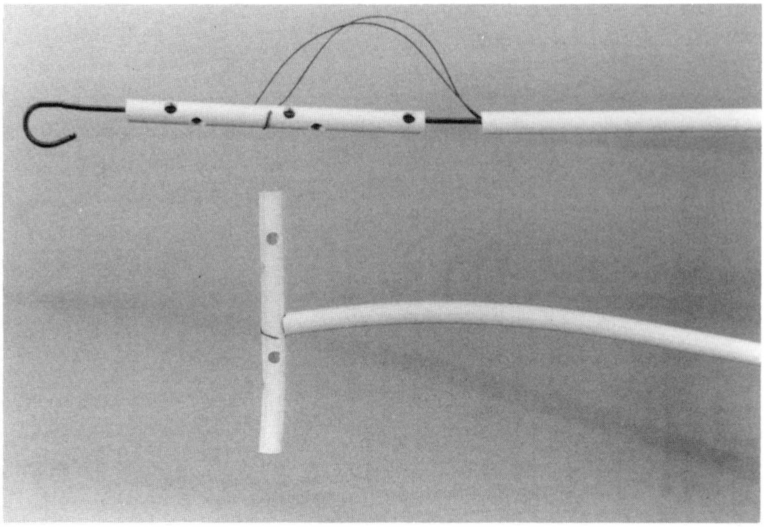

Figure 4. *(above) Soft polyurethane short drain segment with a suture wrapped around its midsection aligned over a guidewire with its accompanying stem, which is threaded internally. (below) After pulling to 2 suture ends, the articulated crosspiece and stem are reformed into a T-tube configuration.*

pull the back end of the cross piece into the common duct and bring about realignment of its centre hole with the distal stem lumen in a T-tube configuration. The suture ends are securely fastened around the distal stem. The articulated T-tube can then be extracted a few days later by pulling on its stem in the same manner as a standard T-tube. When T-tubes are accidentally pulled out, the tract can usually be retrieved within 24 hours either by angiographic catheter techniques or by endoscopy (Fig. 5) [8], if this fails.

Trans-hepatic Choledocholithotomy

Although patients with simple docholithiasis are commonly managed today by retrograde endoscopic sphincterotomy, there are still many occasions when the percutaneous trans-hepatic approach is preferred or necessary, such as when endoscopy is unsuccessful or complicated, or when there is a choledochojejunostomy or a duodenal diverticulum. The interventionist can also assist the endoscopist in some

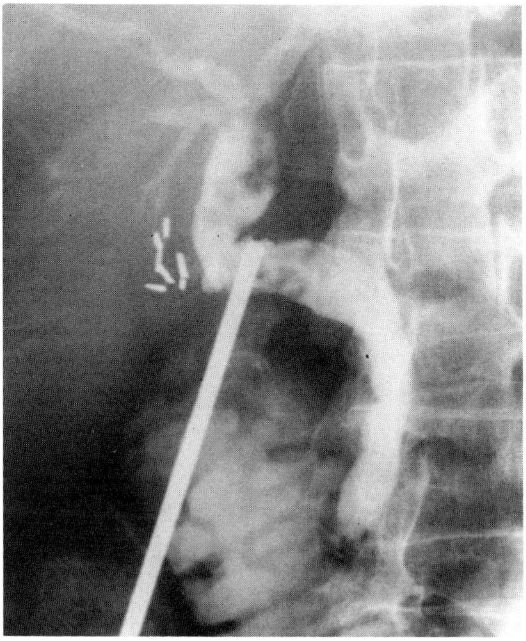

Figure 5. *Following accidental removal of the T-tube one week after surgery, the tract could only be retraced with a small rigid endoscope.*

difficult cases by pulling up baskets and sphincterotomies into the common bile duct through a 5 or 6 French trans-hepatic catheter [9].

Since up to 80% of patients with obstructive choledocholithiasis have infected bile, a course of appropriate cephalosporin antibiotics should be administered intravenously within 6 hours of the procedure and continued for at least 24 hours. Those patients who present with acute cholangitis should likewise be treated vigorously with combination antibiotic therapy for several days until they are afebrile before attempting biliary drainage. Pain is controlled by local anaesthesia and a combination intravenous narcotic and midazolam in simple cases or by epidural anaesthesia if it is anticipated that stone extraction will require prolonged or difficult manipulations. Since peripheral intra-hepatic bile duct radicles may be only minimally dilated because of the intermittent nature of bile duct obstruction, it is wise to use only a skinny 22-gauge needle for exploratory intra-hepatic punctures, rather than a 19-gauge sheathed needle, in order to prevent serious vascular complications [10]. Bending the distal 3-4 cm tip of the needle 5° to 10° by finger pressure can be quite useful by allowing the operator to quickly change the needle direction without having to withdraw it more than a few centimetres, and also to perform a more precise puncture for entering already opacified radicles. The right mid-axillary 9th and 10th intercostal space is the preferred entry site.

Once a suitable bile duct branch has been punctured and opacified under fluoroscopy, the needle tract is dilated over a 0.018 stiff platinum tipped guidewire with a 6.3 French Cope hockey stick introducing dilator. This device allows the operator to aspirate old stasis bile, and then exchange the fine wire for a stiff 0.038" J-guidewire, so that the tract can be further dilated coaxially to allow percutaneous insertion of an 8 or 10 French Cope loop biliary drain. If a large stone completely occludes the ampulla, a 7 or 8 French Cope loop nephrostomy drain is left in the dilatated common bile duct (Fig. 6a). It is usually safer to permit the patient to stabilize on external drainage for 1-2 days before attempting stone extraction, especially in patients who presented with acute cholangitis.

Before stone manipulation can begin, an 8 to 12 French catheter introducing sheath with a check-flow valve is threaded through the trans-hepatic tract to the level of the proximal common hepatic duct and sutured to the skin. The sheath will serve to maintain and protect the tract, to allow irrigation and opacification of the bile ducts, and to facilitate the insertion of catheters and other devices. In order to prevent laceration or perforation of the distal common bile duct and ampulla while driving a stone into the duodenum, the operator is well-advised to pre-dilate the sphincter with an angioplasty balloon to the size of the largest stone, which is usually in the range of 6-12 mm. Stones larger than 10-12 mm should first be broken up into smaller pieces. Stone and stone fragments can be expelled into the duodenum either with an inflated occlusion balloon or with a basket equipped with a flexible guidewire tip guide (Fig. 6b and c) through an 8 French pre-shaped or steerable catheter as previously described.

Following stone extraction, an 8 or 10 French loop catheter is left in the common bile duct for external drainage for 1-2 days to allow oedema of the distal bile duct to resolve (Fig. 6d). The catheter may then be removed, or if there is any doubt about the completeness of stone extraction or bile duct patency, the patient may be sent home for 1-2 weeks with the drain capped and then re-examined as an outpatient and further treated if necessary.

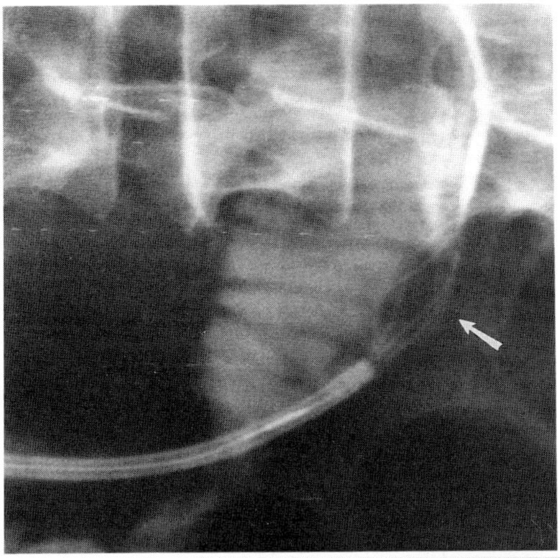

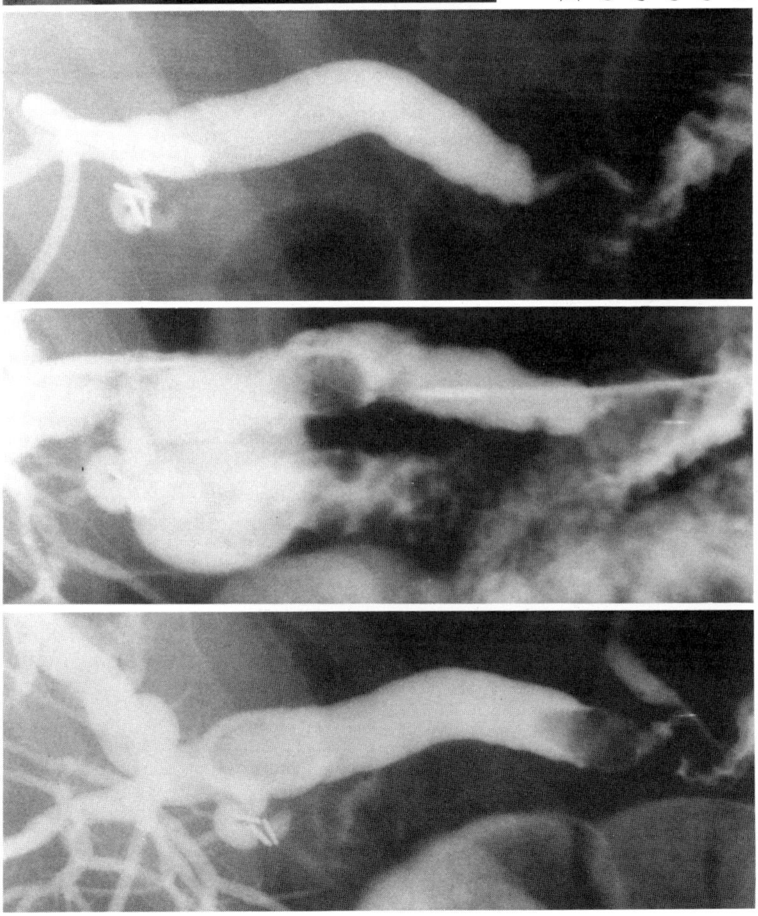

(a) (b) (c) (d)

Figure 6. *(a) Stone impacted in the distal common duct. (b) After sphincter balloon dilatation to 12 mm, the stone is engaged in a long tail basket and (c) pushed into the duodenum. (d) After one week of post-extraction drainage, the ampulla is widely patent.*

Management of Special Problems

Most cases of choledocholithiasis are fairly simple to treat either through a T-tube or a trans-hepatic tract, because the retained stones are usually few in number, congregate in the easily accessible common bile duct, and can be easily retrieved or broken up by standard basket or ballooning techniques.

More sophisticated techniques, however, must be applied in certain special situations.

Balloon Catheters

Fogarty Catheters

Small 2 or 3 French Fogarty latex balloon catheters can easily be passed through pre-shaped 5 or 6 French angiographic catheters and directed into intra-hepatic biliary radicles for retrieving small calculi. When these are lodged at duct bifurcations, they may require to be extracted by the 2-balloon technique to prevent the stone from extruding into one or the other duct.

Large Angioplasty Balloon Catheters

When large stones over 12 mm cannot be broken up within the duct or pulled out through the dilated T-tube tract, they can often be pushed out into the duodenum after overdilating the sphincter to the size of the stone. In the author's experience, and that of others [11], uncomplicated balloon dilatation up to 20 mm can be accomplished safely with successful extrusion of the stones (Fig 7). Surprisingly, when barium studies are done at a later date, no retrograde biliary flow of contrast is seen. Overdilatation is, however, contra-indicated when the bile duct empties into a narrow neck duodenal diverticulum. Angioplasty balloons in tandem can be used to push inaccessible stones located in a main duct outpouching - a useful technique described by Saeed et al [12].

Stone Baskets

Hard stones are difficult to crush, because the basket sheath folds accordion-like when the traction load from the basket becomes too

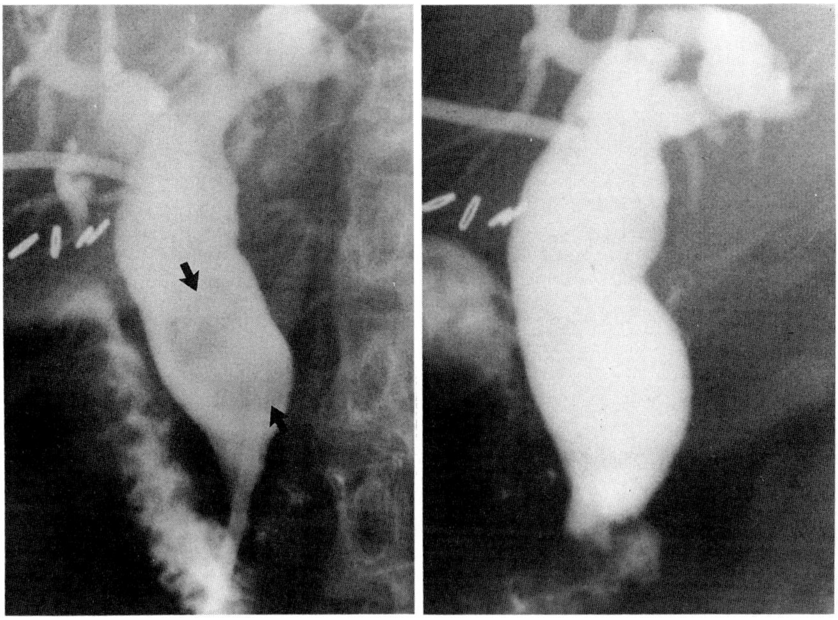

(a) (b)

Figure 7. *(a) A large bi-lobed common duct stone which could not be broken up with a basket; the ampulla was dilated with an angioplasty balloon to 15 mm and the stone passed spontaneously (b) 3 days later, following an episode of severe colic.*

great. The Sohendra basket kit solves this problem by providing a 12 French steel helical spring sheath for the basket which can then support the great traction pressures which are generated by winding the basket wire on the handle assembly (Fig. 8). This device is used with strong, stiff stone-crushing baskets, which are also more efficient in engaging large stones (Fig. 9).

Rigid Forceps

Mazzariello [13] or modified Randall forceps can be used to crush and retrieve common bile duct stones through the T-tube tract. They require a 16 to 18 French entry sheath and are most effective when the stone can be directed close to the distal end of the tract.

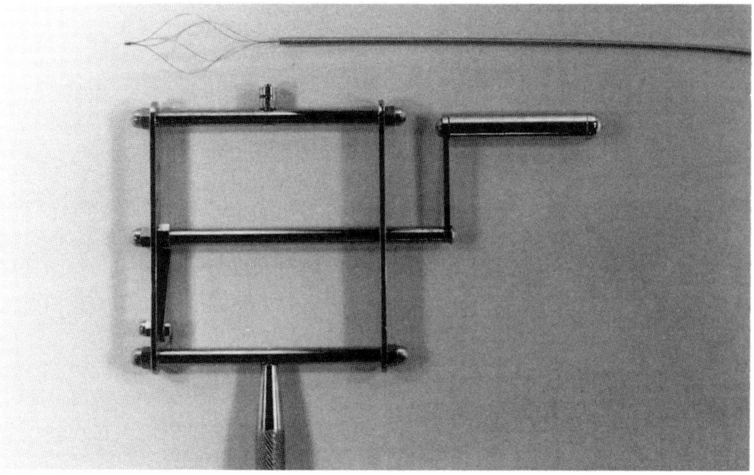

Figure 8. *Sohendra stone-crushing kit. The stone basket sheath is made of stainless steel spring. The winding handle permits great traction forces to be applied to the stone-bearing basket through the 12 French metal sheath.*

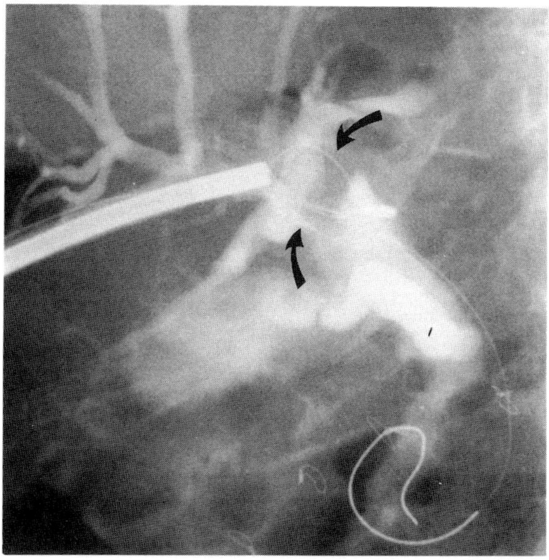

Figure 9. *Large common hepatic duct stone (arrows) being crushed with the Sohendra device. A fine platinum-tipped safety wire extends to the duodenum.*

Litholysis

Mono-octanoin is an inexpensive cholesterol solvent approved for clinical use which has been widely used to manage large bile duct stones via T-tube tract, trans-hepatic tract, and nasobiliary catheter [14]. The course of treatment averages 10 days of irrigation at 3-5 ml/h. Of the 80% of stones that respond, only 30% can be dissolved completely. The majority of stones subjected to mono-octanoin irrigation will either shrink in size or become softer, allowing the operator to more easily break up or retrieve large stones which previously could not be managed by any route. Side effects include diarrhoea, nausea, and vomiting, and biliary colic if the infusion rate is too high. It is usually recommended that a second catheter drain be inserted to keep the bile duct decompressed. Because of the long infusion time that often leads to only incomplete stone dissolution, this drug is usually not used unless other modalities for stone management have failed.

MTBE is a much more efficacious cholesterol solvent than mono-octanoin [15], and has been used successfully to dissolve gallbladder stones, but because of its potential toxicity when absorbed in the duodenum, there has been so far very limited enthusiasm for its use in the common duct.

Percutaneous Biliary Endoscopy and Electrohydraulic Lithotripsy (EHL)

Although percutaneous retrieval or retained duct stones is most commonly performed under fluoroscopy, there are occasions when there is a great need for the accessory use of a flexible endoscope. Endoscopy can be used to distinguish tumour from adherent stones or pseudostones, to capture elusive stones, to reach and extract small intra-hepatic stones, and to biopsy suspicious areas of bile duct mucosa [16]. Small flexible endoscopes with controllable tip angulation and a working instrument channel, today available in sizes of 11 French to 16 French, are being increasingly used to break up stones under direct vision with 3 or 5 French electrohydraulic probes through a trans-hepatic tract [17]. The electrode tip should be placed in direct contact with the stones and the power set usually between

70 and 80. Higher starting voltages may cause exploding stone fragments to perforate the duct wall. The manufacturers recommend that irrigation be performed with one-sixth normal saline for the most efficacious spark production. Although most mixed cholesterol stones can be broken up by intra-ductal EHL, some large diffusely calcified stones may not respond to this modality. Pulsed tunable dye lasers can be effective in these situations [18].

Extracorporeal Shock-Wave Lithotripsy (ESWL)

Large, hard bile duct stones over 1.5-2 cm in diameter are notoriously difficult to break-up or remove by percutaneous or endoscopic techniques, because they cannot be entrapped within a basket and are either not freely movable or impacted. In the past 2 years, ESWL has become an increasingly important modality in managing these cases [19].

Patients first undergo endoscopic sphincterotomy or, if this is not possible, trans-hepatic balloon sphincteroplasty. A catheter is positioned in the bile duct to opacify the biliary tract and render the stones visible under ESWL biplane fluoroscopy. Although most stones will be successfully fractured by ESWL, large fragments will often fail to pass out spontaneously and must be extracted by adjuvant mechanical means (Fig. 10). Overall success rates for complete clearance of stones is in the 60-90% range, with failures in complete extraction occurring most often in older patients and in those with multiple intra-hepatic stones.

Biliary ESWL appears to be a safe procedure which is fast becoming an integral part of the treatment protocol for managing these difficult cases.

Coexisting Bile Duct Strictures and Stones

Stones are commonly formed in the presence of duct strictures because of bile stasis and recurrent cholangitis. Conversely, stones themselves can cause strictures by a process of intermittent duct and ampullary blockage, cholangitis, and pancreatitis (Fig. 11). In this setting, the successful management of stone disease must include the

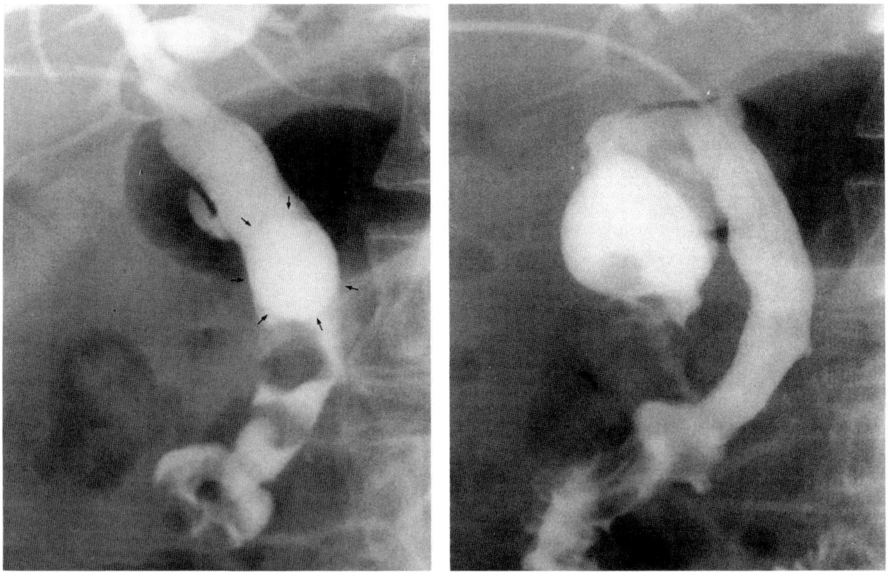

(a) (b)

Figure 10. *(a) Large common duct stone shattered into two large fragments by ESWL. The fragments are being pushed with an occlusion balloon (arrows) into the duodenum, through the sphincterotomy channel (b).*

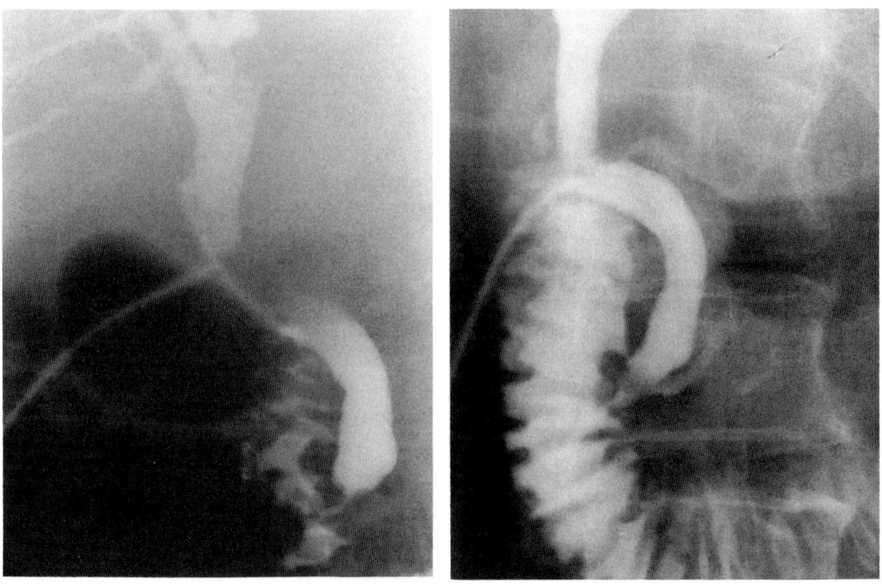

(a) (b)

Figure 11. *(A) Significant papillary stenosis noted after cholecystectomy. (B) Excellent patency established after dilatation with an 8 mm angioplasty balloon.*

eradication of coexisting strictures and recurring infection. When surgical bile duct reconstruction is too hazardous, strictures can be treated by the interventionist percutaneously [20,21] by repeated angioplasty balloon dilatation over either a short period of time, varying from several days to 2-3 weeks, or on an ongoing periodic basis with redilatation at 2-3 month intervals in combination with large internal-external drains. Tough recurring strictures should be dilated under epidural or general anaesthesia. Balloon size averages 6-8 mm for dilatation of intra-hepatic ducts, 8-12 mm for the common duct, and 10-20 mm for choledochoenteric anastomoses or papillary stenoses (Fig. 12).

Generally, papillary stenoses, choledochoenterostomies, and some traumatic bile strictures give good long-term results, while strictures caused by periductal encasement, chronic pancreatitis, sclerosing cholangitis, and oriental cholangiohepatitis require constant attention.

The most common route of access for these procedures is a T-tube or trans-hepatic tract. In the management of stone associated sclerosing cholangitis or oriental cholangiohepatitis, however, the preferred catheterization route is through the T-tube tract because it provides a simple retrograde approach for treating recurrent intra- and extra-hepatic duct strictures and stones (Fig. 13). If this sinus tract is not available, long-term access to the ducts can be facilitated through the construction of a Hutson intestinal loopostomy [22]. Alternatively, a standard choledochojejunostomy can also provide a useful percutaneous approach for bile duct toilet if a knuckle of adjacent jejunum is surgically fixed to the anterior abdominal wall and marked with a radiopaque ring for easily accessing the bowel lumen under fluoroscopy (Fig. 14).

Recently, several types of 8-10 mm expandable metal sleeves have become available to stent strictures which are refractory to standard balloon dilatation techniques. However, it is too early to know at this time whether these devices will lead to long-term patency [23].

Morbidity

The serious morbidity rate for post-operative stone extraction through a surgical biliary-cutaneous fistulous tract is under 5%, but 16% when performed through a trans-hepatic tract [21].

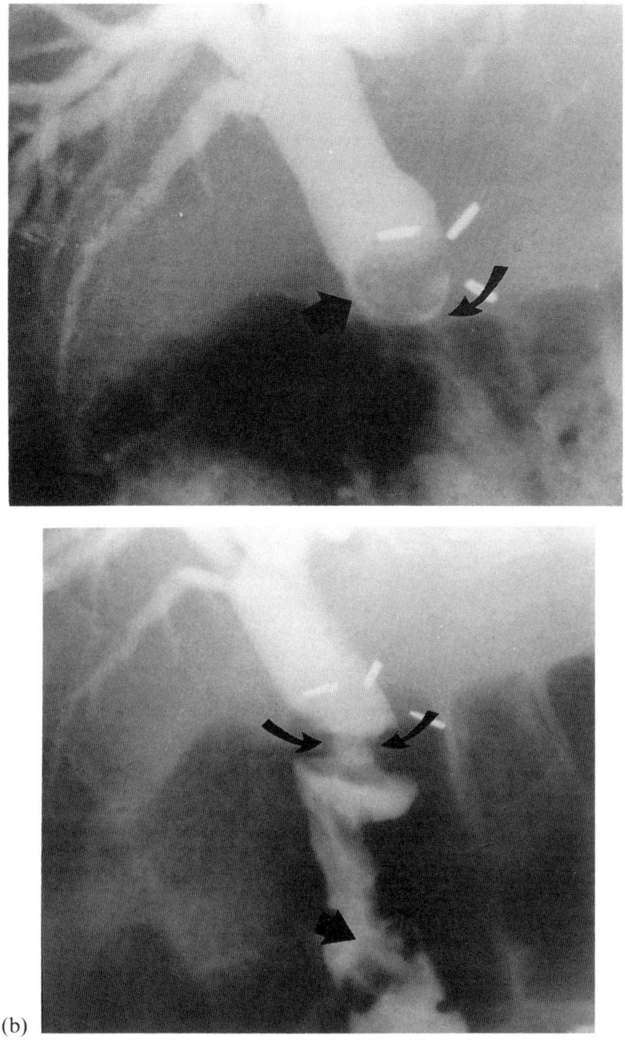

(a)

(b)

Figure 12. *(a) Large common duct stone associated with an anastomotic stricture. (b) Stone passed (arrowhead) after dilatation of stricture (arrows).*

Serious complications common to both approaches include sepsis, duct perforation, and acute pancreatitis; other complications, seen when the trans-hepatic approach is used, comprise subdiaphragmatic and subcapsular collections, hepatic abscesses, and haemobilia due to

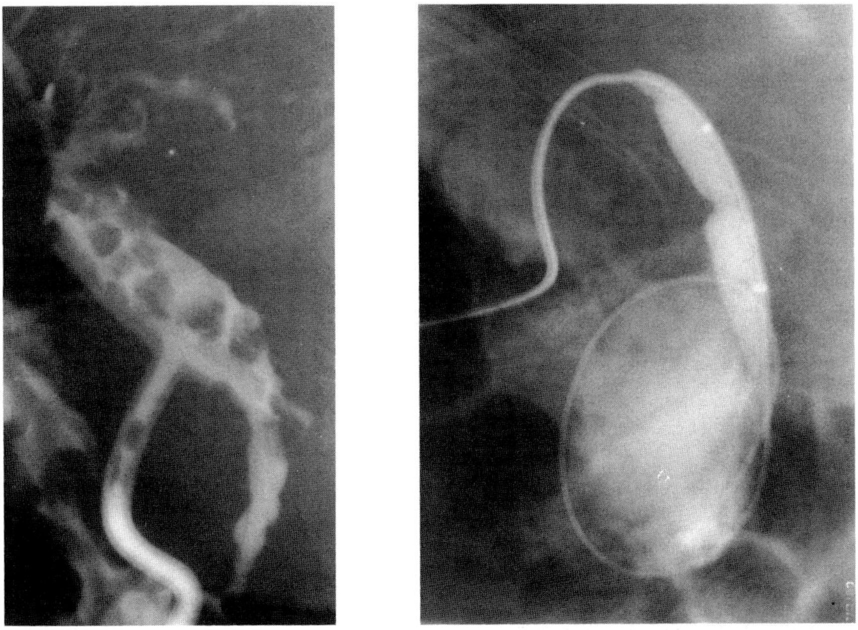

(a) (b)

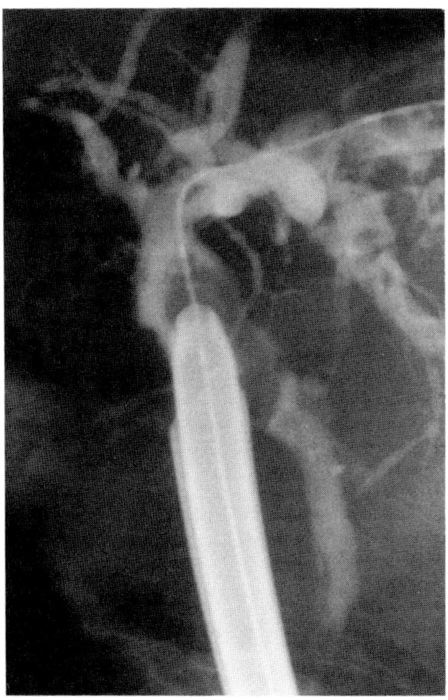

(c)

Figure 13. *(a) Oriental cholangiohepatitis with multiple stones and strictures. (b) Dilatation of common bile duct stricture with an 8 mm balloon. (c) 24-French sheath inserted through T-tube tract to allow dilatation of intra-hepatic duct strictures and extraction of stone material.*

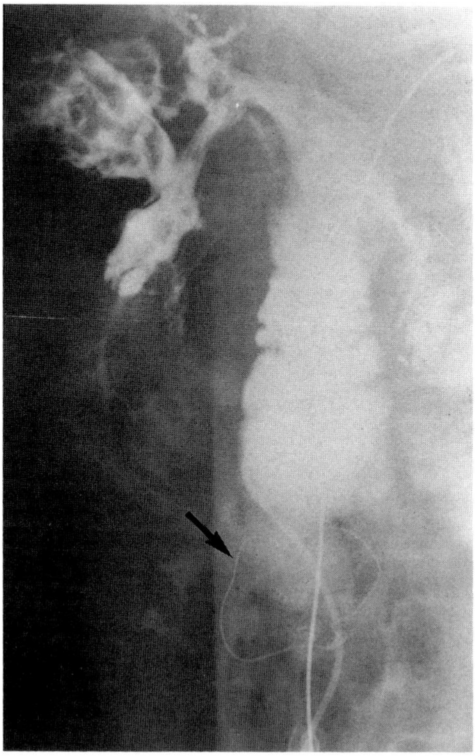

Figure 14. *Patient with stone-associated sclerosing cholangitis. A Radiopaque ring marker (arrow) allows repeated percutaneous access to the jejunum and bile ducts.*

intra-hepatic vascular trauma. Thirty-day mortality of 3% is related to the severity of associated diseases and usually not cause-and-effect of the stone extraction procedures. Stone extraction procedures can be rendered safer by adhering to certain precautions:

1. All manipulations should be gentle.
2. Procedure duration should last about an hour and can be more safely repeated on a daily basis if necessary, rather than being performed at one marathon session.
3. Access to bile ducts should be from as peripheral a trans-hepatic puncture as possible.
4. A plastic sheath should be inserted to protect the trans-hepatic or sinus tract.
5. Broad antibiotic coverage is necessary.
6. Adequate pre-dilatation of the duct sphincter should be performed, to prevent stone impaction and pancreatitis.

When choledocholithiasis is treated by a team approach, with the latest technology available, cure rates by the percutaneous approach can be achieved in as high as 90% over a 31-month average period of follow-up [24].

Percutaneous Cholecystolithomy (PCCL)

We have found that there are many people with symptomatic gallbladder calculi who visit our gallstone treatment centre who prefer to undergo the occasional agony of a gallbladder colic and stay on a fairly tasteless, low fat diet rather than undergo cholecystectomy. The recent advent of new medical modes of therapy for treating gallstones by oral bile acid (UDCA) or extracorporeal shock-wave lithotripsy (ESWL) [25] has raised the hope of many that cholecystectomy would soon be displaced as the primary mode of treatment. For many gallstone sufferers who are not eligible for ESWL, alternate nonsurgical options are now available, such as contact dissolution with methyl-tert-butyl ether (MTBE) [15] or direct percutaneous stone extraction. Since MTBE therapy is not as yet approved by the FDA, suitable patients may be treated by mechanical extraction.

The following categories of patients are felt to be suitable for percutaneous stone extraction:

1. Any symptomatic patient who is not suitable for MTBE or UDCA therapy and who refuses surgery.
2. Patients not suitable for ESWL (e.g., more than three stones, stones larger than 3 cm in diameter, calcified stones, non-functioning gallbladder).
3. Patients who, because of unsatisfactory pulverization of gallstones by ESWL, require extraction of large stone fragments because of continued symptoms.

Contra-indications to PCCL are as follows:

1. Possible gangrenous or perforated gallbladder.
2. Contracted gallbladder with no appreciable lumen on ultrasound examination.
3. Large diffusely calcified stones over 30-40 mm.
4. Unwillingness of the patient to undergo cholecystectomy

should the percutaneous technique fail due to complications.

5. Uncorrectable coagulation disorder.

The technique for PCCL used in the author's department are as follows [26]:

The ambulatory patient is admitted either on the morning of the procedure or the day before with a documented normal coagulation profile. Six oral cholecystography tablets and one dose of Gastrografin are taken the night before so that the gallbladder and the hepatic flexure of the colon will be visible fluoroscopically at the time of PCCL.

Under epidural anaesthesia and antibiotic coverage, the fundus is punctured subhepatically trans-peritoneally with a double needle system consisting of a 22-gauge probing needle for locating the gallbladder lumen under ultrasound and/or fluoroscopy, and a coaxial 17-gauge needle, pre-loaded with a suture anchor, as previously described in detail. Gallbladder bile is aspirated and replaced with dilute contrast medium, the retrievable anchor is discharged into the gallbladder with a guidewire, and the needle is withdrawn so as to allow the centre suture of the anchoring device to be retracted. This manoeuvre, by bringing the gallbladder wall in firm contact with the anterior abdominal wall, will prevent its invagination during subsequent tract dilatation and minimize bile leakage. A 5-French catheter sheath or Cope loop catheter is inserted in order to irrigate the gallbladder, keep it distended, and subsequently flow-direct stones toward the extraction cannula. Using the same insertion anchor technique, a second puncture is made adjacent to the first and the tract is dilated with an angioplasty balloon to allow a 12-French, 16-French, or 24-French stone extraction cannula and a safety wire to be inserted into the gallbladder lumen (Fig. 15a). Stones are then removed through the large sheath by a combination of gravity drainage and irrigation if they are small, or by basketing or extraction with forceps if they are large (Fig. 15b). The use of electrohydraulic lithotripsy catheters to break up stones [17] is rarely needed, since most stones can be crushed by basket techniques. All or as many stones as possible are extracted over a period of 30-60 minutes.

The next day (Fig. 15c), all residual stone fragments are extracted and the debris flushed out. If necessary, the cystic duct may need to be catheterized to expel cystic or common duct retained calculi. The

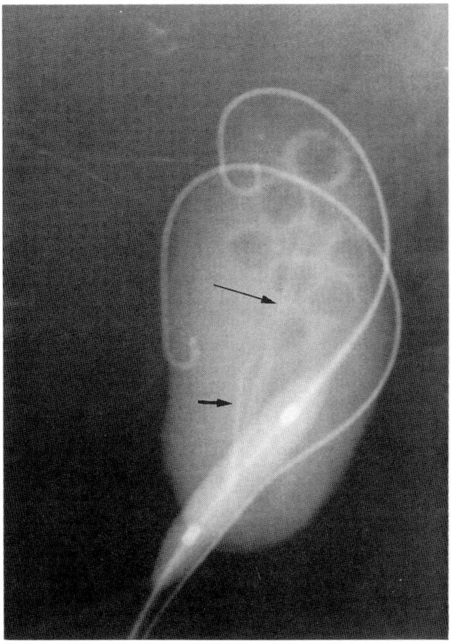

(a)

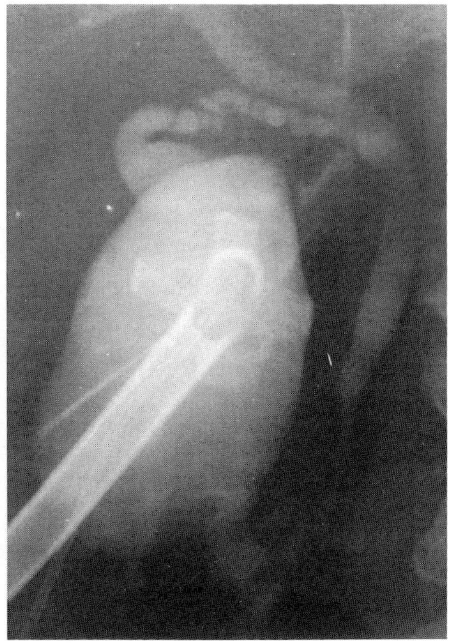

(b)

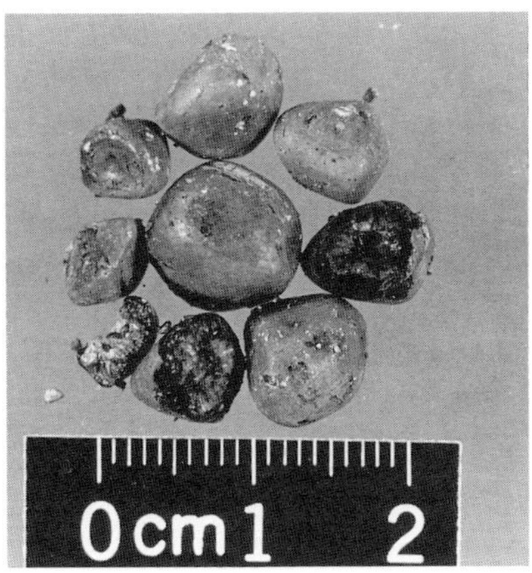

(c)

Figure 15. *(a) Percutaneous extraction of calcified gallstones. 5 French irrigating catheter (long arrow) and metal anchoring device (short arrow). The cholecystostomy tract is being dilated with an 8 mm angioplasty balloon prior to inserting a 24 French stone extraction sheath. There is an introducing and a safety guidewire. (b) 22 French Malecot catheter inserted for external drainage after stone extraction. (c) Extracted stones.*

extraction sheath is then replaced with a Foley catheter of equivalent size, and the irrigation catheter with a 5-French retention loop catheter. The patient, if stable, is discharged the next day on oral antibiotics to be taken for 5 days. The Foley catheter is kept on gravity drainage to a leg bag for 5-10 days and then kept clamped, except for 15-minute drainage periods, morning and evening to decompress the gallbladder and prevent possible leakage.

Two to three weeks after discharge, the patient is examined as an outpatient following intravenous antibiotic administration to ensure that there are no retained stones in the gallbladder, cystic duct, and common duct, as well as no intra-peritoneal leakage when withdrawing the catheter drains. This is done by the interventional radiologist by a combination of careful endoscopy of the gallbladder and cholecystography. A 10.5 French deflecting endoscope or a rigid urethroscope is used. The suture anchors are removed by cutting the centre suture and pulling them out over a 5 French catheter with the end suture. In several cases where the anchor was left in more than 2 weeks, the anchor retrieval suture broke due to tissue ingrowth, and the devices had to be removed with a basket. The patient is subsequently examined by the gastroenterology service at regular intervals for stone recurrence by ultrasound of the gallbladder. UDCA therapy is discontinued 6-8 weeks post-PCCL if the gallbladder is found to be completely stone free.

Results

There have been nine reports describing various techniques and early results of PCCL on a total of 142 patients. [27-34].

Immediate successful gallstone clearance rates vary from 71-100%, but there is as yet insufficient collected data on long-term recurrence rate with PCCL performed under careful endoscopic control. In Akiyama's series of 20 patients [34] followed over a mean period of 3 years with adjuvant chemodesoxycholic acid, there was only one recurrence. In the author's series of over 34 patients, all have been free of stones at 6 months.

Among the 142 patients thought to be good candidates for PCCL 12% required cholecystectomy when the tract could not be properly dilated, when access to the gallbladder was lost, when large stones could not be fragmented, or when calculi could not be retrieved from the cystic duct or phrygian cap. Delayed bile leakage through the trans-hepatic tract necessitated surgery in two other patients, one of whom died of complications. In those patients who had successful percutaneous extraction, morbidity, such as minimal peritoneal leakage, intra-cholecystic bleeding, and superficial infection, was easily controlled.

Status of PCCL

Percutaneous cholecystostomy (PC) has been slow in gaining general acceptance by clinicians because of the fear of complicating biliary peritonitis. This fear has been shown in the last 5-10 years to be generally unfounded, as long as the procedure is performed with small needles and catheters in patients who have no biliary obstruction. The main obstacle in the acceptance of PCCL has been that, in contrast to percutaneous nephrolithotomy, it may be quite difficult to intubate the gallbladder safely with large cannulas because it is a mobile, easily compressible organ. Since the superior surface of the gallbladder is attached to the liver by connective tissue, many interventionalists prefer to go through the liver [27] to prevent bile leakage and gallbladder wall invagination. it should be remembered, however, that this approach is not foolproof, because this bare area of attachment is extremely variable in extent and may not even be present in 5% of cases when the gallbladder is completely ensheathed in peritoneum.

The trans-hepatic route for placement of large 24-French to 30-French cholecystostomy cannula also carries a potential risk of liver laceration and vascular trauma. If the gallbladder fundus could be cannulated subhepatically, as is done in surgical cholecystostomy, the approach could eliminate serious damage to the liver and provide an easier route along the long axis of the gallbladder for extracting stones, for endoscopy, and for catheterizing the common bile duct through the cystic duct. In order to perform subhepatic PCCL safely, however, an anchoring device is helpful to firmly secure and attach the gallbladder fundus to the abdominal wall, especially in long-standing chronic cholecystitis, in order to prevent invagination of the tough fibrotic gallbladder wall, bile leakage during dilatation of the cholecystostomy tract, and loss of access, which can occur when direct cannulation of the free gallbladder fundus is performed [30].

Such an easily introducible suture anchor has been devised and found to be very effective for PC and PCCL in the past 4-5 years. The use of this percutaneous anchoring device represents an additional measure of safety, in that it allows prompt intra-cholecystic introduction of cannulas up to 24 French in size and immediate removal of calculi without having to wait 1-2 weeks for a firm tract to form. The anchors can be removed either at the time of hospital discharge or 2 weeks later on an outpatient basis.

When intra-hepatic gallbladders are present, then a 1-2 cm bridge of liver parenchyma can be found to reach the gallbladder fundus without significant hepatic trauma.

Endoscopy is a necessary step in evaluating the gallbladder, not only to ensure that there are no residual calculi but also to assess the mucosa for fibrosis, cholesterolosis, polyps, as well as to biopsy suspicious areas of malignancy.

Gallbladder endoscopy is very important for localizing residual stone fragments at the time of the 2-week check ups, because 3-6 mm stone fragments may be completely invisible on careful cholecystography. It will, therefore, be interesting to see if, on long-term follow-up, those patients who have had endoscopically clean gallbladders will have a significantly reduced rate of stone recurrence as compared to some widely quoted series in which stone clearance was gauged only by cholecystography or irrigation [35].

All patients, including those with pigment stones, are placed on oral UDCA therapy for 2 months following PCCL in order to potentially dissolve any residual cholesterol crystals within the gallbladder, but this is then discontinued if ultrasound examination of the gallbladder was totally normal.

Although we initially felt that PCCL would be performed mostly on the aged with significant operative risks, we were quite surprised to find that over one third of our patients could not be cajoled into having surgery, despite the fact that they had no medical contraindications to cholecystectomy. Although some were afraid of general anaesthesia, most refused surgery because they could not afford long recuperative periods which would take them away from work or pressing family responsibilities.

New techniques to speed up breaking up gallbladder stones are being evaluated, such as electrohydraulic, ultrasound, and pulsed laser contact probes. A blender-like device, the Kensey-Nash Lithotrite [36], is currently being investigated. It is able to pulverize multiple gallstones to sand-like particles in 15 to 45 minutes. Since it requires only an 11 French sheath for its introduction, it promises to become a safe, significant advance for PCCL (Fig. 16).

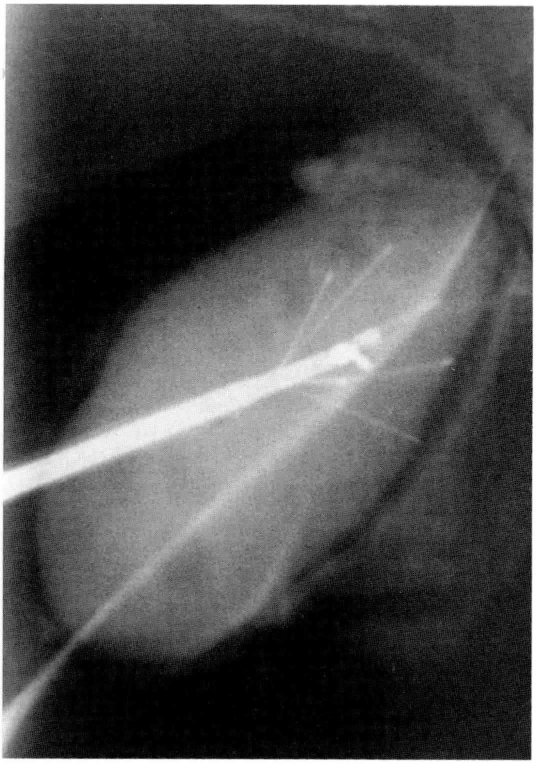

Figure 16. *Kensey-Nash Rotary Lithotrite deployed in the gallstone-bearing gallbladder. The Propeller is in the centre of the strut cone.*

It is evident that PCCL, as it continues to evolve in safety and efficacy, will have an important role in the management of symptomatic gallstone disease, especially in older, inform patients or those with significant associated surgical risks. Younger patients under 65 years of age with no surgical contra-indications should continue to be encouraged to have standard or laparoscopic cholecystectomy.

References

1. Way LW, Pelligrini CA (eds). *Surgery of the Gallbladder and Bile Ducts*. Philadelphia: WB Saunders Co, 1987.

2. Glenn F. Retained calculi within the biliary ductal system. *Ann Surg* 1974;**179:**528-537.
3. Burhenne HJ. Nonoperative retained biliary tract stone extraction: a new roentgenologic technique *AJR* 1973;**117:**388-399.
4. Tadavarthy SM, Hunter DW, Zollikofer CL, et al. Interventional techniques in the hepatobiliary system. In: Castaneda-Zuniga WR, Tadavarthy SM (eds). *Interventional Radiology*. Baltimore: Williams & Wilkins, 1988:649-749.
5. Centola CAP, Stauffer A, Russinovich AE. Balloon dilatation of the papilla of Vater to allow biliary stone passage. *AJR* 1987;**136:**613-614.
6. Guelrud MS, Mendoza S, Viera L. Does somatostatin prevent acute pancreatitis after pancreatic duct sphincter hydrostatic balloon dilatation? *Gastrointest Endosc* 1987;**33:**148-151.
7. Meranze SG, Stein EJ, Burke DR, et al. Removal of retained common bile duct stones with angiographic occlusion balloons. *AJR* 1986;**146:**383-385.
8. Cope C. Endoscopic replacement of drain catheters. *AJR* 1981;**137:**626-627.
9. Shorvon PJ, Cotton PB, Mason RR, et al. Percutaneous transhepatic assistance for duodenoscopic sphincterotomy. *Gut* 1985;**26:**1373-1376.
10. Cope C. Percutaneous biliary decompression. In: Cope C, Burke DR, Meranze SG. *Atlas of Interventional Radiology*. Philadelphia: JB Lippincott, 1989:13.1-133.40.
11. Graziani L, Fabrizzi G, Manfrini E, et al. Percutaneous transhepatic ODD: Sphincter dilatation for bile duct stone removal. *AJR* 1989;**152:**73-75.
12. Saeed M. Newman GE, Dunnick NR. Use of angioplasty balloons in the percutaneous management of biliary calculi: tandem-balloon method. *AJR* 1987;**148:**745-746.
13. Mazzariello R. Review of 220 cases of residual bile tract calculi treated without reoperation: an eight-year study. *Surgery* 1973;**73:**299-306.
14. Haskin P, Teplick SK. Percutaneous management of biliary stones. *Semin Intervent Radiol* 1985;**2:**81-96.
15. Thistle JL, May GR, Bender CE, et al. Dissolution of cholesterol gallbladder stones by methyl tert-butyl ether administered by percutaneous transhepatic catheter. *N Engl J Med* 1989;**320:**633-639.
16. Jakimowicz JJ, Mak B, Carol EJ, vanBaalen JM. Post-operative choledochoscopy. *Arch Surg* 1983;**118:**810-812.
17. Picus D, Weyman PJ, Marx MV. Role of percutaneous intracorporeal electrohydraulic lithotripsy in the treatment of biliary tract calculi. *Radiology* 1989;**170:**989-993.
18. Kozarek RA, Low DE, Ball TH. Tunable dye laser lithotripsy: in vitro studies and in vivo treatment of choledocholithiasis. *Gastrointest Endosc* 1988;**34:**418-420.
19. Rawat B, Burhenne H. Biliary extracorporeal shockwave lithotripsy. *Cardiovasc Intervent Radiol* 1990;**13:**258-263.
20. Jueller PR, vanSonnenberg E, Gerrucci JT, et al. Biliary stricture dilatation: Multicenter review of clinical management in 73 patients. *Radiology* 1986;**160:**17-22.
21. Stokes KR, Clouse ME. Biliary duct stones: percutaneous transhepatic removal. *Cardiovasc Intervent Radiol* 1990;**13:**240-244.
22. Russell E, Hutson EG, Guerra JJ Jr, et al. Dilatation of biliary strictures through stomatized jejunal limb. *Acta Radiol Diagn* 1985;**26:**283-287.
23. Coons HG. Self-expanding stainless steel biliary stents.*Radiology* 1989;**170:**979-983.
24. Gandini G, Righi D, Regge D, et al. Percutaneous removal of biliary stones. *Cardiovasc Intervent Radiol* 1990;**13:**245-251.
25. Sackmann M, Delius M, Sauerbruch T, et al. Shock wave lithotripsy of gallbladder stones: the first 175 patients. *N Engl J Med* 1988;**318:**393-397.
26. Cope C, Burke DR, Meranze SG. Percutaneous extraction of gallstones in 20 patients. *Radiology* 1990;**176:**19-24.
27. Picus D, Marx MV, Hicks ME, et al. Percutaneous cholecystolithotomy: preliminary experience and technical considerations. *Radiology* 1989;**173:**487-491.

28. Kerlan RK, LaBerge JM, Ring EJ. Percutaneous cholecystolithotomy: preliminary experience. *Radiology* 1985;**157**:653-656.
29. Hwang MH, Mo LR, Chan LR, et al. Percutaneous transhepatic cholecystic ultrasonic lithotripsy. *Gastrointest Endosc* 1987;**33**:301-302.
30. Kellett MJ, Russell RCG, Wickham JEA. Percutaneous cholecystolithotomy. *Endoscopy* 1989;**21**:365-366.
31. Wenk H, Thomas ST, Schmeller N, et al. Percutaneous transhepatic cholecystolithotripsy. *Endoscopy* 1989;**21**:221-222.
32. Hruby W, Stackl W, Urban M, et al. Percutaneous endoscopic cholecysto-lithotripsy. *Radiology* 1989;**173**:477-479.
33. Bogan ML, Hawes RH, Kopecky KK, Goulet RJ. Percutaneous cholecystolithotomy with endoscopic lithotripsy by using a pulsed-dye laser: preliminary experience. *AJR* 1990;**155**:781-784.
34. Akiyama H, Ozazaki T, Takashima I, Satoh S, et al. Percutaneous treatments for biliary diseases. *Radiology* 1990;**176**:25-30.
35. Norrby S, Schoneback J. Long-term results with cholecystolithotomy. *Acta Chir Scand* 1970;**136**:711-713.
36. Miller FJ, Rose SC. Intervention for gallbladder disease. *Cardiovasc Intervent Radiol* 1990;**13**:264-271.

Diagnosis of pancreatic tumours with ultrasound, computed tomography and endoscopic retrograde cholangiopancreatography

A.L. Baert and H. Rigauts
Department of Radiology, University Hospitals K.U. Leuven, Belgium

Tumours of the Exocrine Pancreas

Epithelial tumours of the exocrine pancreas originate in the ductal cells (95%), in the acinar cells (1.5%) or are of uncertain histogenesis. Non-epithelial tumours of the pancreas are extremely rare [1].

Ductal Adenocarcinoma

Ducal adenocarcinoma represents more than 90% of all pancreatic tumours. The majority of ductal adenocarcinomas (60-70%) are located in the head of the pancreas. Their diameter is usually about 2.5-3.5 cm at the time of operation and they produce early clinical symptoms because of their proximity to the common bile duct. Tumours of the body and tail of the pancreas measure between 5 and 7 cm at the time of diagnosis and produce clinical symptoms at a more advanced stage.

Ductal adenocarcinoma frequently extends through the thin fascial layer covering the organ and quickly infiltrates the peripancreatic loose fibrous and lipomatous tissue following the course of the perineural sheaths as well as lymphatic and venous pathways. Perineural propagation explains why pain is the most frequent clinical symptom of tumours located in the body and tail.

The prognosis for ductal adenocarcinoma of the pancreas is very poor, especially for tumours of the body and tail. Complete surgical resection is the only durative procedure. Although some authors have reported survival rates of 30% for tumours not exceeding 2 cm in diameter, most results of surgery, regardless of the type of resection employed, indicate a 5-year survival of only 5% [2,3].

One could therefore raise the question of whether we should make an effort to attain correct diagnosis and staging of these tumours. Here we consider two groups of patients where pancreatic imaging is frequently performed:

(1) Patients with a pancreatic tumour. These patients will greatly benefit in terms of comfort and cost with non-invasive imaging methods, allowing rapid diagnosis in most cases. Moreover, it is important to avoid unnecessary attempts at curative resection in patients whose tumours can be proven to be unresectable by radiological staging methods.

(2) Patients who present clinical symptoms suggesting the possibility of a pancreatic tumour but who eventually will be proven not to present with tumours will also benefit. Indeed, noninvasive imaging methods allow accurate demonstration that the pancreas is normal or will reveal another disease or a cause of the symptoms. Thus explorative laparotomy can now be avoided totally.

Diagnosis

Radiological examination of pancreatic ductal adenocarcinoma will reveal focal parenchymal changes induced by the tumour and the effects, secondary to the space-occupying lesion, on the calibre of the pancreatic and/or the bile ducts. Segmental or global changes in volume of the organ are more rate [4].

Ultrasonography

Optimal visualization of the pancreas by ultrasonography - even after applying the special manoeuvres for eliminating overlying bowel gas such as scanning in the erect position or stomach distension - is not always possible. While the head and proximal portion of the body may be well visualized in 85-90% of patients, the remainder of the body as well as the tail of the pancreas may be delineated only in 60-70% [5].

Ductal adenocarcinoma will show on ultrasonography (Fig. 1) mainly as a hypoechoic mass, relative to the normal pancreatic parenchyma. In patients with lipomatous infiltration, the tumour mass will even appear more hypoechoic relative to the hyperechoic fatty infiltrated pancreas. Anechoic areas due to intratumoural necrosis are rarely seen and suggest the possibility of pancreatitis associated with a cystic tumour of the pancreas, or of a rare pancreatic neoplasm.

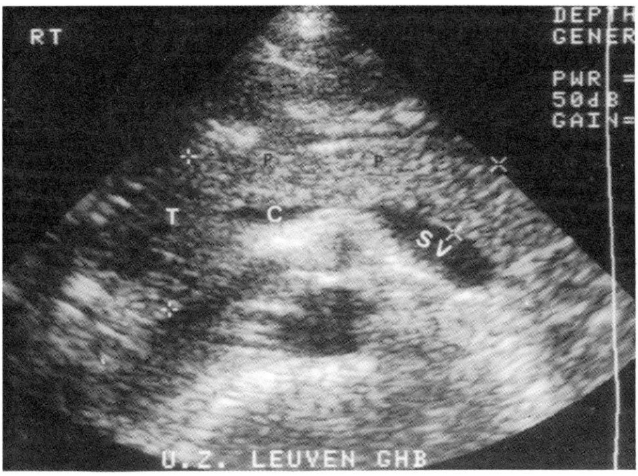

Figure 1. *ADENOCARCINOMA IN THE HEAD OF THE PANCREAS. US IN THE TRANSVERSE PLANE. The hyperreflective area represents lipomatous pancreas (P). The hyporeflective area represents tumour (T) in the head of the pancreas. SV=splenic vein. C=confluence of spleen and superior mesenteric vein.*

Abnormal dilatation of the pancreatic duct is present when the inner diameter of the duct measure more than 2.5 mm in the head and more than 1 mm in the tail, but may be due to chronic pancreatitis as well as to tumour. However, as a tumour causes dilatation by obstruction of the duct, the dilatation in this instance tends to be more uniform and to have parallel walls.

Abnormal dilatation of the bile ducts is very common in carcinoma of the pancreatic head [6]. An internal diameter of more than 7 mm in the common bile duct or the common hepatic duct is considered to be abnormal. The right hepatic duct proximal to the common hepatic duct can frequently be seen by ultrasonography and should not measure more than 2-3 mm in internal diameter. Abrupt termination of a dilatated common bile duct at the level of the upper margin of the head, or within the head itself, is highly suggestive of tumour. Scanning along the longitudinal plane of the dilatated common bile duct will frequently allow identification of the exact site and cause of the obstruction [7]. If ultrasonography fails to identify a mass at the site of the obstruction, this suggests a primary tumour originating in the bile duct or the ampullary region rather than a pancreatic origin. Dilated intrahepatic bile ducts are typically identified as double channels representing dilated branch ducts adjacent to portal vein segments.

When the common bile duct becomes strongly dilated it may follow a more transverse course and thereby assume a tortuous shape.

The sensitivity of ultrasonography for diagnosis of pancreatic ductal adenocarcinoma is 80% [8,9]. The accuracy of the method, however, may be as high as 94% [10,11].

Computed Tomography

Technique

The pancreas should be scanned at contiguous levels using a slice thickness of 8-10 mm starting at level L2-L3 and proceedings cephalad to include the liver. Scan times should preferably be 2 seconds or less.

Oral administration of diluted iodinated or barium sulphate contrast media is considered to be most helpful in delineating the duodenum and the small bowel. Scanning is performed in the supine position but the right lateral decubitus position may occasionally be helpful for better filling of the duodenal loop. Antiperistaltic drugs will help to eliminate streak artefacts and to obtain a better dilatation of the duodenum but are less frequently used with the faster scanners that are now available. Air or water can also be used to fill the stomach and the duodenum. Both have the advantage of eliminating beam hardening artefacts. In addition, they will, if combined with an antiperistaltic drug, better distend the stomach and thus displace the jejunal loops so that the pancreatic tail becomes better visualized. Stomach distension will also slightly displace the pancreatic tail caudally so that it follows a more horizontal course which accords better with the transversal plane of CT. A fat density oral contrast regimen has also been advocated. Enhancement by i.v. iodinated contrast media greatly increases the diagnostic information obtained from CT study of pancreatic tumours [12,13]. A total of 70-120 ml of a 70% (350 mgI/ml) solution is injected at a rate of 4-5 ml/sec through an 18G or 20G needle placed preferentially within an antecubital vein. Automatic power injection is now used more and more frequently than normal injection. Complications related to its use such as paravasal injection or extravasation may occur in 0.1% of patients. These may be avoided by careful monitoring of the injection site in order to stop the process immediately at any sign of inappropriate injection. Power injection results in a more reliable high iodine concentration in the blood vessels and thus in a better contrast enhancement of normal and abnormal visceral structures as well as of the blood vessels.

The i.v. contrast medium injection can be given immediately in combination with the oral contrast material or can be performed during a second series of scans. The advantages of performing a pre-i.v. contrast series are, first, a better identification of pancreatic calcifications and, second, a better selection of the level(s) where post-contrast scans should be performed in order to obtain an optimal depiction of the suspect area.

Indeed, marked enhancement of the pancreatic parenchyma occurs during the capillary phase at about 20 seconds following the start of the i.v. bolus injection but will persist only for 60-120 seconds. Not only short scanning times (less than 5 seconds), and rapid sequential scanning with table incrementation, but also careful selection of the area of maximal diagnostic interest are necessary in order to obtain all the benefits of i.v. contrast administration. Non-ionic iodinated contrast media will not result in an improved pancreatic contrast enhancement but because of their lower osmolarity will provoke less pain in case of extravasation and will also produce less heat sensation during the rapid injection.

Findings

Direct signs. Most ductal adenocarcinomas are visible on CT as focal and abrupt changes of the size or the contour of the organ. Segmental or diffuse enlargement is uncommon. A mass arising in the centre of the gland must measure at least 2.5 cm in diameter in order to produce a change in contour or be visible on CT. A tumour arising on the periphery of the pancreas may already be visible at a smaller size because of the disruption of the normal lobular outer contour of the pancreas - readily visible in some individuals.

The attenuation value of most ductal adenocarcinomas of the pancreas is quite similar to that of the normal parenchyma. If they do not provoke contour deformation they will not be visible on the pre-i.v. contrast scan. A slight decrease in density may be occasionally seen which may be due to associated focal pancreatitis or secondary desmoplastic peritumoural changes.

In fatty-infiltrated pancreas, the attenuation value of a ductal adenocarcinoma will evidently be more elevated than the surrounding parenchyma, rendering it easily visible on the pre-v.i. contrast images. These focal changes in the lipomatous pancreatic texture ('marbling') allow the detection of small intrapancreatic tumours (Fig. 2a).

In some patients with lipomatous pancreas, a 'skip' area of normal pancreatic tissue may be preserved in the region of the uncinate process. The transition line between normal and lipomatous pancreas is situated at the level of the fusion line between the ventral and dorsal embryonal portion of the organ. This normal area of tissue can be easily differentiated from a small tumour because of the preserved triangular shape of the uncinate process (Figs. 3 and 4) [15].

It is difficult to define the normal size of the pancreas in view of the very important individual variations and the atrophy related to age.

The tissue of ductal adenocarcinoma is hypovascular when compared to the normal (non-lipomatous) pancreatic tissue. After i.v.-contrast enhancement the tumour will not enhance to the same degree as the normal adjacent parenchyma, resulting in a more evident delineation of the focal mass (Fig. 5). However, this feature will only be adequately visualized if a sufficiently high degree of intravascular iodine concentration has been reached and will persist only during the short capillary phase following i.v. bolus injection (60-120 seconds). Careful analysis of the pre-i.v. contrast images will allow to concentrate the early post-i.v. contrast slices to the suspected area of the organ indicated by contour deformity.

If no contour deformity is visible on the pre-i.v. contrast images the scanning will be performed on a level immediately caudal to the inferior end of the dilated biliary and/or pancreatic duct.

If no dilatation is present the choice of the level as well as the direction in which the scanning will be performed will be based on

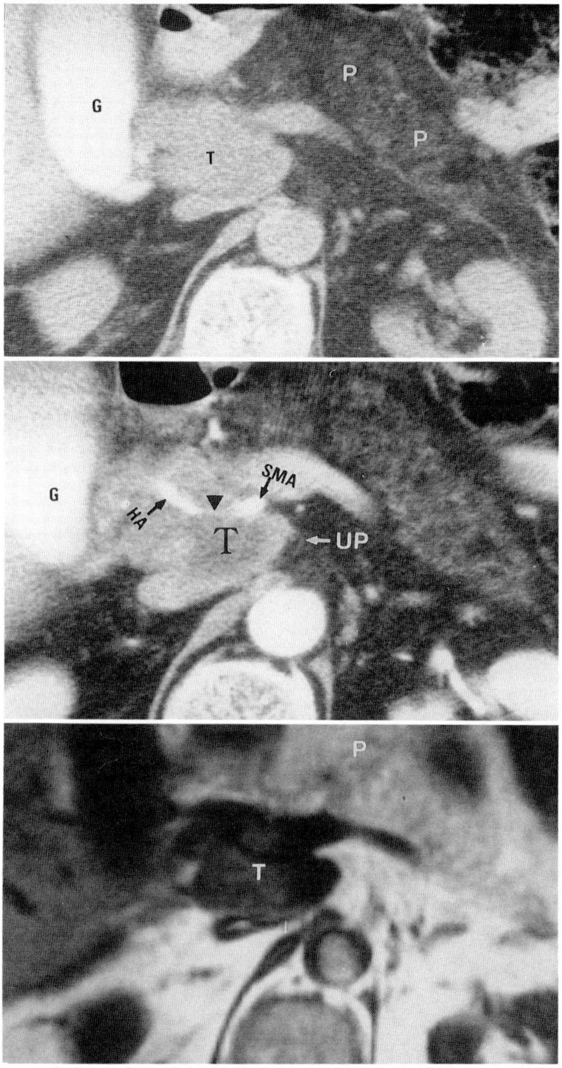

(a)
(b)
(c)

Figure 2. *ADENOCARCINOMA OF THE HEAD OF A LIPOMATOUS PANCREAS. (a) Precontrast CT. The tumour (T) is evident as a 'hyper-dense' mass relative to the lipomatous body and tail of the pancreas (P). The gall-bladder (G) is opacified due to preceeding ERCP. (b) Post-contrast CT. The tumour (T) is less enhancing than the small remaining portion of normal pancreatic parenchyma in the uncinate process (UP). The replaced hepatic artery (HA) originating from the superior mesenteric artery (SMA) is narrowed (▲) by the tumour. (c) MRI T_1-weighted sequence. The tumour (T) has a lower signal intensity than the lipomatous body and tail of the pancreas (P).*

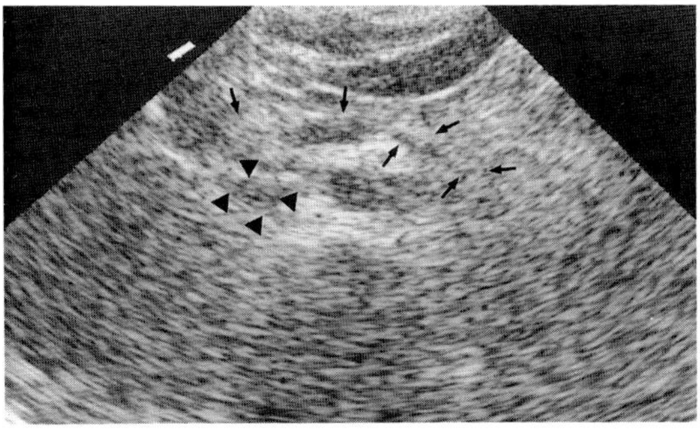

Figure 3. *INCOMPLETE LIPOMATOSIS OF THE PANCREAS. SKIP AREA IN THE PANCREATIC HEAD. US of the pancreas in the transverse plane showing hypoechoic aspect of the pancreatic body and tail (↑) and normal reflectivity of the pancreatic head: skip area (▴).*

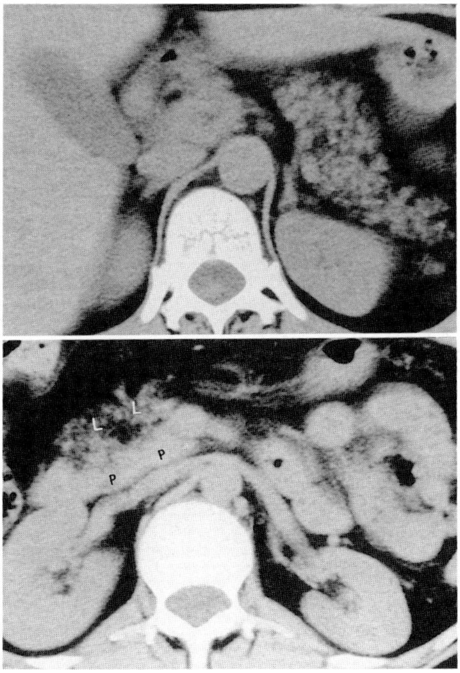

Figure 4. *INCOMPLETE LIPOMATOSIS OF THE PANCREAS. CT slices through tail (a) and head (b) of pancreas. (a) Moderate degree of lipomatous involvement of pancreatic tail. (b) Lipomatous involvement is limited to the ventral portion of the uncinate process (L) while normally enhancing homogeneous pancreatic parenchyma (P) is visible in the dorsal portion.*

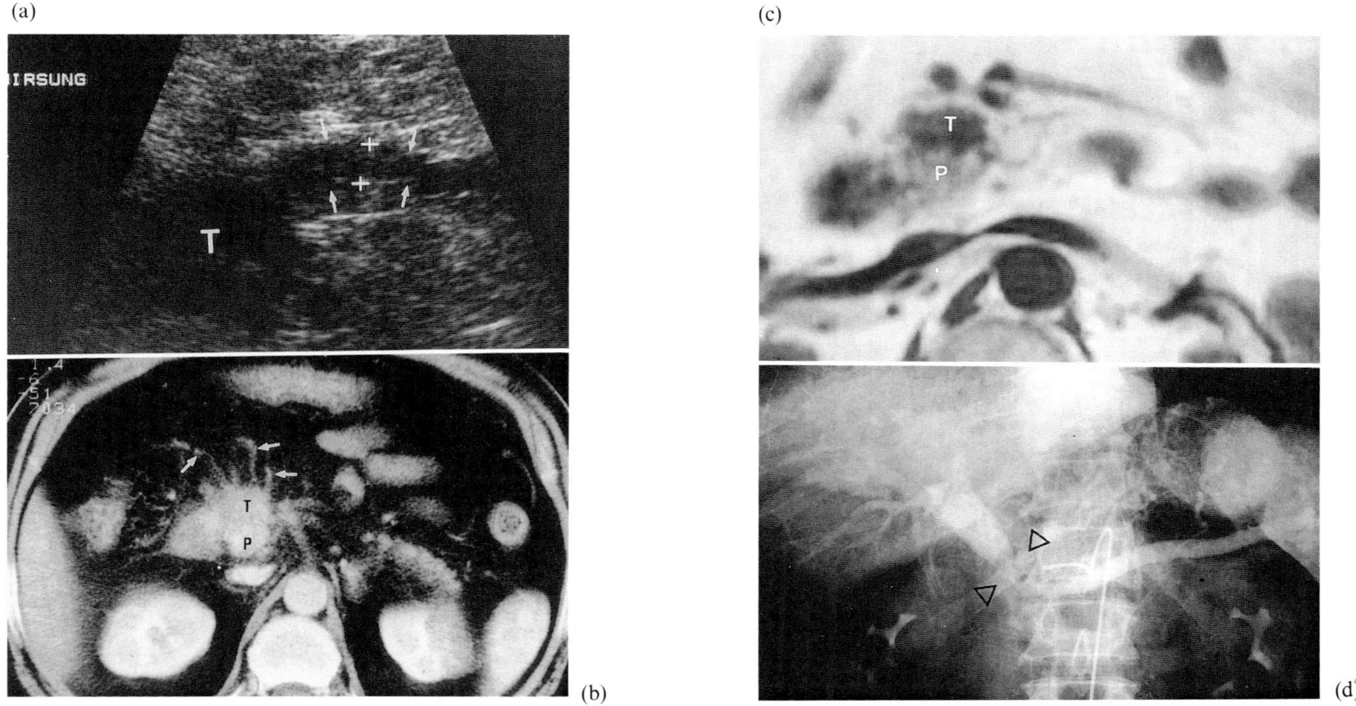

Figure 5. *ADENOCARCINOMA HEAD OF THE PANCREAS. (a) Ultrasound. The hyporeflective area represents tumour (T) and dilatation of the pancreatic duct(→←) is seen. (b) Post-contrast CT. The tumorous ventral portion (T) of the pancreatic head is less enhancing than the dorsally situated normal parenchyma (P). Linear strands represent peripancreatic tumour extension. (c) MRI. MRI T_1-weighted sequences. The tumour (T) has a lower signal intensity than the normal parenchyma (P). (d) Angiography venous phase. Narrowing (▵) of the splenomesenteric confluence indicates vascular invasion by tumour.*

the clinical situation: if jaundice is present the post-contrast slices should be centred on the inferior portion of the head of the pancreas and proceed in a cephalad direction.

Indirect signs. Indirect CT signs are secondary to the ductal obstruction. *Pancreatic duct dilatation* is considered to be present if the diameter exceeds 3 mm in the head and 2 mm in the body and tail of the pancreas. It is present in approximately 50% of patients if 8 or 10 mm collimation is used. By applying 5 mm collimation, a higher frequence of pancreatic dilatation may be seen. It is more frequently seen in the head than in the body and tail of the pancreas. The dilated duct will not always lie centrally. Eccentric localization can be explained by the orientation of the transversal plane relative to the pancreas. The duct may dilate to a large calibre with smooth parallel walls. Chronic obstruction of the pancreatic duct leads to *atrophy of the parenchyma* distal to the obstruction which may be more or less pronounced according to the duration of the obstruction. Sometimes only a small rim of pancreatic parenchyma remains, surrounding the dilated pancreatic duct. Although not specific, the combined CT findings of a focal mass, pancreatic duct dilatation and parenchymal atrophy are highly suggestive of ductal adenocarcinoma. They may, however, occasionally be seen in chronic pancreatitis (see differential diagnosis). Chronic ductal obstruction by ductal adenocarcinoma can also lead to small intrapancreatic *pseudocyst* formation distal to the tumour site. These post-obstructive pseudocysts will be seen in about 10% of patients.

Biliary duct dilatation. Biliary dilatation is frequently present in ductal carcinoma of the pancreatic head due to direct involvement of the intrapancreatic portion of the common bile duct. A diameter of more than 8 mm is considered to be abnormal, although diameters up to 10 mm are occasionally seen in older patients without underlying tumour or in patients with prior cholecystectomy.

Common bile duct dilatation is both more frequent and more pronounced than intrahepatic duct dilatation [16]. This may be due to physical reasons (LaPlace's law stating that the force required to dilate a closed elastic cylinder is inversely proportional to its diameter) or may be related to some degree of hepatic fibrosis or to the duration of the obstruction. In the case of minimal dilatation, the main bile duct will be seen on CT as a small round radiolucency in the liver hilus situated in front of the portal vein and medial to the proper hepatic artery. It can then be traced caudally on successive slices down to the level of obstruction. In the case of advanced dilatation, the suprapancreatic portion of the common bile duct can assume a tortuous and transverse course and will be visible on CT not as circular but as a band-like longitudinal structure. If a ductal adenocarcinoma of the head of the pancreas causes contiguous involvement of both the common bile duct and the pancreatic duct, two adjacent round dilated structures known as the 'double duct' sign are visible on the pancreatic head.

Isolated dilatation of the biliary and/or pancreatic duct without mass lesion is present in a small minority of patients with ductal adenocarcinoma of the pancreas. Adjunctive procedures such as ERCP are indicated here.

Intrahepatic duct dilatation is considered to be present when the intrahepatic ducts are visible in the peripheral portion of the liver or if the diameter exceeds 4 mm in the region of the liver hilus. Distinction between intrahepatic bile ducts and branches of the portal vein can easily be made after i.v. contrast enhancement.

Intrahepatic biliary dilatation in ductal adenocarcinoma originating either in the head or the body of the pancreas may also be due to enlarged metastatic lymph nodes in the liver hilus.

Dilatation of the gall-bladder is most often associated with bile duct dilatation if the level of the biliary obstruction is distal to the cystic duct but may be absent in case of chronic inflammation and fibrosis.

Value

CT is considered to be the most sensitive non-invasive diagnostic method for the diagnosis of ductal adenocarcinoma of the pancreas with a sensitivity reaching 90-99% depending on whether only direct CT signs or both direct and indirect signs are taken into account [4].

False negative findings are mainly due to faulty dynamic contrast studies, small tumour size or, in rare instances, to the 'isovascularity' of the tumour relative to normal pancreatic parenchyma (Fig. 6).

False positive findings are explained by focal masses due to chronic pancreatitis [17], atypical pseudocysts, peripancreatic adenopathies (due to lymphoma or metastasis) [18,19], intrapancreatic lymphoma localization [20,21] or metastasis to the pancreas [22,23] or pancreatic sarcoidosis [24].

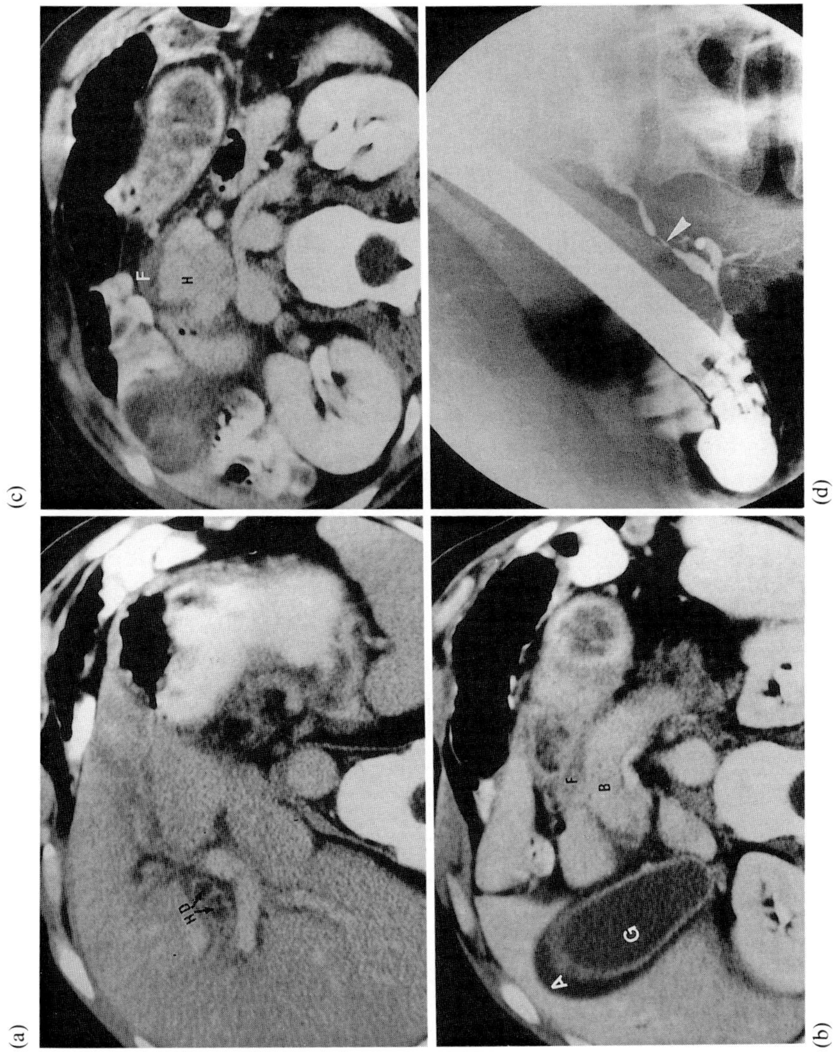

Figure 6. *ADENOCARCINOMA OF THE PANCREATIC HEAD. FALSE NEGATIVE CT. (a), (b) and (c): CT slices from cranial (a) to caudal (c) aspect. (a) Dilatation of the left and right hepatic ducts (HD). (b) and (c) Normal and homogeneous enhancement of pancreatic body (B) and head (H) of pancreas. No tumour visualized. Limited fluid collection (F) ventral to the pancreas. Distend gallbladder (G) surrounded by ascites (A). (d) ERCP. Severe stenosis of the pancreatic duct* (▲) *by tumour.*

Differential Diagnosis

Acute or chronic pancreatitis with focal mass and ampullary carcinoma are the main pathological conditions to be considered in the differential diagnosis of ductal adenocarcinoma of the pancreas by CT. The following CT findings are in favour of pancreatitis:

- Irregular and less pronounced dilatation of the pancreatic duct with a non-parallel and beaded aspect of the walls.
- Presence of dilated duct(s) or small pseudocysts within the mass.
- Intraductal or parenchymal calcifications.
- Less pronounced degree of atrophy of the pancreatic parenchyma surrounding the dilated pancreatic duct.
- Gradual, not abrupt, obstruction of the dilated pancreatic and/or bile duct. Rather than the sudden transition from a dilated duct to the absence of duct as seen in abrupt obstructive tumour caused by a gradual obstruction, CT will show a series of progressively smaller, circular areas of low attenuation.

Ampullary carcinoma is an irregular polypoid intraluminal mass obstructing the distal common bile duct. CT will often show abrupt obstruction of the common bile duct and the pancreatic duct without associated mass lesion. Opacification of the duodenal loop with positive contrast medium will show a small defect within the duodenal lumen. If air or water is used, the protruding mass lesion itself may be visible (Fig. 7). However, the smooth bulge into the duodenal lumen seen in such cases can be in part due to the distal portion of the dilatated common bile duct protruding within the duodenum.

MRI

This is presently of limited value in the diagnosis of ductal adenocarcinoma because of its low spatial resolution due to its low matrix size and respiratory movement (Fig. 8) [25,26].

In fatty infiltration of the pancreas, the tumour may be quite well visualized on T_1-weighted images as an area of lower signal intensity compared with higher signal intensity of the fatty tissue.

In the future, shorter scanning times as well as the use of i.v. contrast agents may improve the results of MRI and lead to an adjunctive role for this modality, for instance for patients with doubtful findings on US and CT.

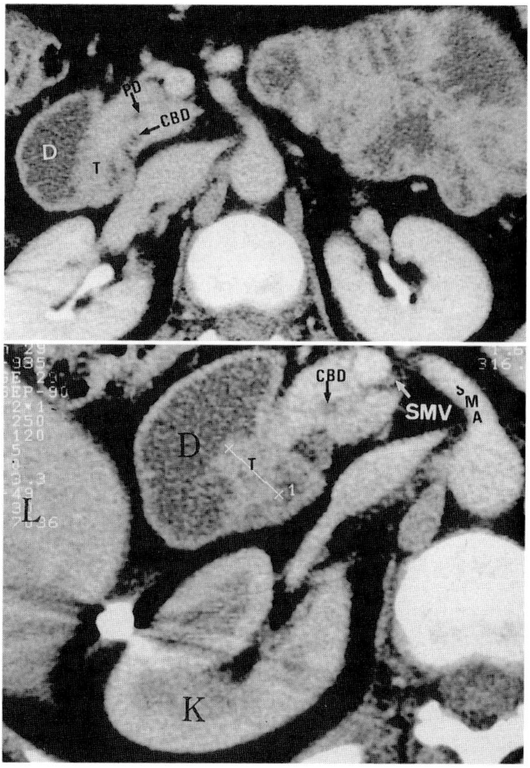

Figure 7. *AMPULLARY CARCINOMA. (a) CT slice at the level of papil of Vater. (b) Detail from (a). Small (diameter 1 cm) intraluminal tumour (T) protruding into the duodenal lumen (D) and causing obstruction of the pancreatic duct (PD) and common bile duct (CBD). L=caudal portion right liver lobe, K=right kidney.*

Endoscopic Retrograde Cholangiopancreatography (ERCP)

ERCP findings in ductal adenocarcinoma include: complete obstruction or narrowing of the pancreatic duct due to tumour encasement, and duct erosion by tumours with extraductal contrast accumulation.

Although highly sensitive for the diagnosis of ductal adenocarcinoma which causes early changes in the ductal anatomy, ERCP is used less frequently because of its invasive nature and the risk of complications. It is now used mainly as an adjunctive method when US and CT findings are equivocal, for instance when ductal dilatation is present without evidence of mass lesion.

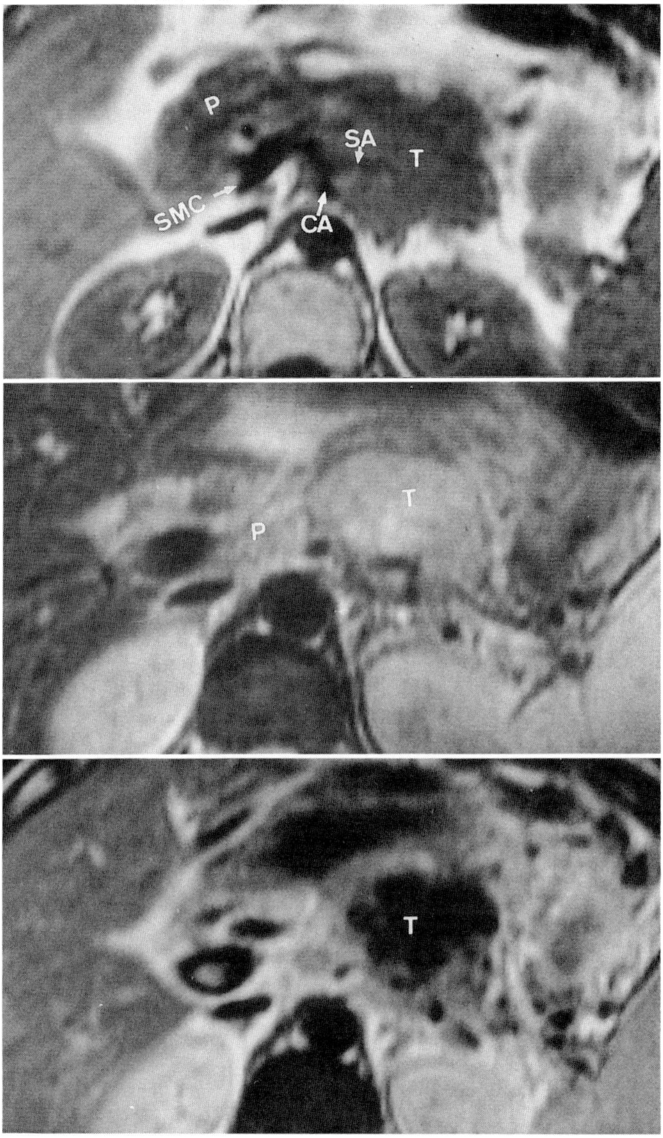

(a)

(b)

(c)

Figure 8. *ADENOCARCINOMA OF THE TAIL OF THE PANCREAS. MRI. (a) T_1-weighted sequence. Large tumour (T) slightly hypo-intense relative to normal pancreatic parenchyma (P). The tumour surrounds the splenic artery (SA). CA=coeliac artery. SMC=confluence of splenic and mesenteric vein. (b) T_2-weighted sequence. The tumour (T) is isointense compared to the normal pancreatic parenchyma (P). (c) T_1-weighted sequence after i.v. gadolinium DTPA. The tumour (T) is visible as an area of low intensity.*

Radiologically Guided Fine Needle Aspiration Biopsy

Patients with focal masses where surgery is not performed but another treatment, for instance chemotherapy, is planned, should be evaluated with this method. Indeed, false positive CT findings due to chronic pancreatitis or lymphoma may otherwise lead to an incorrect therapeutic approach (Fig. 9) [27].

Staging

It is important to determine the extent of the tumour by non-operative means in order to avoid unnecessary attempts at resection.

CT is able to provide a much wider range of diagnostic information than ultrasonography and is therefore the method of choice for radiological staging of ductal adenocarcinoma. Indeed, CT is the single best modality in evaluating extrapancreatic tumour extension (invasion of retroperitoneal space, mesentery, vascular encasement or occlusion), contiguous organ invasion (stomach-duodenum, colon, spleen), regional lymph node involvement or distant metastasis (peritoneal space-liver).

Invasion of the retropancreatic space is indicated by loss of the normal posterior fat planes. Soft density streaks and strands in the retroperitoneal fat or thickening of the perirenal fascia may also be seen. These signs are more difficult to evaluate in thin or cachectic patients. Moreover, they are aspecific and can also occur in pancreatitis.

Perivascular extension is indicated by thickening due to a soft tissue sheath surrounding, the proximal portion of the coeliac artery or superior mesenteric artery [28,29]. Encasement of these arteries as well as of the splenic artery, will be readily visible on the bolus enhanced images (Fig. 10). Superior mesenteric vein invasion can also be well demonstrated (Fig. 11).

Splenic vein narrowing and complete occlusion with associated splenomegaly and collateral venous circulation are also easily demonstrated after i.v. contrast enhancement.

CT signs of mesenteric extension are abnormal streaky soft tissue densities extending from the tumour into the small bowel mesentery in a radial fashion.

Enlarged lymph nodes due to metastatic involvement will be seen on CT as abnormal nodular structures of more than 1 cm diameter, in

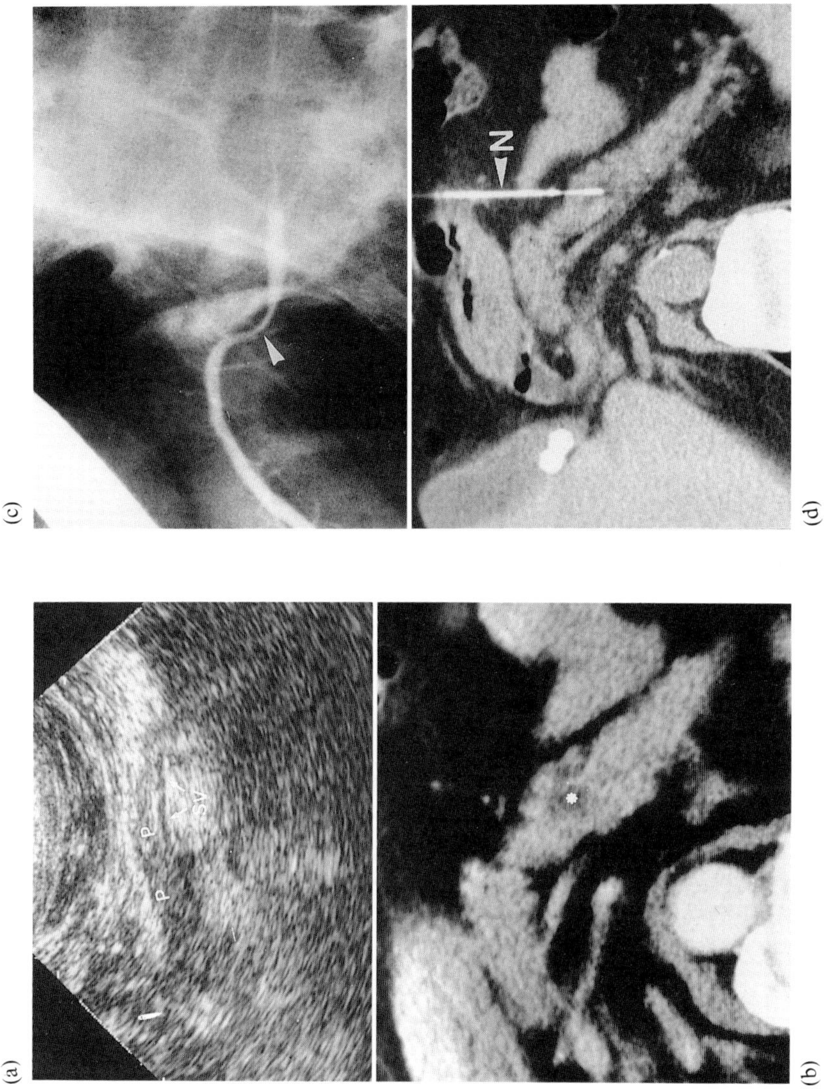

Figure 9. *SMALL ADENOCARCINOMA OF THE BODY OF THE PANCREAS. False negative US. (a) Ultrasonography: normal pattern of reflectivity of the pancreas. (P). SV=splenic vein. (b) Post-contrast CT. Small (diameter 10 mm) non-enhancing area (*) in body of the pancreas. No associated contour deformity. (c) ERCP. Segmental narrowing of pancreatic duct (▲) in body of the pancreas. (d) CT guided fine needle puncture. The needle (N) is seen entering the lesion.*

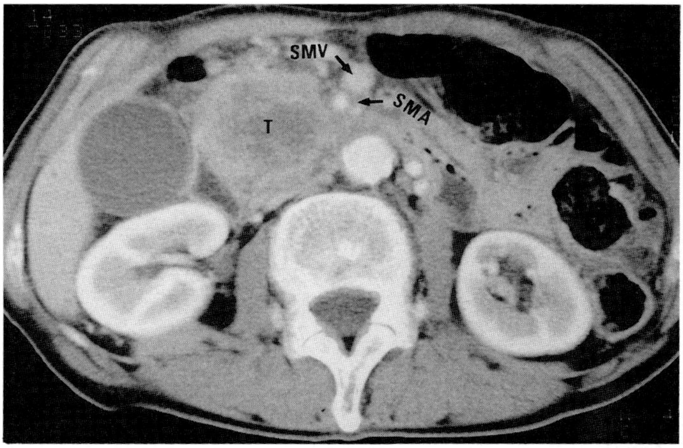

Figure 10. *ADENOCARCINOMA OF THE HEAD OF THE PANCREAS. MESENTERIC ARTERY INVASION. Large tumour (T) invading the perivascular lipomatous tissue surrounding the superior mesenteric artery (SMA). The superior mesenteric vein (SMV) is displaced to the left.*

the periaortic and pericaval area as well as in the suprapancreatic region (Fig. 12).

The contiguous organs most frequently invaded by ductal adenocarcinoma of the pancreas are the stomach, duodenum and colon. Although barium studies may also demonstrate invasion, direct visualization of the tumoral extension is often striking on CT (Figs. 13 and 14).

Distant metastasis occurs early and very frequently to the liver. They are hypovascular and visible as areas of lower attenuation relative to the liver parenchyma after i.v. contrast enhancement.

Peritoneal metastatic spread is less frequent. CT will depict even small amounts of ascites while the peritoneal metastatic implants are only rarely visualized. Ascites may also be due to tumoural vein invasion.

CT criteria for non-resectability of ductal adenocarcinoma of the pancreas are: a diameter of 3 cm or more of the tumour which is contiguous with the surface of the gland or with adjacent structures, signs of extrapancreatic extension or contiguous organ invasion. Vascular involvement is the most common sign of non-resectability.

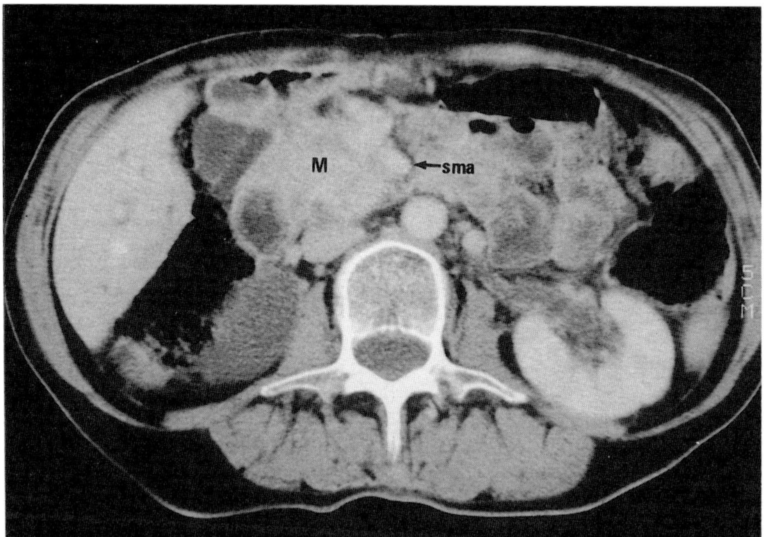

(a)

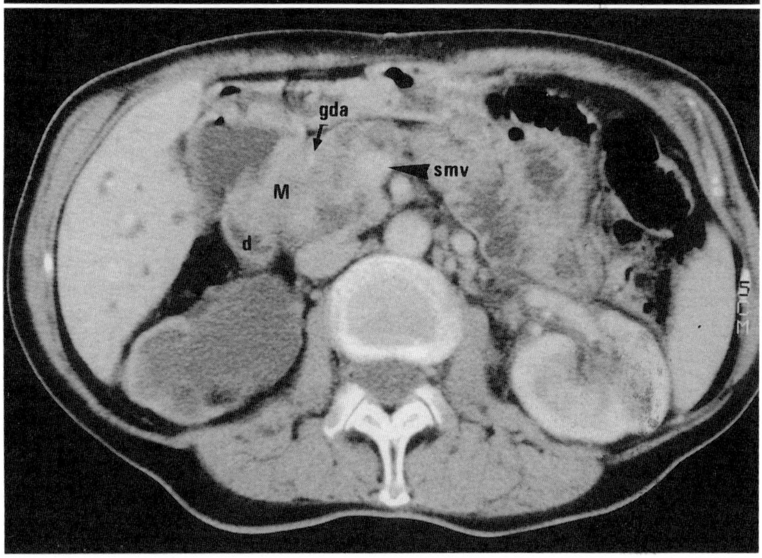

(b)

Figure 11. *ADENOCARCINOMA OF THE HEAD OF THE PANCREAS. MESENTERIC VEIN INVASION. (a) Tumoural mass (M) extends into the fatty tissue surrounding the superior mesenteric artery (SMA). (b) Slice 2 cm more cranially. The water-filled second part of duodenum (d) is compressed by tumour mass (M) Tumour completely surrounds the gastro-duodenal artery (GDA) and partially surrounds the superior mesenteric vein (SMV).*

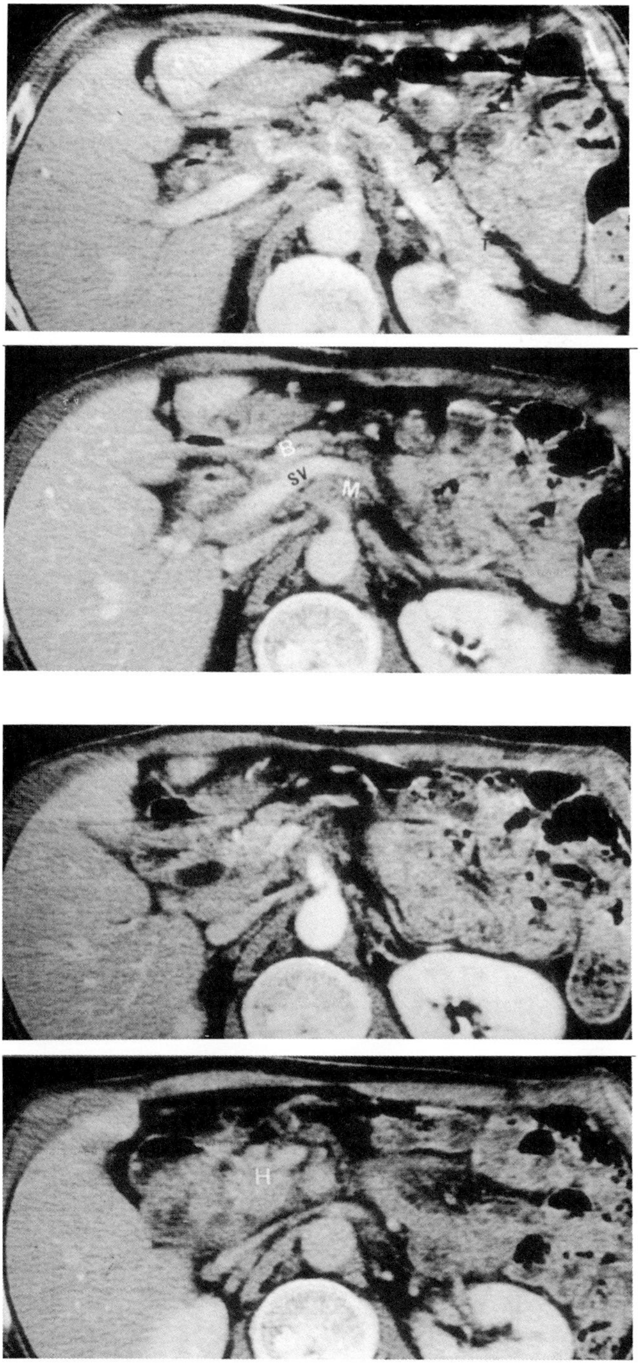

(a)

(b)

(c)

(d)

(e)

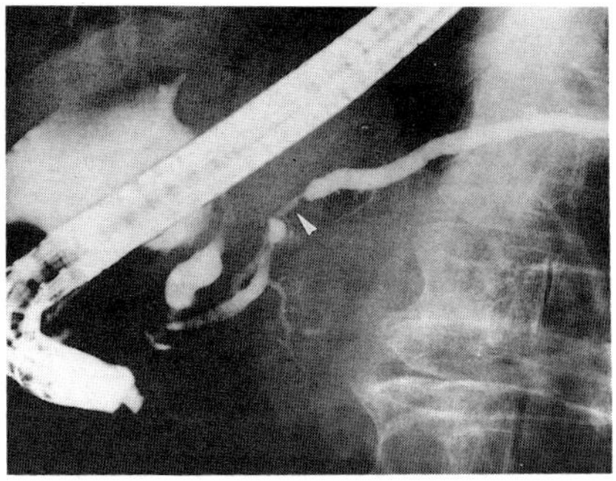

(f)

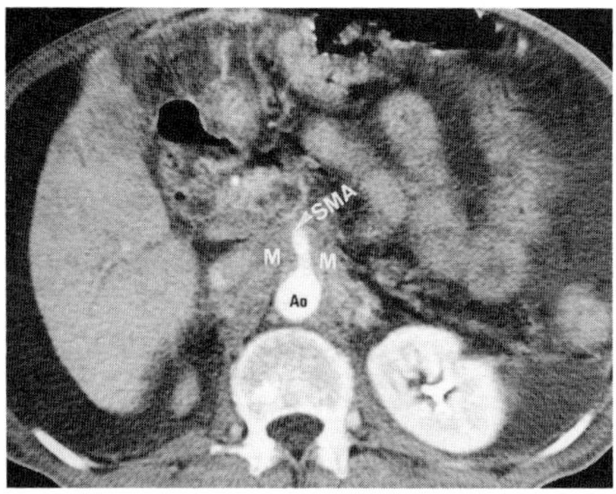

Figure 12. *ADENOCARCINOMA OF THE PANCREAS. FALSE NEGATIVE CT. (a) Four adjacent dynamic bolus incremental scans extending from pancreatic head (H) to pancreatic body (B) and tail (T): no tumour lesion is visualized although metastasis (M) is seen dorsal to the splenic vein (SV). Minimal dilatation of pancreatic duct. (b) ERCP. Severe stenosis of the junction of the pancreatic head and body. (c) CT performed 8 months later. Massive ascites is now present. Metastatic (M) tumour extension surrounds the superior mesenteric artery (SMA) and abdominal aorta (AO).*

Other Epithelial Tumours of Ductal Origin

Colloid Carcinoma (mucinous adenocarcinoma)

The clinical symptoms as well as the prognosis of this tumour are identical to ductal adenocarcinoma. These tumours are characterized by the presence of cystic intratumoural spaces which can well be visualized by US and CT.

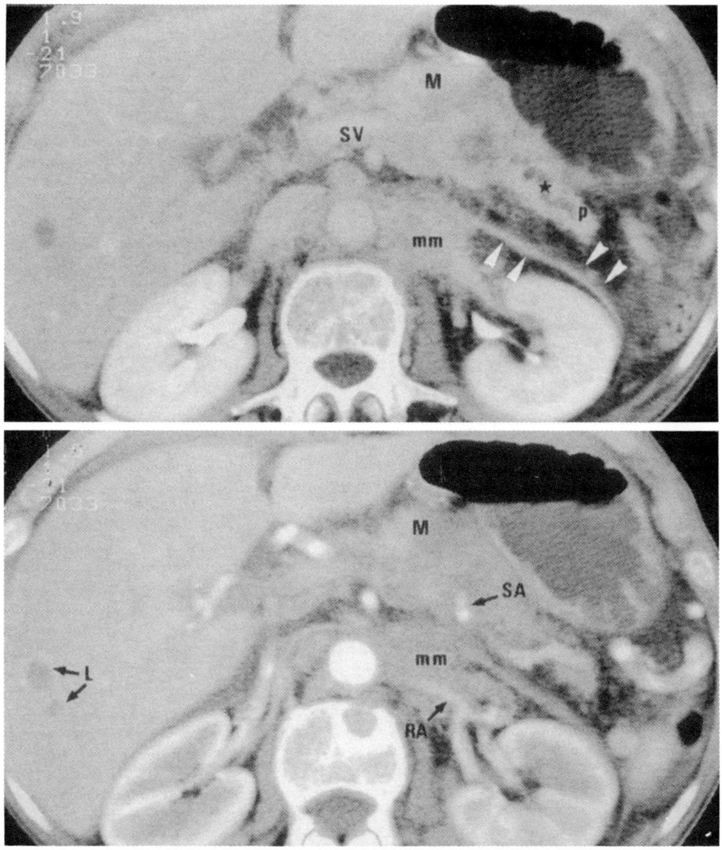

Figure 13. *UNRESECTABLE ADENOCARCINOMA OF THE BODY OF THE PANCREAS. (a) Tumoural mass (M) surrounding the splenic vein (SV). Retro-obstructive dilatation of Wirsungian duct (*) and atrophy of the pancreatic parenchyma (p). Metastatic mass (mm) in left para-aortic area. Thickening of Gerota's fascia (→). (B) Tumoural mass (M) also surrounds the splenic artery (SA). Metastatic mass (mm) surrounds the left renal artery (RA). Two small liver metastases (L).*

Colloid Carcinoma with Ductasia and Hypersecretion of Mucoid Substances

This tumour is characterized by clinical symptoms resembling acute pancreatitis and has a favourable diagnosis.

Morphologically, the tumours present either in a flat form with papillary surface or with polypoid proliferation [30].

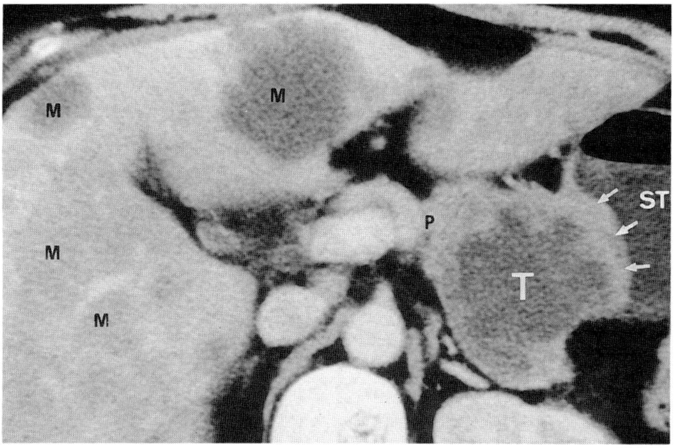

Figure 14. *UNRESECTABLE ADENOCARCINOMA OF THE TAIL OF THE PANCREAS. INVASION OF STOMACH. Large tumour (T) of pancreatic tail (P) invading the stomach (St) with multiple metastatic deposits in the liver (M).*

Both lead to an extreme degree of dilatation of the main pancreatic duct as well as of the side branches. This tumour has also been classified as a non-aggressive form of the mucinous adenocarcinoma or as a mucinous ductectatic adenocarcinoma [31-34]. Radiological diagnosis is based on the demonstration of an extremely dilated pancreatic duct with intraluminal structures and debris. US and CT can suggest the diagnosis but proof should be provided by ERCP which will better demonstrate the dilatation of the canal and the lacunar images caused by the accumulation of mucoid substance.

Muco-epidermoid Carcinoma

This rare tumour can not be differentiated from ductal adenocarcinoma by radiological methods. In some instances CT may demonstrate intratumoural areas of decreased attenuation due to necrosis of the epidermoid component of the tumour [35,36].

Anaplastic Carcinoma with Large Pleiomorphic Cells

These tumours are characterized by rapid growth, large size at the time of diagnosis and a very poor prognosis [37,38].

This diagnosis can be suggested if US or CT demonstrate the

presence of a large pancreatic tumour with multiple areas of decreased reflection or attenuation due to tissue necrosis associated with multiple enlarged abdominal adenopathies [39]. Differential diagnosis should involve pancreatic sarcoma and lymphoma.

Cystic Tumours

Cystic neoplasms of the pancreas comprise two groups: [40,41]

1. Serous cystadenoma (microcystic adenoma-cystadenoma) rich in glucogen. This tumour occurs predominantly in aged women but may also be seen in men [42].
2. Mucinous cystic neoplasms comprising the mucinous cystadenoma (macrocystic adenoma) and the mucinous cystadenocarcinoma. There is a strong predominance for females.

It is important to differentiate both entities: the cystic mucinous neoplasm has a malignant potential while the serous cystadenoma is always benign. The different macroscopic features of both groups can in some instances be visualized by radiological imaging: [43-45].

Serous Cystadenoma

This tumour consists of a solid area and very small cysts separated by thin septa which may contain calcifications. Ultrasonography may show these cysts as small anechoic structures if they reach a minimum diameter of 2-5 mm [46].

Computed tomography without i.v. contrast enhancement will mostly show a rather homogeneous mass: the cystic components being too small to be identified. A stellar central large calcification has been described but is rare. More frequently, numerous punctiform calcifications disseminated throughout the mass will be visible. The solid components of the tumour as well as the septa are moderately or strongly vascularized. After i.v. contrast administration, enhancement of the tumour becomes evident. If the cysts are sufficiently large, a 'honeycomb' aspect may therefore be seen on the contrast enhanced images. Otherwise, the tumour will show a homogeneous contrast enhanced aspect quite similar to the well vascularized large non-active endocrine tumours. If the cystic components are very large, the CT aspect may resemble very much that of mucinous cystic neoplasm. In a recent report, MRI imaging was considered equal or slightly superior to CT in the overall diagnosis of cystic neoplasms of the pancreas [47]. It was more sensitive to differences between compartments and showed the outer contour of cystic masses more clearly, especially on T_2-weighted images. Therefore, in the future, MRI may have a useful role in the differentiation of microcystic adenoma from mucinous cystic neoplasm.

Cystic Mucinous Neoplasm

The cystic mucinous neoplasm can be either uni- or multilocular. About two-thirds are located within the tail and one-third in the body of the pancreas [48]. Localization in the head is very rare. Punctiform or crescent shaped calcifications are sometimes present within the fibrous capsula. The tumour is furthermore characterized by the presence of papillary endocavitary proliferation originating in the septal wall separating the cysts. The epithelial lining of the cyst secretes mucin. Macroscopically, it is impossible to distinguish between the benign and the malignant form of cystic mucinous tumours. Ultrasonography as well as CT are able to visualize the important morphological features: peripheral calcifications, cystic cavities of relatively large size separated by septa and the endocystic proliferations. CT after i.v. contrast administration in addition demonstrates that the solid components as well as the septa are moderately enhancing (Fig. 15).

Neither ultrasonography nor CT are able to make the differential diagnosis between mucinous cystadenoma or cystadenocarcinoma [49]. If the solid component is large or if there are signs of extrapancreatic extension, a malign tumour may be suspected.

A subentity, namely mucinous ductectatic cystadenoma or cystadenocarcinoma, is characterized by dilatation of the main pancreatic duct as well as of the branches, frequently located within the uncinate process [32,31]. The dilated ducts are covered by atypical epithelial cells identical to those seen in cystadenoma and cystadenocarcinoma, secreting a mucin-like substance.

Ultrasonography and CT will demonstrate a spherical or multinodular cystic structure situated within the uncinate process. ERCP will demonstrate the communication between the cystic cavities and the pancreatic duct and thus allow a firm diagnosis.

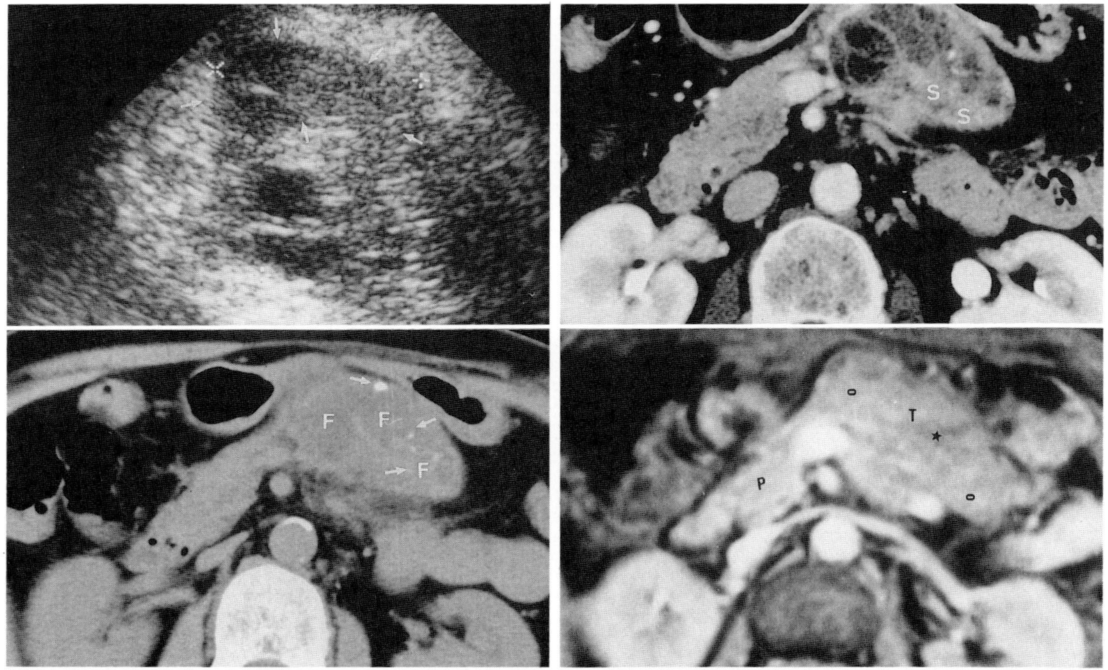

Figure 15. *MUCINOUS CYSTADENOCARCINOMA OF THE TAIL OF THE PANCREAS. (a) Ultrasonography. Hypoechoic mass (↑) involving pancreatic tail. (b) Precontrast CT. Space occupying lesion of pancreatic tail with area of fluid density (F) separated by septa containing punctate calcification (→). (c) Post-contrast CT. The solid components (S) as well as the septa are strongly enhancing. The multilocular aspect of the lesion is more visible (d) MRI. T_1-weighted spin echo sequence; after injection of Gd-DTPA. The space occupying lesion (T) is slightly hypointense relative to the cranial pancreas parenchyma (P). The lesion itself contains areas more hypointense (*) relative to the rest of the tumour (o).*

Tumours of Acinar Origin

Acinar Cell Carcinoma

This rare pancreatic carcinoma is possibly induced by external carcinogens. It is seen preferentially in elder men. The clinical features are similar to those of acute pancreatitis with metastatic foci of steatonecrosis due to the systemic release of lipase. The tumour has mostly metastasized at the time of diagnosis [50].

The radiological features of the rare published cases are non-specific: most tumours are very large with a central necrotic area.

Pancreatoblastoma

This is also a rare tumour occurring in children younger than 7 years. It can arise in the ventral pancreas and is probably caused by a disturbance in organogenesis due to a failure of communication between the duct of Santorini and the ampulla of Vater [51,52].

Ultrasonography shows a large echogenic well delineated mass with small hypoechoic areas. CT demonstrates an inhomogeneous solid tumour.

Tumours of Uncertain Origin

This category of rare pancreatic tumours includes micro-adenocarcinoma, anaplastic carcinoma and papillary and solid epithelial tumours. Radiological features have been described only for the latter [53-56].

The papillary and solid epithelial tumour is found mainly in young females with a predilection for blacks. This tumour is sometimes diagnosed incidentally on abdominal trauma or by a clinical syndrome provoked by the intravascular release of lipases. It has a low degree of malignancy and most patients are cured after tumour ablation.

Ultrasonography will demonstrate a well delineated mass with hypoechoic areas due to the presence of necrosis or haemorrhage. Hyperechoic reflection may be due to calcifications situated in the periphery of the lesion.

On CT, the attenuation value of the radiolucent areas is higher than clear fluid indicating the presence of haemorrhage or debris. The solid portions of the tumours are well vascularized and will enhance after i.v. contrast.

In case of extensive necrosis, ultrasonography and CT will both visualize a thick walled 'cystic' mass with irregular internal contour.

Tumours of Non-epithelial Origin

Mesenchymal benign and malignant tumours of the pancreas are rare and show characteristics similar to those arising in other organs. The very few case reports available in the radiological literature do not allow describe specific radiological features.

Metastasis and Lymphoma

The radiological features of pancreatic metastatic involvement are similar to ductal adenocarcinoma [22,23].

If multiple intrapancreatic lesions associated with multiple and invasive lymph node enlargement are present, lymphoma is more likely [20,21]. It may, however, be very difficult to differentiate peripancreatic lymph node involvement by lymphoma from intrapancreatic lymphoma localization [19].

Tumours of the Endocrine Pancreas

Tumours arising from the endocrine cells of the pancreas can be classified into two groups: clinically inactive and active tumours.

Clinically inactive tumours or non-functioning tumours are frequently large at the time of diagnosis and have often already metastasized to the liver [57,58].

The important CT features which allow inactive endocrine tumours to be differentiated from an adenocarcinoma are clacifications (present in 20% of the cases) [59], the large volume and the hypervascular enhancing aspect of the primary tumours as well as the liver metastasis.

Active tumours of endocrine origin or pancreatic islet tumours are classified according to the hypersecretion of the specific peptides. Most are very small - 70% of insulinomas are less than 1.5 cm in diameter and 38% of gastrinomas are less than 1 cm in diameter.

On ultrasonography, islet cell tumours of the pancreas mostly appear hypoechoic relative to the normal pancreatic parenchyma.

Success rate for the detection of insulinoma by ultrasonography varies from 25-65% [60-62], while results for gastrinoma average

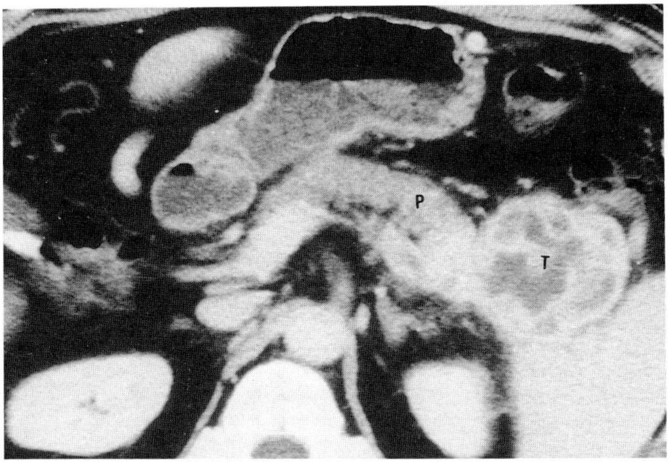

Figure 16. *GLUCAGONOMA OF THE TAIL OF THE PANCREAS. POST-CONTRAST CT. Inhomogeneously enhancing tumour (T) originating from the pancreatic tail. The solid components of the lesion are iso-enhanced relative to the normal pancreatic parenchyma (P).*

only 20%. Active islet cell tumours can be visualized on CT as small, strongly enhancing intrapancreatic nodular structures (Fig. 16). Intrahepatic metastatic deposits from malignant islet tumours are also frequently hypervascular and therefore visible as intrahepatic solitary or multiple area enhancing areas [62-65].

MRI has been reported to be able to demonstrate insulinoma as a hypointense area on T_1-weighted images and a hyperintense area on T_2-weighted images [66].

Concerning the detection of extrahepatic and hepatic gastrinomas, MRI has been reported to be as effective as abdominal US but less effective than either CT scanning or abdominal angiography [67-70].

The role of radiological imaging in active endocrine tumours of the pancreas is primarily to localism them exactly and to detect metastatic deposits.

Because of the low sensitivity of ultrasonography, radiological study should start with CT. Arteriography should be performed if CT is negative. In the future, MRI may preceed arteriography.

Intraoperative ultrasonography is now used widely in pancreatic surgery for small endocrine tumours. The sensitivity has been reported to be very high (85-100%) [71-74].

References

1. Chen J, Baithun SI. Morphologic study of 391 cases of exocrine pancreatic tumours with special reference to the classification of exocrine pancreatic carcinoma. *J Pathol* 1985;**146:**17-29.
2. Edis AJ, Kiernan PD, Taylor WF. Attempted curative resection of ductal carcinoma of the pancreas: review of Mayo Clinc experience, 1951-1975. *Mayo Clin Proc* 1981;**55:**531-536.
3. Van Heerden JA, ReMine WH, Weiland LH, et al. Total pancreatectomy for ductal adenocarcinoma of the pancreas. Mayo Clinic experience. *Am J Surg* 1981;**142:**308-311.
4. Freeny PC, Marks WM, Ryan JA, et al. Pancreatic ductal adenocarcinoma: diagnosis and staging with dynamic CT. *Radiology* 1988;**166:**125-133.
5. Op den Orth JO. Sonography of the pancreatic head aided by water and glucagon. *Radiographics* 1987;**7:**85-100.
6. Laing FC, Jeffrey RBJr, Wing VW, et al. Biliary dilatation: defining the level and cause by real-time ultrasound. *Radiology* 1986;**160:**39-42.
7. Robledo R, Prieto ML, Pérez M, Camunez F, Echenagusia A. Carcinoma of the hepaticopancreatic ampullar region: role of US. *Radiology* 1988;**166:**409-412.
8. Iish H, Yamamura H, Tatsuta M, Okuda S, Kitamura T. Value of ultrasonographic examination combined with measurement of serum tumour markers in the diagnosis of pancreatic cancer of less than 3 cm in diameter. *Cancer* 1986;**57:**1947-1951.
9. Ormson MJ, Charboneau JW, Stephens DH. (1987) Sonography in patients with a possible pancreatic mass shown on CT. *AJR* 1987;**148:**551-555.
10. Päiansalo M et al. US and CT in pancreatic malignancy. *Acta Radiol* 1988;**29:**343-344.
11. Garra BS, Shawker TH, Doppman JL, Sindelar WF. Comparison of angiography and ultrasound in the evaluation of the portal venous system in pancreatic carcinoma. *J Comput Assist Tomogr* 1988;**15:**83.
12. Marchal G, Baert A, Wilms G. Intravenous pancreatography in computed tomography. *J Comput Assist Tomogr* 1979;**3:**727-732.
13. Rossi P, Baert A, Marchal G, et al. Multiple bolus technique versus single bolus or infusion of contrast to obtain prolonged contrast enhancement of the pancreas. *Radiology* 1982;**144:**929.
14. Raptapoulos V, et al. CT of the pancreas with a fat density oral contrast regimen. *AJR* 1988;**150:**1303-1306.
15. Marchal G, Verbeken E, Van Steenbergen W, Baert A, Lauweryns J. Uneven lipomatosis: a pitfall in pancreatic sonography. *Gastrointest Radiol* 1989;**14:**233-237.
16. Gibson RN, Yeung E, Thompson JN, et al. Bile duct obstruction: radiologic evaluation of level, cause and tumour resectability. *Radiology* 1986;**160:**39-42.
17. Lin JT, et al. Pancreatic carcinoma associated with chronic calcifying pancreatitis in Taiwan: a case report and review of the literature. *Pancreas* 1988;**3:**111-114.
18. Zeman RD, Schiebler M, Clark LR, Jaffe MH, Paushter DM, Grant EG, Choyke PL. The clinical and imaging spectrum of pancreaticoduodenal lymph node enlargement. *AJR* 1985;**144:**1223-1227.
19. Costello P, Duszlank EJJr, Kane RA, et al. Peripancreatic lymph node enlargement in Hodgkin's disease, non-Hodgkin's lymphoma, and pancreatic carcinoma. *CT* 1984;**8:**1-11.
20. Sktamlu B, et al. Primary lymphoma of the head of the pancreas. *J Surg Oncol* 1988;**38:**48-51.
21. Teefey SA, Stephens DH, Sheedy PF. CT appearance of primary pancreatic lymphoma. *Gastrointest Radiol* 1986;**11:**41-43.
22. Wernecke K, Peters PE, Galanski M. Pancreatic metastases: US evaluation. *Radiology* 1986;**160:**399-402.

23. Rumancik WM, Megibow AJ, Bosniak MA, et al. Metastatic disease to the pancreas: evaluation by computed tomography. *J Comput Assist Tomogr* 1984;**8:**829-834.
24. Sagalow BR et al. Pancreatic sarcoidosis mimicking pancreatic cancer. *JCU* 1988;**16:**131-134.
25. Steiner E, et al. Imaging of pancreatic neoplasms: comparison of MR and CT. *AJR* 1989;**152:**487.
26. Tscholakoff D, Hricak H, Thoeni R, et al. MR Imaging in the diagnosis of pancreatic disease. *AJR* 1987;**148:**703.
27. Taavitsäinen M, et al. US guided fine needle aspiration biopsy in focal pancreatic lesions. *Acta Radiol* 1987;**28:**541-543.
28. Megibow AJ, Bosniak MA, Ambos MA, et al. Thickening of the celiac axis and/or superior mesenteric artery: a sign of pancreatic carcinoma on computed tomography. *Radiology* 1981;**141:**449-453.
29. Mitchell DG, et al. The superior mesenteric artery fat plane: is obliteration pathognomonic of pancreatic carcinoma? *J Comput Assist Tomogr* 1987;**11:**247-253.
30. Suyama M, Ariyama J, Shimagu S. Clinicopathology of mucin producing cancer of the pancreas. *Diagn Imaging Abdomen* 1985;**5:**289-296.
31. Agostini S, Choux A, Payan MJ, Sastre B, Sahel J, Clément JP. Mucinous pancreatic ductectasia in the body of the pancreas. *Radiology* 1989;**170:**815-816.
32. Itai Y, Ohhashi K, Nagai H, et al. 'Ductectatic' mucinous cystadenoma and cystadenocarcinoma of the pancreas. *Radiology* 1986;**161:**697-700.
33. Itai Y, Kokubo T, Atomi Y, et al. Mucin-hypersecreting carcinoma of the pancreas. *Radiology* 1987;**165:**51-55.
34. Ohhashi K, Murakami Y, Takekoshi T, Takagi K, Yanagisawa A, Katoh Y. Mucin producing pancreatic cancer. *I to cho* 1986;**21:**755-756 (Japanese: abstract in English).
35. Cihak RW, Kawashima T, Steer A. Adenoacanthoma (adenosquamous carcinoma) of the pancreas. *Cancer* 1972;**19:**1133-1140.
36. Fajardo LC, et al. CT findings in squamous cell carcinoma of the pancreas. *J Comput Assist Tomogr* 1988;**12:**138-139.
37. Guillan RA. Pleomorphic adenocarcinoma of the pancreas. An analysis of five cases. *Cancer* 1968;**21:**1072-1079.
38. Wolfman NT, Karstaedt N, Kawatomo EM. Pleomorphic carcinoma of the pancreas: Computed tomographic, sonographic and pathologic findings. *Radiology* 1985;**154:**329-332.
39. Radin DR, Collitti PM, Forrester DM, et al. Fine needle aspiration of pleomorphic giant-cell carcinoma of the pancreas: case report with ultrastructural observations. *Act Cytol* 1986;**30:**430-434.
40. Friedman AC, Lichtenstein JE, Dachman AH. Cystic neoplasms of the pancreas: radiological-pathological correlation. *Radiology* 1983;**149:**1290-1291.
41. Yamaguchi K, Enjoli M. Cystic neoplasms of the pancreas. *Gastroenterology* 1987;**92:**1934-1943.
42. Shorten SD, Hart WR, Petras RE. Microcystic adenomas (serous cystadenomas) of pancreas. A clinicopathologic investigation of eight cases with immunohistochemical and ultrastructural studies. *Am J Surg Pathol* 1986;**10:**365-372.
43. Johnson CD, Stephens DH, Charbonneau JW, Carpenter HA, Welsh TJ. Cystic pancreatic tumours: CT and sonographic assessment. *AJR* 1988;**151:**1133-1138.
44. Itai Y, Moss AA, Ohtomo K. Computed tomography of cystadenoma and cystadenocarcinoma of the pancreas. *Radiology* 1982;**145:**419-425.
45. Vilgrain V, Menu Y, Lorphelin JM, Nahum H. Cystadénomes pancreatiques. Pièges et limites du diagnostic radiologique. *J Radiol* 1987;**68:**455-463.
46. Compagno J, Oertal JE. Microcystic adenomas of the pancreas: a clinicopathologic study of 34 cases. *Am J Clin Pathol* 1978;**69:**289-298.

47. Minami M, Itay Y, Ohtomo K, Yoshida H, Yoshikawa K, Masahiro I. Cystic neoplasms of the pancreas: comparison of MR Imaging with CT. *Radiology* 1989;**171**:53-56.
48. Compagno J, Oertel JE. Mucinous cystic neoplasms of the pancreas with overt and latent malignancy (cystadenocarcinomas and cystadenomas). A clinicopathologic study of 41 cases. *Am J Clin Pathol* 1978;**69**:573-580.
49. Hodgkinson DJ, Remine WH, Weiland LH. A clinicopathologic study of 21 cases of pancreatic cystadenocarcinoma. *Ann Surg* 1978;**188**:679-684.
50. Cantrell BB, Cubilla AL, Erlandson RA, et al. Acinar cell cystadenocarcinoma of human pancreas. *Cancer* 1981;**47**:410-416.
51. Drut R, et al. Congenital pancreatoblastoma in Beckwith-Wiedemann syndrome: an emerging association. *Paediatr Radiol* 1988;**8**:331-339.
52. Horie A, Yano Y, Kotoo Y, et al. Morphogenesis of pancreatoblastoma, infantile carcinoma of the pancreas. *Cancer* 1977;**39**:247-254.
53. Choi BI, Kim KW, Han MC, Kim YI, Kim CW. Solid and papillary epithelial neoplasms of the pancreas: CT findings. *Radiology* 1988;**166**:413-416.
54. Balthazar EJ, Subramanyam BR, Lefleur RS, et al. Solid and papillary epithelial neoplasm of the pancreas. Radiographic, CT, sonographic, and angiographic features. *Radiology* 1984;**150**:39-40.
55. Friedman AC, Lichtenstein JR, Fishman EK, et al. Solid and papillary epithelial neoplasm of the pancreas. *Radiology* 1985;**154**:333-337.
56. Kim SY, Lim JH, Lee JD. Papillary carcinoma of the pancreas: findings of US and CT. *Radiology* 1985;**154**:338.
57. Eelkema EA, Stephens DH, Ward EM, Sheedy PF. CT features of non-functioning islet cell carcinoma. *AJR* 1984;943-948.
58. Simpsom WF, et al. Nonfunctioning pancreatic neuroendocrine tumours presenting as pancreatitis: report of four cases. *Pancreas* 1988;**3**:223-231.
59. Imhof H, Frank P. Pancreatic calcifications in malignant islet cell tumours. *Radiology* 1977;**122**:333.
60. Galiber AK, Reading CC, Charboneau JW, et al. Localization of pancreatic insulinoma: comparison of pre and intraoperative ultrasound with CT and angiography. *Radiology* 1988;**166**:405.
61. Gunther RW, Klose KJ, Ruckert K. Islet cell tumours: detection of small lesions with CT and US. *Radiology* 1983;**148**:485.
62. Gunther RW, Klose KJ, Ruckert K, et al. Localization of small islet cell tumours. Preoperative and intraoperative US, CT, arteriography, DSA and pancreatic venous sampling. *Gastronintest Radiol* 1985;**10**:145.
63. Breathnach ES, Han SY, Rahatzad MT, Stanley RJ. CT evaluation of glucagonomas. *J Comput Assist Tomogr* 1985;**9**:25-29.
64. Rossi P, Baert A, Passariello R, et al. CT of functioning tumours of the pancreas. *AJR* 1985;**144**:57.
65. Krudy AG, Doppman LJ, Jensen RT. Localization of islet-cell tumours by dynamic CT: comparison with plain CT, arteriography, sonography and venous sampling. *AJR* 1984;**143**:585.
66. Pavone P, et al. Small pancreatic insulinomas: detection by MR imaging. Presented at the *RSNA meeting 1989*.
67. Doppman JL, Miller DL, Chang R, Maton PN, London JF, Gardner JD, Jensen RT, Norton JA. Gastrinomas: localization by means of selective intraarterial injection of secretin. *Radiology* 1990;**174**:25-29.
68. Dunnick NR, Doppman JL, Mills SR, et al. CT detection of nonbeta pancreatic islet-cell tumours. *Radiology* 1980;**135**:117.

69. Frucht H, Doppman JL, Norton JA, Miller DL, Dwyer AJ, Frank JA, Vinayek R, Maton PN, Jensen RT. Gastrinomas: comparison of MR Imaging with CT, angiography, and US. *Radiology* 1989;**171**:713-717.
70. Wank, SA, Doppman JL, Miller DL, et al. Prospective study if the ability of CT to localize gastrinomas in patients with Zollinger Ellison syndrome. *Gastroenterol* 1987;**92**:905.
71. Norton JA, Cromack DT, Shawker TH, et al. Intraoperative ultrasonographic localization of islet cell tumours (a prospective comparison to palpation). *Ann Surg* 1987;**207**:160.
72. Shawker TH, Doppman JL. Intraoperative US. *Radiology* 1988;**166**:568-569.
73. Gorman B, Charbonneau JW, James EM et al. Benign pancreatic insulinoma: preoperative and intraoperative sonographic localization. *AJR* 1986;**147**:929.
74. Grant CS et al. Insulinoma. The value of intraoperative ultrasonography. *Arch Surg* 1988;**123**:843-848.
75. Klotteer HJ, Ruckert K, Kummerle F, et al. The use of intraoperative sonography in endocrine tumours of the pancreas. *World J Surg* 1987;**11**:635.

Recommended Reading

Siegelman SS (ed.), *Computed tomography of the pancreas*, Edinburgh: Churchill Livingstone, 1983.

Friedman AD (ed.), *Radiology of the liver, biliary tract, pancreas and spleen.* Baltimore: Williams & Wilkins, 1987.

Freeny PC, Lawson ThL (eds.), *Radiology of the pancreas.* Heidelberg: Springer Verlag, 1982.

Freeny PC (ed.), *Radiology of the pancreas.* Radiologic Clinics of North America, Volume 27, 1989.

Cubilla A, Fitzgerald PJ (eds.). *Tumours of the exocrine pancreas.* Washington: Armed Forces Institute of Pathology, 1984.

Diagnosis of liver tumours by ultrasonography, computed tomography and magnetic resonance imaging

A. L. Baert, H. Rigauts and G. Marchal
Department of Radiology, University Hospitals K.U. Leuven, Belgium

Technique

Ultrasonography

Ultrasonography of the liver is a sensitive method for the detection of focal lesions. This method is non-invasive and allows a real time evaluation of the entire organ. Sections in transverse, coronal, sagittal or paraxial planes can be made without any restrictions. This allows a good evaluation of the relation between liver lesions and surrounding vascular or biliary structures [1].

Additional information on vascular flow can be obtained using Duplex Doppler or Color Doppler modalities. These allow measurement of flow rates and flow directions in either liver or neoplastic vessels. The combination of real time bidimensional imaging and flow analyses can be very useful [2].

Disadvantages of ultrasonography are its operator dependency (the experience of the examiner is crucial), and to a lesser degree the dependence on patient cooperation.

Large air containing collections or aero-enterie make ultrasonography impossible.

Computed Tomography

Distinction should be made between techniques aimed at screening the liver and metastasis and techniques aimed at characterizing lesions.

Screening Techniques

Non-contrast CT

This technique is usually utilized in patients with renal impairment or in conjunction with a contrast enhanced CT examination.

Non-contrast scans are helpful in detecting metastasis from hypervascular tumours (carcinoid, pancreatic islet cell tumours, renal cell carcinoma) because they tend to become iso-dense relative to the normal liver parenchyma following i.v. contrast and therefore become less conspicuous.

Post-contrast Incremental Dynamic CT

Following i.v. bolus injection. A bolus injection of 50 ml 60% iodinated is performed at a rate of 2 ml/sec for 25 seconds followed by rapid infusion of 120-125 ml of 60% (290 mgI/ml) CM over 90-120 seconds. After a 30-second delay following the start of the injection incremental dynamic scanning is performed using contiguous 1-cm sections with a goal of scanning the entire liver within 2-3 minutes (corresponding to the period of maximal enhancement of normal liver parenchyma) [4].

CT during hepatic arteriography (CT-HA). The catheter tip is positioned in the proper hepatic artery distal to the gastroduodenal artery or in a replaced hepatic artery originating from the SMA. Multiple small boluses of 7-10 ml 60% iodinated are then infused at a rate of 2 ml/sec followed by a series of incremental dynamic scans [5].

CT during arterial portography (CT-AP). The catheter tip is positioned in the proximal SMA distal to any replaced hepatic branch. Infusion of 30-40 ml 60% iodinated is followed by incremental dynamic scanning through the entire liver [6-9].

Delayed high dose iodine CT. Following an i.v. bolus enhanced CT, or a CT-HA, or a CT-AP dynamic scan, additional CM up to a total dose of 60 g iodinated is administered. The liver is rescanned after 4-6 hours. As 10% of the injected CM will be eliminated by the normal hepatocytes, a maximal density difference between lesion and normal liver parenchyma will be seen on the delayed scanning [10].

Post-contrast Non-dynamic CT

This technique is most often utilized when the liver has been included at the end of an examination of another organ or body site. The i.v. contrast is then administered several minutes before the region of the liver is scanned.

Several studies have demonstrated the superiority of CT angiography over other CT techniques in the detection of focal hepatic lesions [11,12]. CT angiography is especially advantageous in detecting small lesions. The sensitivity of this method in studies with operative confirmation is approximately 81-86%.

The main pitfalls related to CT angiography are perfusion abnormalities, especially with CT-HA, because of anomalies in the hepatic arterial distribution. It is important to use a minimum amount of contrast material during positioning of the catheter in order to obtain maximal lesion to liver contrast [13-15].

Selection of the technique to be utilized to evaluate the liver will depend on the clinical situation. Most authors agree that for an initial screening study for metastatic lesions, the bolus incremental dynamic scan is the most efficient. Based on studies from patients with colorectal carcinoma, this will result in detecting 72-85% of patients with liver metastasis (compared with a 50% detection rate with non-contrast enhanced CT). The lesion detection rate, however, is much lower and probably in the range 40-55%. If therapeutic decisions will change depending on the number of lesions found, further evaluation beyond the screening study is necessary. Delayed high dose CT will detect additional lesions in 27% of patients. CT-HA and CT-AP will detect additional lesions in 40-55% of patients.

While CT-AP has a slightly higher sensitivity for detecting lesions, early comparison studies showed it has a higher false positive rate than CT-HA.

CT Technique for Characterization of Focal Liver Lesions

This should always include a non-contrast series in order to visualize the intrinsic morphological features as well as the attenuation values of the lesion.

The post-contrast series is performed after i.v. bolus injection of 60 ml 76% iodinated at a rate of 5-6 ml/sec followed by stationary dynamic scanning initiated at 15-20 seconds after the start of the injection of CM. Scanning is performed at a frequency of 4-6 scans/minute for the first 2 minutes followed by cuts at 3, 4 and 5 minutes. More delayed scans at the same level may be obtained at progressively greater intervals until no further change in the pattern of the contrast enhancement is observed.

MR Imaging

The liver is usually imaged with a slice thickness of 8-10 mm and a gap of 2-5 mm, without respiratory or cardiac gating. Transverse views are obtained in all cases. Coronal or sagittal images are obtained in selected cases to define the relationship of an hepatic mass to the diaphragm, surrenals or other adjacent organs, and to evaluate lesions involving the vena cava inferior [16].

MR images in which tissue signal intensity is based on T_1-relaxation time (T_1-weighted images) can be acquired with spin-echo (SE) and inversion recovery (IR) pulse sequences. Selection of the shortest possible TE is essential for maximal T_1-weighting. With short TR/short TE, SE pulse sequence signal averaging is used to reduce artefacts that arise due to physiologic motion.

The best image quality for hepatic imaging is obtained using T_1-weighted images (short TR and short TE). This spin-echo sequence provides excellent anatomic detail and is less affected by motion artefacts [17]. On T_1-weighted images, liver neoplasms - both benign and malignant - appear hypo-intense relative to normal liver. Because of flow void, vascular structures also appear hypo-intense. Thus on these images it may be difficult to distinguish between small hepatic masses whose size approaches that of blood vessels seen in cross-section and the blood vessels themselves. Image contrast is the best in T_2-weighted images (long TR and long TE). T_2-weighted images are used to confirm lesions identified or suspected on T_1-weighted images because on T_2-weighted pulse sequences, hepatic masses appear hyper-intense relative to normal liver and can be readily distinguished from vascular structures, which remain hypo-intense due to flow void. Another use of T_2-weighted pulse sequences is tissue characterization.

Inversion recovery techniques, in which contrast secondary to T_1 and T_2 differences are additive, can result in good lesion detectability.

However inversion recovery techniques have poorer signal-to-noise ratio than spin-echo techniques [18].

Several techniques that use a very short TR (15-50 msec) and a reduced flip angle (<90°) have been developed. These allow single- or multi-slice sectioning in a very short period of time. Artefacts related to respiratory motion can be reduced. However, this method is more susceptible to magnetic-field differences and ferromagnetic artefacts than the conventional spin-echo technique.

Paramagnetic contrast agents in MRI have been used - results with Gd-DPTA enhanced MRI do not demonstrate any improvement in lesion detectability over non-enhanced fast scan or spin-echo techniques [16].

Tumours

Benign Tumours

Cavernous Haemangioma

Hepatic cavernous haemangiomas are the most common benign tumours of the liver with a frequency at autopsy of up to 7.3%. These tumours can be found at any age and it is estimated that 70-95% occur in women [19]. They are usually solitary but are multiple in 10% of cases. They are typically located in the subcapsular region or near to a liver fissure. Size is mostly less than 3 cm in diameter but they may become very large. The large majority of liver haemangiomas will not change in size over a period of several years.

Histologically hepatic haemangiomas consist of blood-filled spaces lined by a single layer of endothelium. These spaces are separated by fibrous septa which commonly proliferate centrally and extend peripherally to a variable degree. Calcifications or phlebolithes are rare. Central thrombosis is common and leads to fibrosis.

Hepatic haemangiomas are usually asymptomatic, although larger tumours may result in liver enlargement and abdominal discomfort. They may enlarge during pregnancy. Spontaneous haemorrhage has been reported but is rare.

US Features

The typical ultrasound features of liver haemangioma are a well defined, homogeneously hyper-echoic mass with acoustic shadowing posteriorly and without an hypo-echoic peripheral border [20].

The anatomic basis for the typical echogenic appearance of an haemangioma is thought to be due to multiple interfaces between the walls of the cavernous sinuses and the blood contained within.

A minority (15-20%) of hepatic haemangiomas will present as an iso-echoic or hypo-echoic mass relative to the liver parenchyma. When the lesion exists within a liver with diffuse steatosis, it may be evidently hypo-echoic relative to the hyper-reflective fatty liver parenchyma [21].

Some haemangiomas, especially if they are large (more than 5-6 cm in diameter) present a heterogeneous ultrasound echo pattern (Fig. 1). The anatomical basis for these alterations in the echogenicity of liver haemangioma is not well understood but degeneration and fibrosis, thrombosis or haemorrhagic necrosis may produce these changes. It has been demonstrated that the echo pattern of liver haemangiomas may change over a period of several years. During manual compression, the echogenicity of liver haemangiomas may also decrease due to some degree of suppression of the blood flow within the lesion. This feature will not be observed in primary or secondary liver tumours.

Computed Tomography

On the pre-contrast scan, small to medium-sized haemangiomas are visible as being round and hypo-dense compared to the normal liver parenchyma.

After i.v. bolus contrast-enhancement, the following features are seen in typical cases:

- visualization of small vascular structures at the periphery of the lesion on the early scan (15-45 seconds after the start of the i.v. bolus injection). This is the single most specific CT finding in liver haemangioma.
- progressive centropetal opacification of the lesion, the lesion becoming iso-attenuating between 4 to 30 minutes following contrast injection.

Most (25-80%) haemangiomas will present this opacification pattern [22].

The CT pattern of large hepatic haemangiomas may be different on the pre-contrast scan. A stellate or cleft-like area of lower attenuating

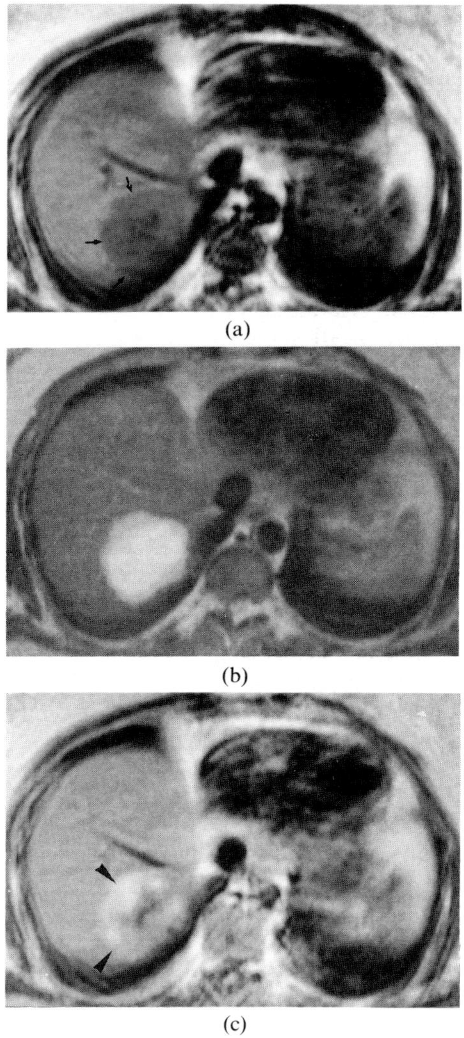

Figure 1. *MRI of a cavernous haemangioma. (a) T_1-weighted sequence. The lesion (→) shows a hypo-intense appearance when compared to the liver parenchyma. (b) T_2-weighted sequence. Notice the homogeneous hyper-intense aspect of the lesion. (c) Gadolinium-enhanced T_1-weighted sequence. The hyper-intense aspect of the peripheral portion (▸) of the lesion.*

value than the remainder of the haemangioma is frequently visible. After contrast administration, this area will not show a complete iso-attenuating fill-in, even on the delayed scans (Fig. 1) [23].

As with all focal lesions, the relative degree of attenuation of the lesions versus the liver parenchyma before contrast administration will depend on the degree of fatty liver changes. Liver haemangiomas may therefore appear iso- or even hyper-dense in case of liver steatosis. Most cavernous haemangiomas will be detected by CT if the technique for lesion characterization can be used. If no pre-contrast series is performed or if multiple lesions are present, stationary dynamic scanning at the correct level is not always possible. In these circumstances, the sensitivity and specificity of CT for the diagnosis of liver haemangioma may be lower.

MRI

Hepatic haemangiomas demonstrate variable degrees of lengthening of T_1 and T_2 values. Haemangiomas are hypo-intense of T_1 weighted images. The lengthening of T_2 is generally greater for haemangiomas, than for malignant tumours regardless of field strength. As a result, haemangiomas demonstrate the so-called light-bulb sign: a round or elliptic mass that usually has smooth and distinct margins and whose largely homogeneous contents have a very high signal intensity, similar to that of the gallbladder or CSF (Fig. 2) [24,25]. However, the specificity of the light-bulb sign is not 100% since it has also been observed with hyper-vascular metastatic lesions such as islet cell tumours or carcinomas and with metastases from sarcomas and adenocarcinomas of the pancreas and uterus [26,27].

Gradient-echo sequences combined with i.v. gadolinium DTPA (Gd-DTPA) administration will demonstrate the typical sequential enhancement similar to iodide enhanced CT of liver haemangiomas.

Compared with ^{99m}Tc Rblc scanning with SPECT, MR imaging will demonstrate superior sensitivity in the detection of haemangiomas smaller than 2.5 cm and adjacent to major intra-hepatic blood vessels and the heart. The overall accuracy of MR is also greater than SPECT. On the other hand, MR can not categorically differentiate haemangiomas from hyper-vascular metastasis while SPECT is able to do so.

Most radiologists admit that a focal liver lesion with a typical appearance or a combination of two imaging modalities (US, CT, MRI, SPECT) does not require any further diagnostic work-up.

Cysts (Fig. 3)

Ultrasonography is ideally suited to studying cystic liver lesions. Simple, non-complicated liver cysts (congenital and biliary origin) will present as sharply delineated anechoic round or slightly lobulated areas with strong dorsal acoustic shadowing. Internal scattered or

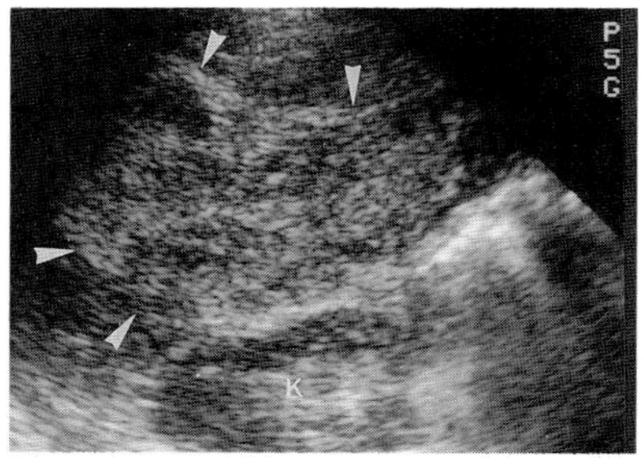

(a)

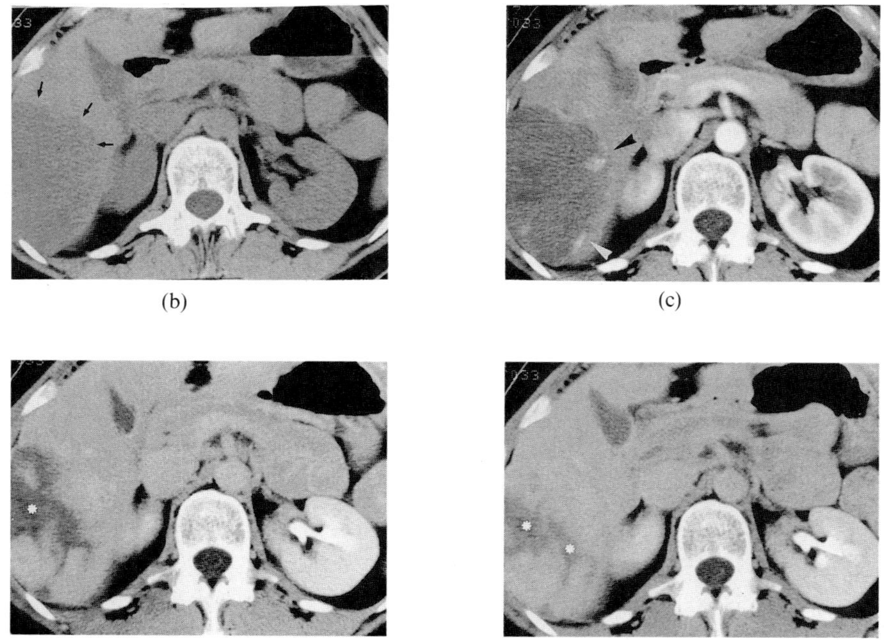

(b) (c) (d) (e)

Figure 2. *Large cavernous haemangioma. (a) Ultrasound. A very large area of inhomogeneous reflectivity (▸) is apparent in the lower aspect of right liver lobe. K=right kidney. (b)-(e) Computed tomography. (b) Pre-contrast CT. The haemangioma is visible as a large hypo-dense area (←) relative to the surrounding liver parenchyma. (c) Postcontrast CT. Arterial phase (15 minutes after i.v. bolus injection). Two strongly enhancing small structures (▸) are visible in the peripheral portion of the lesion. (d) Post-contrast CT. Late phase (7 hours after i.v. bolus injection). Some sections of the lesion are now contrast enhanced but the lateral portions (*) do not take up the contrast material. (e) Post-contrast CT. Late phase (25 hours after i.v. bolus injection). Further contrast uptake into the lesion but two small portions (*) are still not enhanced.*

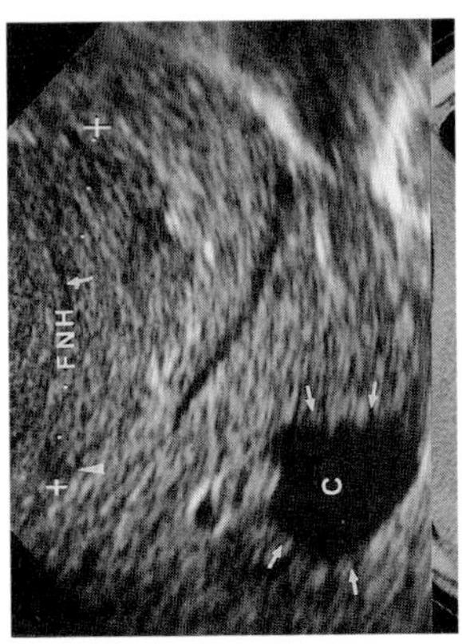

(a)

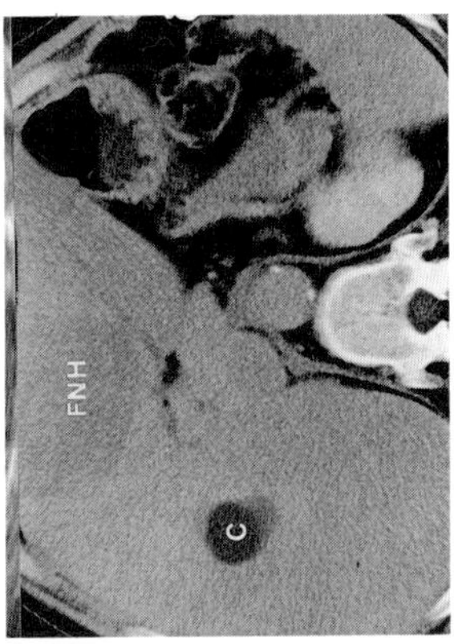

(b)

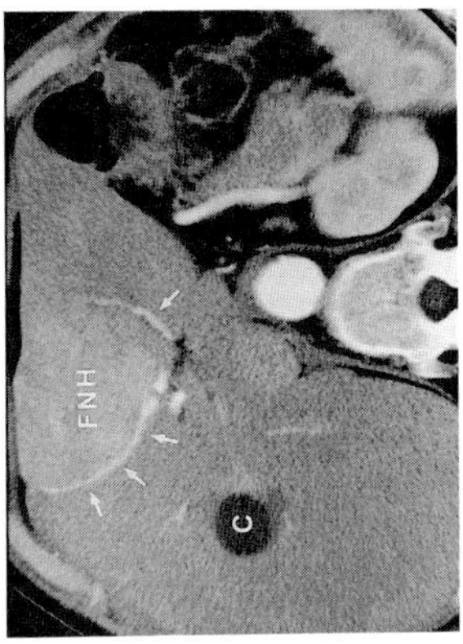

(c)

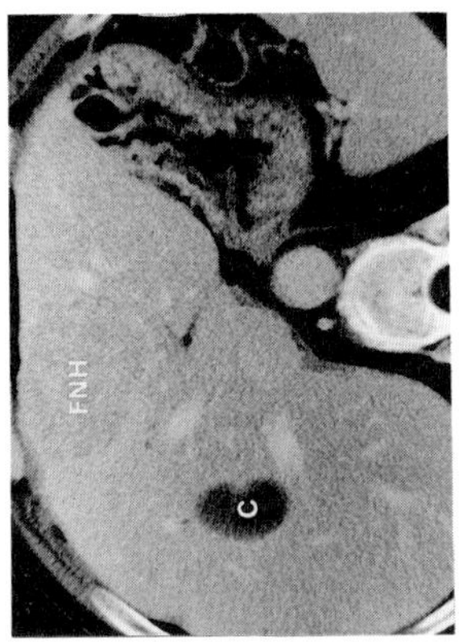

(d)

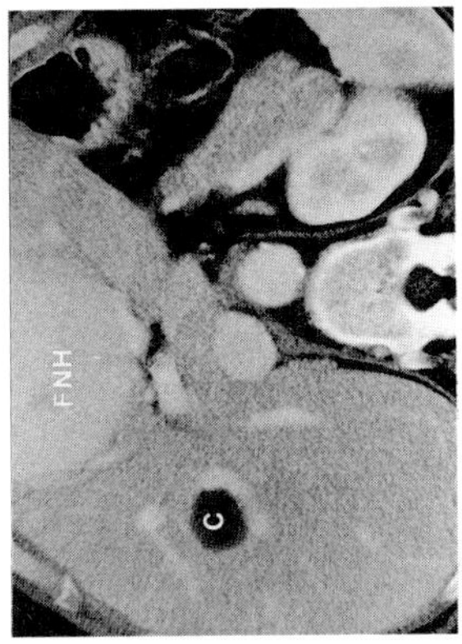

(e)

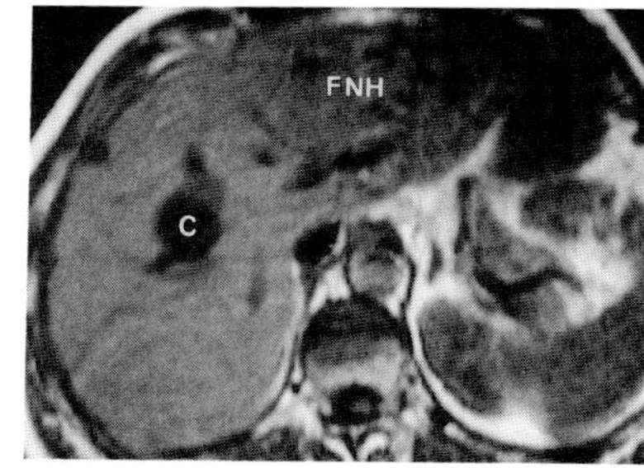

(f)

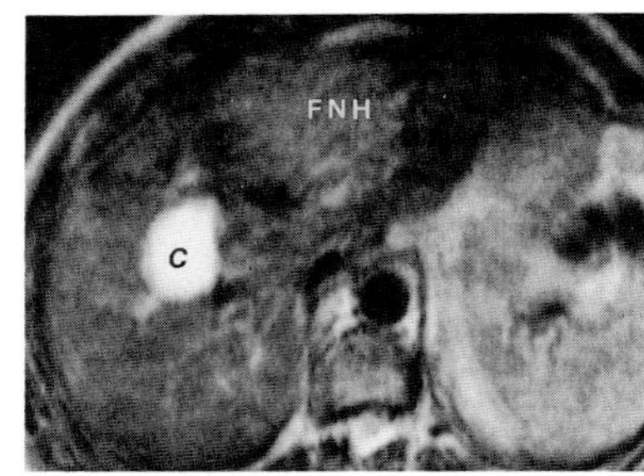

(g)

Figure 3. *Benign cyst and focal nodular hyperplasia (FNH). (a) Ultrasound. Area of decreased reflectivity (+.......+) in left liver lobe, sharply demarcated from surrounding liver parenchyma. Central (↑) and peripheral (▸) small tubular areflective zones are detected. A polygonal areflective zone is seen anteromedial in the right liver lobe. (b)-(d) Computed tomography. (b) Pre-contrast scan. The FNH mass (FNH) has an attenuation coefficient of 45 HU compared with 62 HU of the normal surrounding liver parenchyma. The cyst (C) has an attenuation coefficient of water. (c) Post-contrast scan 15 minutes after i.v. bolus of CM. The FNH mass (FNH) is strongly enhancing. A circular artery (→) closely following the outer contour of the lesion is clearly visible. There is total absence of contrast enhancement and no visible wall in the cyst (C). (d) Post-contrast scan 30 minutes after i.v. bolus of CM. The FNH mass (FNH) remains homogeneously more strongly enhanced compared to the surrounding liver parenchyma (C=cyst). (e) Post-contrast scan 45 minutes after i.v. bolus of CM. The FNH mass (FNH) now shows the same degree of enhancement as the normal liver parenchyma. (f) and (g) MRI. (f) T_1-weighted sequence. The FNH mass (FNH) shows a slightly lower signal and the cysts (C) a very low signal when compared to the liver parenchyma. (g) T_2-weighted sequence. The FNH mass (FNH) shows a slightly increased signal compared to the liver parenchyma. A very strong signal intensity can be seen in the cyst (C).*

dependent echos moving during positional changes of the patient indicate infection or the presence of intra-cystic blood.

CT features of simple liver cysts are attenuation values between 0 and +10 HU, total lack of contrast enhancement, sharp demarcation and no visible wall. The attenuating valves may be higher in an infected cyst and rim enhancement may be present.

A slight increase in attenuation values, visible after contrast injection, is artefactual, usually due to marked increase in attenuation of surrounding normal liver parenchyma.

On MRI, simple liver cysts may feature the same spectrum of findings as haemangiomas. They are of homogeneously low intensity on T_1 weighted images and high intensity on T_2 weighted images. Although hepatic cysts usually can be distinguished from haemangiomas, because the former have even longer T_1 and T_2 values, the distinction between small cysts and haemangiomas (<1.5 cm) may be difficult because of partial volume averaging.

Adenoma and Focal Nodular Hyperplasia

Although these tumours have similar features on US, CT and MRI (Figs. 3 and 4), there is a need to distinguish one from the other as they are managed differently.

Hepatic adenoma is a benign epithelial tumour which is partially or completely encapsulated and strongly vascularized. They are frequently of large size at the time of diagnosis and subcapsular in location. A certain number will present intra-tumoural haemorrhage and/or necrosis.

An adenoma is composed of normal hepatocytes but without lobular architecture - thus without bile ducts, portal triads or centrolobular veins. Kupffer cells are mostly absent.

Hepatic adenomas occur predominantly (90-95%) in young women and have a strong association with the use of oral contraceptives based on oestrogens. They will cause clinical symptoms more frequently than focal nodular hyperplasia. Pain which is often secondary to intra-tumoural or intra-peritoneal haemorrhage is present in 40-50% of patients. They may rarely occur in men, mostly with a history of androgen-use. Children with type I glycogen storage disease may present multiple adenomas.

Focal nodular hyperplasia also occurs predominantly in women but the mean age is higher than for adenoma. There is still some controversy about the causal role of contraceptives but most authors support

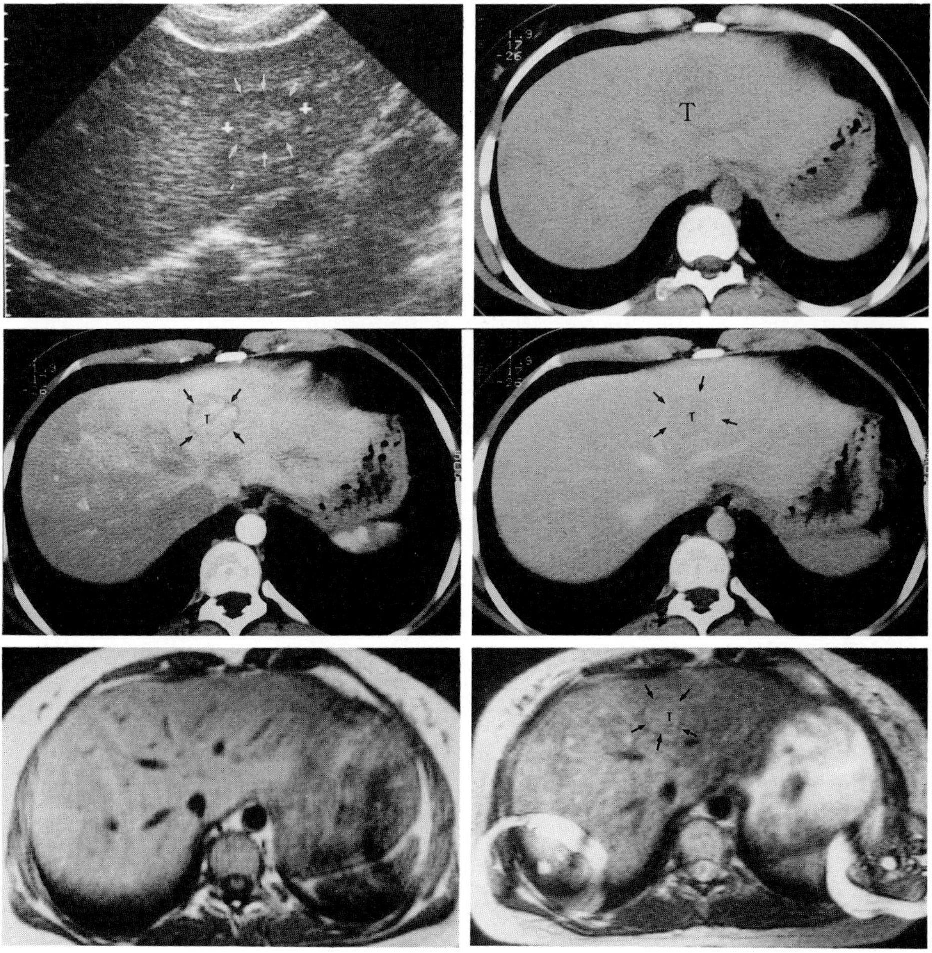

Figure 4. *Adenoma of the left lobe. (a) Ultrasonography. Rounded area of heterogeneous reflectivity bordered by very thin hypo-reflective line (←). (b)-(d) Computed tomography. (b) Pre-contrast CT. The tumour (T) is nearly iso-dense relative to the surrounding liver parenchyma. (c) Post-contrast CT phase (15 minutes after i.v. bolus injection). The tumour (T) is slightly hyper-vascular and slightly more enhancing than the liver parenchyma. The tumour capsula (→) is clearly less enhancing. (d) Post-contrast CT portal phase (42 minutes after i.v. bolus injection). The tumour (T) has rapidly become iso-dense relative to the liver parenchyma. The tumour capsula (→) is now slightly enhanced. (e) and (f) MRI. (e) T_1-weighted sequence. The lesion is iso-intense with the liver parenchyma and not visible. (f) T_2-weighted sequence. The tumour capsula (→) is slightly hypo-intense relative to the liver parenchyma and to the tumour. This feature allowed identification of the tumour itself (T), which remains iso-intense.*

the view that there is no aetiological relationship, although their use by patients with focal nodular hyperplasia may increase an haemorrhagic tendency.

Macroscopically, focal nodular hyperplasia is an unencapsulated lobular mass with septations and a central stellate structure. Connective tissue radiates towards the periphery. Within the central scar and the radial fibrous septa hyperplastic vessels are present. The tumour is frequently subcapsular and may be pedunculated.

Microscopically the lesion is composed of units of hepatocytes, Kupffer cells with sinusoids and bile duct structures.

About 90% of patients with focal nodular hyperplasia have no clinical symptoms. Rupture or bleeding occurs in only 1.5% of cases.

Ultrasound

Hepatic adenomas are usually echogenic but may occasionally be hypo-echoic. In symptomatic patients, sonolucent areas within the lesion may be due to haemorrhage. The echogenicity of focal nodular hyperplasia is extremely variable: hyper-echoic, iso-echoic and hypo-echoic aspects have been described. The central scar may be visible as a central strongly hyper-reflective area.

Computed Tomography

On the pre-contrast image, adenomas and focal nodular hyperplasia may be iso-dense relative to the normal liver parenchyma. Haemorrhage in an adenoma may be identified as areas of heterogenous attenuation with high attenuation components if bleeding has been recent. The central scar in focal nodular hyperplasia may be visible or have a stellate hypo-dense central area. After stationary dynamic bolus CT both lesions will show an intense but very transient enhancement due to their hyper-vascularity [28]. They will, however, become iso-dense relative to the surrounding liver parenchyma after 1-2 minutes following contrast injection. In adenoma, the fibrous capsule may be visible as an enhancing rim on the more delayed scans. The central fibrous tissue in focal nodular hyperplasia will become more visible on the post-contrast images. As with ultrasonography, differentiation between adenoma and focal nodular hyperplasia may be impossible even with high quality CT.

MRI

The MRI appearance of adenoma may be indistinguishable from that of primary hepatocellular carcinoma [29].

A majority of focal nodular hyperplasia cases have the following features: the lesions are homogeneous and almost iso-intense, with the adjacent liver parenchyma on all pulse sequences. The margins of the lesions are either ill-defined or non-visible. The central scar when present is hypo-intense on T_1 weighted images [30-32]. However, central scars, hyper-intense on T_2, have also been described in other primary liver tumours such as hepatocellular carcinoma and large cavernous haemangioma [33].

Hepatocellular Carcinoma (Fig. 5)

Ultrasound

Large (>2-3 cm) nodular HCC, either single or multiple, are mostly hyper-echoic compared to the surrounding liver parenchyma. They are surrounded by a thin hypo-echoic rim corresponding to the tumour capsule. Small (<2 cm) HCC may present a mixed echogenicity (mosaic pattern). This mosaic pattern is probably due to the compartimentalization caused by the fibrous septa dividing the tumour.

These typical US findings will pose no diagnostic problem especially in patients with liver cirrhosis and elevated α-fetoprotein. Unfortunately these findings may be absent, especially in small HCC which may present also as hypo-echoic lesion without mosaic appearance or hypo-echoic rim. These hypo-echoic HCC can not be differentiated from regenerative nodules occurring in cirrhosis.

Rarely, nodular HCC will be iso-echoic with the surrounding liver parenchyma and may only be detected on the basis of an hypo-echoic rim.

The diffuse form of HCC will be visible on ultrasound as multiple areas of increased or decreased echogenicity without conspicuous nodular structure.

The sensitivity of US in the detection of HCC is very high. With adequate equipment the detection rate for large HCC should be near to 100% but it may be as low as 50% for lesions between 1-2 cm.

Recent evidence seems to indicate that in the future colour Doppler echography may be important for the US diagnosis of HCC. The

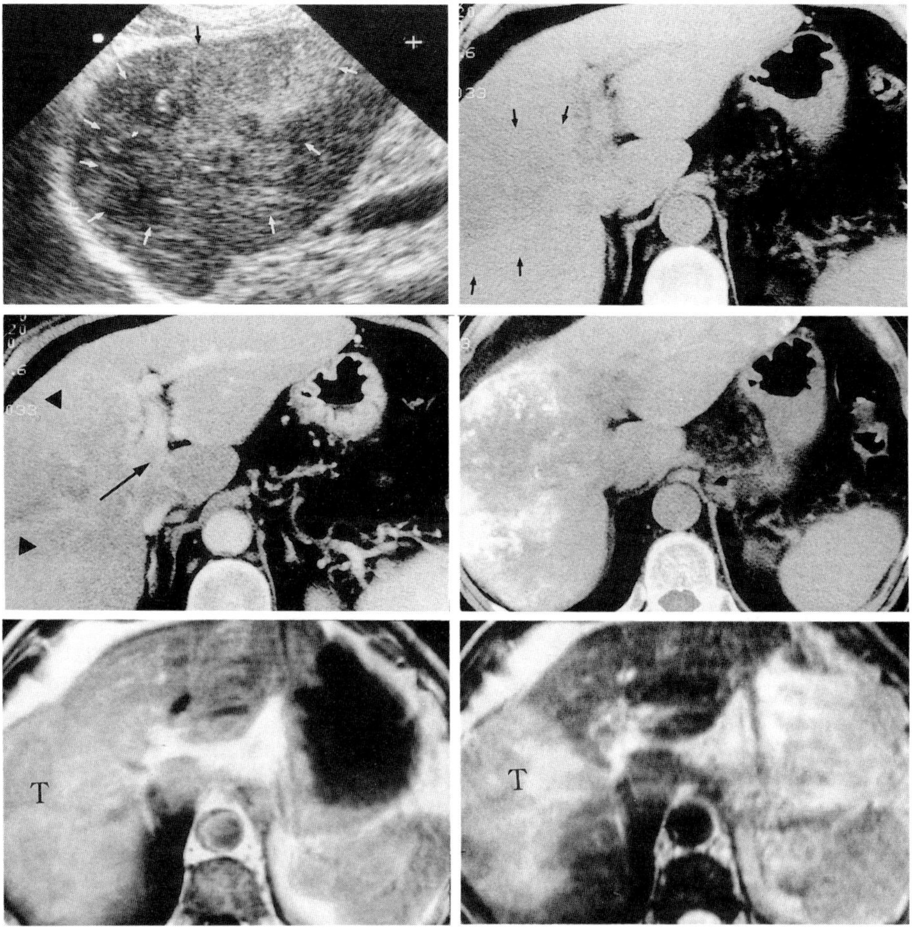

(b)

(d)

(f)

Figure 5. *Hepatocellular carcinoma. (a) Ultrasonography. Large inhomogeneous - partially hyper-reflective, partially hypo-reflective - mass (↑) on the right liver lobe. There is no sharp delineation between ill-defined and normal liver parenchyma. (b) Pre-contrast CT. Large, slightly hypo-dense irregular area with unclear borders in the right liver lobe (→). (c) Post-contrast CT. The tumour shows a moderate degree of contrast enhancement, especially in its peripheral portion (▲). Notice invasion by tumour into the left portal vein (→). (d) CT 24 hours after intra-arterial lipiodol injection. Elective accumulation of lipiodol in the tumour but preferentially in the peripheral portion. (e) MRI, T_1-weighted sequence. The tumour (T) is iso-intense relative to liver parenchyma. (f) MRI, T_2-weighted sequence. The tumour (T) is easily identified as a hyper-intense area.*

presence of arterioportal shunting in HCC leads to high frequency Doppler signals (>5 kHz). Metastatic lesions will either show no signal or signals up to a maximum of 4 kHz [2].

Computed Tomography

The nodular form of HCC will present on pre-contrast scan mostly as an hypo-dense or iso-dense lesion with a peripheral narrow hypo-dense layer. Calcifications are present in 10% of HCC. On bolus dynamic scan, a pronounced but transient heterogeneous contrast captation will be visible. Arterioportal shunts cause early and prolonged portal vein enhancement and transiently increased attenuation of contralateral lobes or segments. Dilated abnormal vessels or irregular enhancing areas may be visible outside the tumour. These various patterns of contrast enhancement are related to the degree of arterioportal shunting and venous obstruction as well as to the anatomic location of the tumour within the liver.

Diffuse forms of HCC will produce alternations that are less well circumscribed and difficult to differentiate from the diffuse changes occurring in liver cirrhosis.

Lipiodol ultrafluid accumulates within hyper-vascular hepatic tumours when it is injected in a catheter in the appropriate hepatic artery (lipiodol-CT). The contrast medium is retained for several weeks to over a year. The lack of reticulo-endothelial system and lymphatic flow may inhibit decomposition and absorption of oil and probably contributes to its long-term retention [34].

CT obtained 2-3 weeks after intra-arterial injection of lipiodol may be useful for the detection of small secondary tumour nodules in HCC, although it has been shown that lipiodol also accumulates in hyper-vascular metastatic liver lesions as well as in cavernous haemangiomas. Transient, but not long-term, accumulation has been noted in regenerative nodules.

MRI

Fifty per cent of nodular HCC appears on T_1-weighted images as iso- or hyper-intense compared with adjacent liver parenchyma. A hypo-intense rim is often present peripherally and corresponds to the fibrous capsula. On T_2-weighted images, 90% of nodular HCC are hyper-intense. With T_2-weighting, the fibrous capsula continues to appear hypo-intense and may be surrounded by a second thin hyper-intense rim [35-37].

Fatty degeneration and recent haemorrhage might be causal factors of hyper-intensity of HCC on T_2-weighted images. Tumours which are hypo-intense on T_2-weighted images present coagulation necrosis. Fatty degeneration of HCC is a common pathological finding. It will lead to an increased lesion/liver signal ratio on the T_1-weighted images [38].

HCC will show a variety of contrast enhancement patterns following Gd-DTPA injection, depending on the tumour vascularity. The peripheral rim is non-enhancing on the early images but will display a high signal intensity on the delayed images [39,40].

Vascular invasion by tumour thrombus is seen as an area of increased signal within a normally signal-free lumen of the vessel.

Fibrolamellar Hepatocellular Carcinoma (Fig. 6)

This separate entity has different clinical features to and a better prognosis than HCC.

Pathologically, the tumour is always partially or completely encapsulated and may even be pedunculated. A central stellate fibrous scar, similar to that seen in focal nodular hyperplasia is frequently present.

The radiological features are as follows:

- on ultrasound, the lesion is moderately echogenic and well circumscribed.
- on CT a central stellate or trabecular calcification will be seen on 30-40% of patients. On pre-contrast images the lesion is hypodense relative to adjacent liver parenchyma. On post-contrast images moderate or strong transient enhancement will occur in the tumour with the exception of the central scar. The scar may, however, enhance on the more delayed images and becomes less visible.
- on MRI the central scar may appear hyper-intense both on T_1- and T_2-weighted images if the scar is predominantly collagenous. If inflammatory scar tissues presents it will be hypo-intense on T_1 and hyper-intense on T_2-weighted images [41].

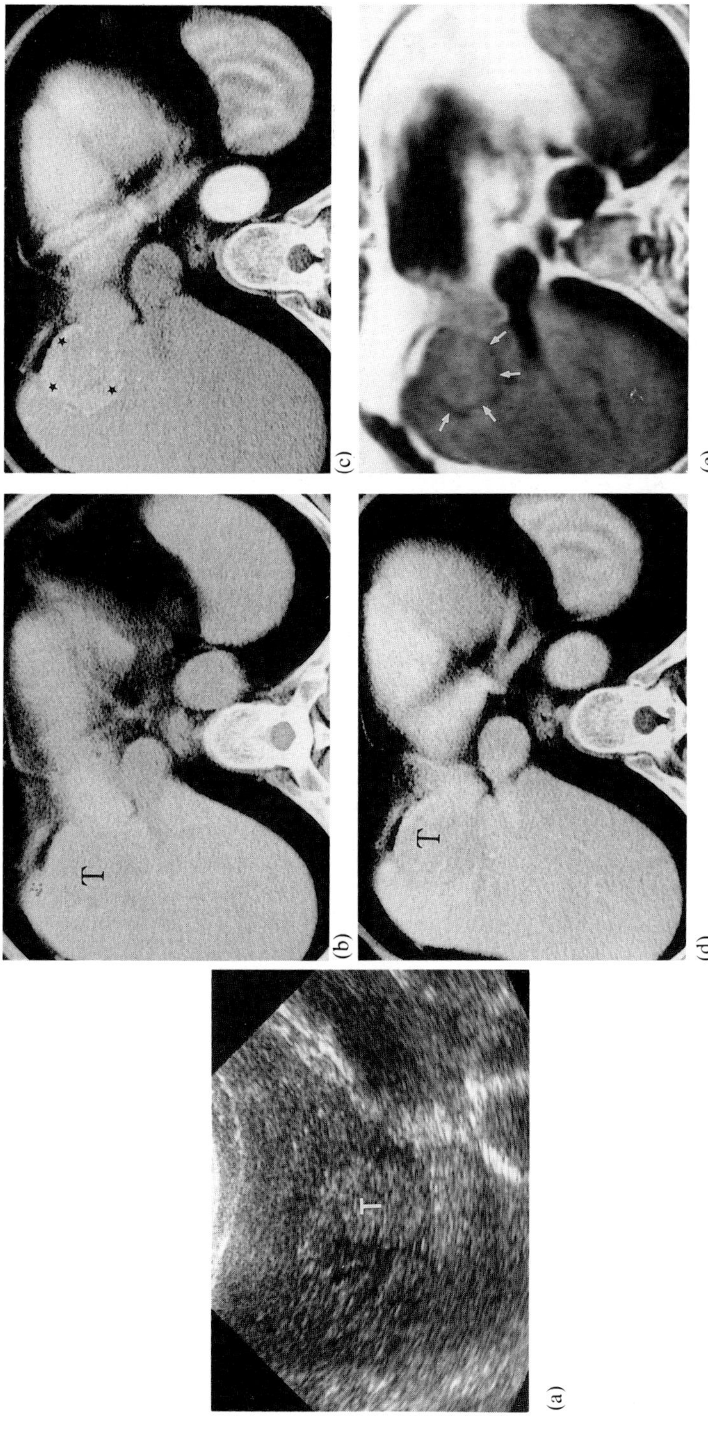
(c)
(e)
T
(b)
T
(d)
T
(a)

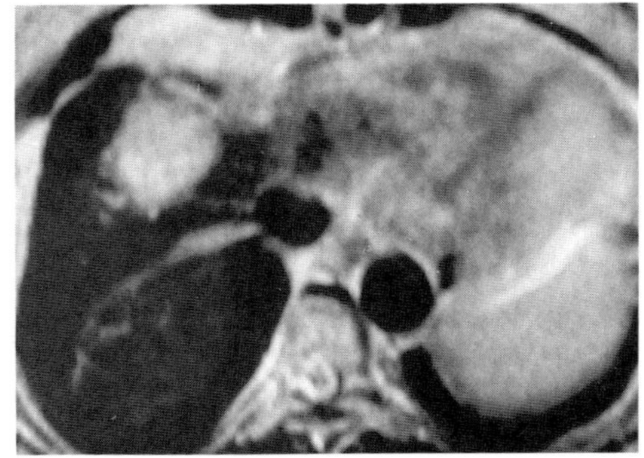

(f)

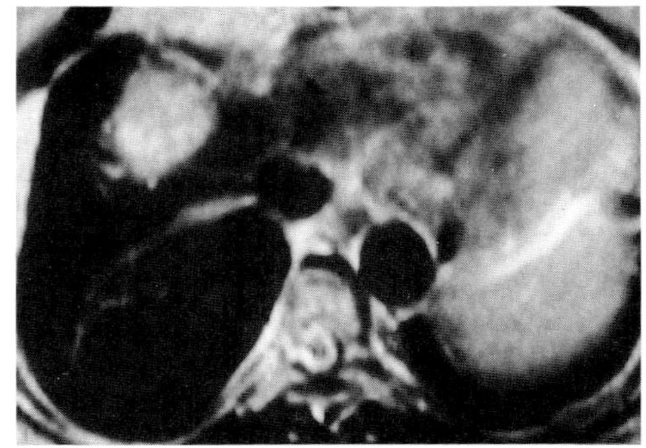

(g)

Figure 6. *Fibrolamellar hepatocellular carcinoma.* *(a) Ultrasound.* *The tumour (T), situated in the ventral portion of the right liver lobe, is moderately hyper-reflective compared to the liver parenchyma.* *(b)-(d) Computed tomography.* *(b) Pre-contrast scan. The tumour (T) is visible as a very sharply defined hypo-dense (+49 HU) area relative to the liver parenchyma (+69 HU). (c) Post-contrast scan 15 minutes after i.v. bolus of CM. Moderate degree of enhancement (+87 HU) of the peripheral portions (*) of the lesion. (d) Post-contrast scan 30 minutes after i.v. bolus of CM. The degree of contrast enhancement of the tumour has already decreased to +67 HU. The liver parenchyma has reached its peak contrast enhancement at +117 HU. Thus the tumour (T) again shows as a hypo-dense area.* *(e)-(g) MRI.* *(e) T_1-weighted sequence; TR:650, TE:15. The lesion itself is iso-intense compared to the liver parenchyma but is surrounded by a thin more hypo-intense rim (→). (f) T_2-weighted sequence; TR:2296, TE:60. The tumour has an evident hyper-intense but non-homogeneous aspect. (g) T_2-weighted sequence; TR:2296, TE:120. On this more heavily T_2-weighted sequence, the signal intensity of the lesion is further increased.*

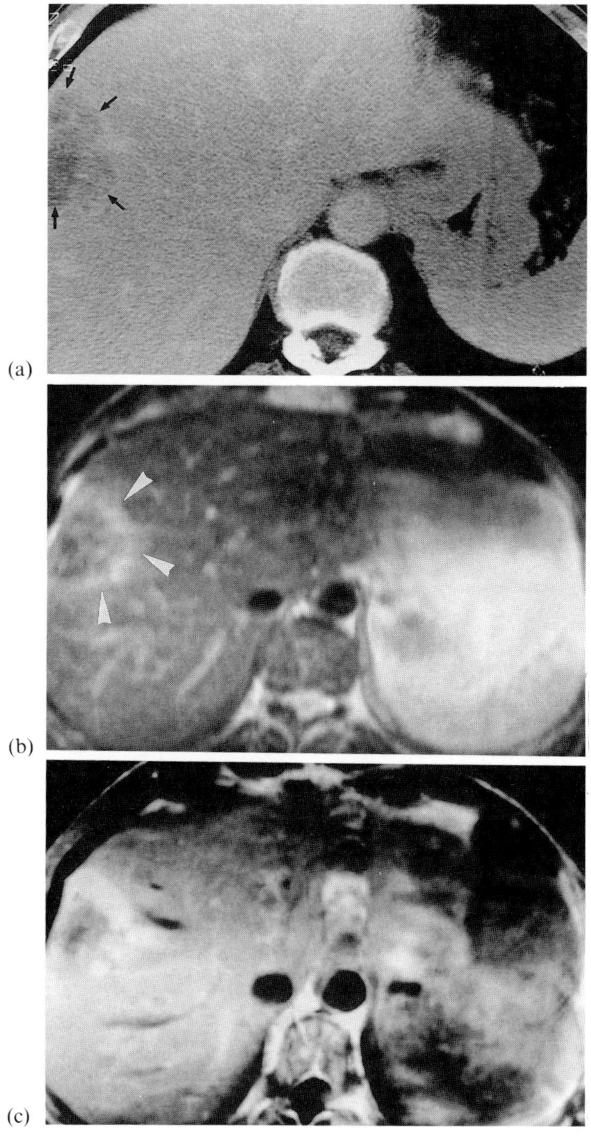

Figure 7. *Liver metastasis from a primary bronchogenic carcinoma. (a) Computed tomography. Post-contrast scan. Irregularly bordered non-homogeneous area of lower enhancement (→) in right liver lobe. (b) and (c) MRI. (b) T_2-weighted sequence. The peripheral portions (▲) of the lesion show an increased signal intensity compared to the surrounding liver parenchyma, while the central core of the metastasis is iso-intense. (c) Gadolinium-enhanced T_1-weighted sequence. The peripheral portion (▲) of the lesion shows an increased uptake of contrast medium.*

Metastasis (Fig. 7)

Ultrasound

Nodular forms of metastatic lesions may rarely appear as hypo-reflective circular areas. Much more common metastatic lesions will be seen as hyper-echogenic areas. Frequently there exists around a reflective nodule a circular hypo-echoic rim. This appearance has been termed bull's eye.

Necrotic liver metastasis may present a liquid pattern with mostly irregular borders. If situated superficially, metastatic lesions will cause a contour deformity of the organ.

In diffuse forms of liver metastasis a more diffuse change in echogenicity of the liver parenchyma will be seen. Diagnosis by ultrasound is much more difficult and special attention should be paid to the study of liver contours to detect contour deformity.

Computed Tomography

On pre-contrast images most metastatic lesions will appear hypodense relative to the normal liver parenchyma. They may appear iso- or hyper-dense in fatty livers. Borders may be sharp or ill-defined. The shape is mostly round but may be ovular or irregular. Punctate or amorphous calcifications may be present, especially in metastases originating from primary tumours of the gastrointestinal tract or breast.

On the post-contrast images, most metastatic lesions remain hypo-attenuating relative to liver parenchyma but a peripheral enhancing ring is frequently seen. Sometimes two or three concentric bands or variable attenuation are visible. Metastasis from hyper-vascular tumours, such as from carcinoid, islet cell tumours or renal cell carcinoma, will show an early strong but transient contrast enhancement, but may become iso-dense relative to the liver on images taken 3-5 minutes following contrast injection. Pre-contrast scans are essential for their detection.

Diffuse metastatic involvement will lead to an overall inhomogeneous aspect and distortion of the vascular pattern. These more subtle findings can be better visualized by narrowing the window settings.

Although CT is often the imaging technique of choice in screening the liver for metastatic disease, small liver cysts may be mistakenly diagnosed as metastatic disease by CT as the liquid lesions appear solid as a result of volume averaging. Ultrasound is particularly helpful in diagnosing these lesions correctly.

MRI

The most important diagnostic finding in metastatic disease is a bright halo surrounding the lesion on mildly T_2-weighted images. It is believed that this aspect reflects microscopic peritumoural oedema or tumour neovascularity. Other features of metastases are less specific. With longer echo-delay T_2-weighted sequences solid tumours show gradual loss of hyper-intensity and image sharpness [42].

Metastasis from hyper-vascular tumours or tumours with central necrosis may show an homogeneous bright signal on T_2-weighted images similar to the 'light-bulb' appearance of haemangiomas and cysts.

Most metastasis will be hypo-intense relative to liver on the T_1-weighted images. Rarely, a bright signal may be seen due to the paramagnetic effect of recent intra-lesional haemorrhage.

As stated above, tumour encapsulation, steatosis and a proclivity for vascular invasion are signs characteristic of HCC, especially when present in combination. These signs are usually absent in metastatic lesions. The central tumour scar identified in fibrolamellar hepatocellular carcinoma is another useful differential sign. The central necrotic area of a metastatic lesion is usually found. Concerning the value of MRI versus CT preliminary experience suggested that T_2-weighted images (SE 2000/700) obtained at 1.5T are significantly superior to bolus enhanced CT.

The use of Gd-DTPA is now being explored in combination with rapid scanning. Emerging information would indicate that Gd-DTPA enhanced MRI does not offer any advantages in terms of liver lesion detection. As regards characterization, metastatic lesions do not present a consistent pattern of contrast enhancement different from hepatocellular carcinoma as some other focal liver lesions.

The use of reticulo-endothelial iron oxide agents is still in the earliest phase of evaluation. At mid-field strength, an important increase in the number of lesions detected was noted. At high-field strength, lesion detection was not significantly improved compared to the long TR/TE sequence, although in all cases the contrast enhanced images showed improved lesion to liver contrast [43].

References

1. Needleman L, Kurtz AB, Rifkin MD, Cooper HS, Pasto ME, Goldberg BB. Sonography of diffuse benign liver disease: accuracy of pattern recognition and grading. *AJR* 1986;**164:**1011-1015.
2. Taylor KJW, Ramos I, Morse SS, Fortune KS, Hammers L, Taylor CR. Focal liver masses: differential diagnosis with pulsed doppler US. *Radiology* 1987;**164:**643-647.
3. Baron RL. Imaging metastatic hepatic disease. SBCT. *Annual Meeting Monterey* 1988.
4. Tyrrel RP, Bernardino ME. La tomodensitométrie du foie avec injection. *J Radiol* 1990;**5:**317-323.
5. Nakao N, Miura K, Takayasu Y, Wada Y, Miura T. CT angiography in hepatocellular carcinoma. *J Comput Assist Tomogr* 1983;**7:**780-787.
6. Matsui O, Takasjima T, Kadoya M, Ida M, Suzuki M, Kitagawa K, Kaminura R, Inoue K, Konishi H, Itoh H. Dynamic computed tomography during arterial portography: the most sensitive examination for small hepatocellular carcinomas. *J Comput Assist Tomogr* 1985;**9:**19-24.
7. Matsui O, Takashima T, Kadoya M, Suzuki M, Hirose J, Kameyama T, Choto S, Konishi H, Ida M, Yamaguchi A, Izumi R. Liver metastases from colorectal cancers: detection with CT during arterial portography. *Radiology* 1987;**165:**65-69.
8. Tyrrell RT, Kaufman SL, Bernardino ME. Straight line sign: appearance and significance during CT portography. *Radiology* 1989;**173:**635-637.
9. Nelson RC, Chezmar JL. Diagnostic approach to hepatic hemangiomas. *Radiology* 1990;**176:**11-13.
10. Bernardino ME, Erwin BC, Steinberg HV, Baumgartner BR, Torres WE, Gedgaudas-McClees RK. Delayed Hepatic CT Scanning: increased confidence and improved detection of hepatic metastases. *Radiology* 1986;**159:**71-74.
11. Heiken JP, Weyman PJ, Lee JKT, Balfe DM, Picus D, Brunt EM, Flye MM. Detection of focal hepatic masses: prospective evaluation with CT, delayed CT, CT during arterial portography, and MR imaging. *Radiology* 1989;**171:**47-51.
12. Nelson RC, Chezmar JL, Sugarbaker PH, Bernardino ME. Hepatic tumours: comparison of CT during arterial portography, delayed CT and MR Imaging for pre-operative evaluation. *Radiology* 1989;**172:**27-34.
13. Freeny PC, Marks WM. Hepatic perfusion abnormalities during CT angiography: detection and interpretation. *Radiology* 1986;**159:**685-691.
14. Doppman JL, Dwyer A, Vermess M, Girton M, Sugarbaker P, Miller D, Cornblath M. Segmental hyperlucent defects in the liver. *J Comp Assist Tomogr* 1984;**8:**50-57.
15. Itai Y, Moss A, Goldberg J. Transient hepatic attenuation difference of lobar or segmental distribution detected by dynamic computed tomography. *Radiology* 1982;**144:**835-839.
16. Marchal G, Demaerel P, Vanhoenacker P, Van Ongeval C, Aerts P, Rigauts H, Bosmans H, Van Hecke P, Baert AL. Recent developments in liver imaging. *Curr Opin Gastroenterol* 1990;**6:**427-433.
17. Chezmar JL, Rumancik WM, Megibow AJ, Hulnick DH, Nelson RC, Bernardino ME. Liver and abdominal screening in patients with cancer: CT versus MR Imaging. *Radiology* 1988;**168:**43-47.
18. Curati WL, Halevy A, Gibson RN, Carr DH, Blumgart LH, Steiner RE. Ultrasound, CT and MRI comparison in primary and secondary tumours of the liver. *Gastrointest Radiol* 1988;**13:**123-128.
19. Marchal G, Baert AL, Fevery J, Kint E, Peeters S, Van Dijck X, De Maeyer P, Usewils R, Wilms G. Ultrasonography of liver hemangioma. *Fortschr Röntgenstr* 1983;**2:**201-207.

20. Nelson RC, Chezmar JL, Sugarbaker PH, Murray DM, Bernardino ME. Pre-operative location of local liver lesions to specific liver segments. Utility of CT curing arterial portography. *Radiology* 1990;**176:**89-94.
21. Marsch IJ, Gibney RG, Li DKB. Hepatic hemangioma in the presence of fatty infiltration: an atypical sonographic appearance. *Gastrointest Radiol* 1989;**14:**262-264.
22. Ashida C, Fishman K, Zerhouni EA, Herlong FH, Siegelman SS. Computed Tomography of Hepatic Cavernous Hemangioma. *J Comp Assist Tomogr* 1987;**11:**455-460.
23. Scatarige JC, Kenny JM, Fishman EK, Herlong FH, Siegelman SS. CT of giant cavernous hemangioma. *AJR* 1987;**149:**83-85.
24. Li KC, Glazer GM, Quint LE, Francis IS, Aisen AM, Ensminger WD, Bookstein FL. Distinction of hepatic cavernous hemangioma from hepatic metastases with MR imaging. *Radiology* 1988;**169:**409-415.
25. Ohtomo K, Itai Y, Yoshikawa K, Kokubo T, Iio M. Hepatocellular carcinoma and cavernous hemangioma: differentiation with MR Imaging. Efficacy of T_2 values at 0.35 and 1.5 T. *Radiology* 1988;**168:**621-623.
26. Ferrucci JT. Liver Tumour Imaging. *Current Concepts Radiolog* 1990;**155:**473-484.
27. Wittenberg J, Stark DD, Forman BH, Hahn PF, Saini S, Weissleder R, Rummeny E, Ferrucci JT. Differentiation of hepatic metastases from hepatic hemangiomas and cysts by using MR Imaging. *AJR* 1988;**151:**79-84.
28. Lüning M, Simon G, Dewey CH, Decker T, Sperling P. CT diagnosis of hepatic adenoma. *Eur J Radiol* 1987;**7:**30-36.
29. Nokes SR, Baker ME, Spritzer CE, Meyers W, Herfkens RJ. Case Report: hepatic adenoma: MR appearance mimicking focal nodular hyperplasia. *J Comput Assist Tomogr* 1988;**12:**885-887.
30. Butch RJ, Stark DD, Malt RA. Case Report: MR Imaging of hepatic focal nodular hyperplasia. *J Comp Assist Tomogr* 1986;**10:**874-877.
31. Mattison GR, Glazer GM, Quint LE, Francis IR, Bree RL, Ensminger WD. MR Imaging of hepatic focal nodular hyperplasia: characterization and distinction from primary malignant hepatic tumours. *AJR* 1987;**148:**711-715.
32. Schiebler ML, Kressel HY, Saul SH, Yeager BA, Axel L, Gefter WB. MR Imaging of focal nodular hyperplasia of the liver. *J Comput Assist Tomogr* 1987;**12:**651-654.
33. Wilbur AC, Gyi B. Hepatocellular carcinoma: MR appearance mimicking focal nodular hyperplasia. *AJR* 1987;**149:**721-722.
34. Merine D, Takayoshu K, Wakao F. Detection of hepatocellular carcinoma: comparison of CT during arterial portography with CT after intra-arterial injection of iodized oil. *Radiology* 1990;**175:**707-710.
35. Ebara M, Ohto M, Watanabe Y, Kimura K, Saisho H, Tsuchiya Y, Okuda K, Arimizu N, Kondo F, Ikehira H, Fukuda N, Tateno Y. Diagnosis of small hepatocellular carcinoma: correlation of MR imaging and tumour histologic studies. *Radiology* 1986;**159:**371-377.
36. Itoh K, Nishimura K, Togashi K, Fujisawa I, Noma S, Minami S, Sagoh T, Nakano Y, Itoh H, Mori K, Ozawa K, Torizuka K. Hepatocellular carcinoma: MR imaging. *Radiology* 1987;**164:**21-25.
37. Matsui O, Kadoya M, Kameyama T, Yoshikawa J, Arai K, Gabata T, Takashima T, Nakanuma Y, Terada T, Ida M. Adenomatous hyperplastic nodules in the cirrhotic liver: differentiation from hepatocellular carcinoma with MR Imaging. *Radiology* 1989;**173:**123-126.
38. Rummeny E, Saini S, Wittenberg J, Compton C, Hahn PF, Mueller PR, et al. MR Imaging of liver neoplasms. *AJR* 0000;**152:**493-499.
39. Ohtomo K, Itai Y, Yoshikawa K, Kokubo T, Yashiro N, Iio M, Furukawa K. Hepatic Tumours: dynamic MR Imaging. *Radiology* 1987;**163:**27-31.

40. Yoshida H, Itai Y, Ohtomo K, Kokubo T, Minami M, Yashiro N. Small hepatocellular carcinoma and cavernous hemangioma: differentiation with dynamic FLASH MR Imaging with Gd-DTPA. *Radiology* 1989;**171**:339-342.
41. Rummeny E, Weissleder R, Sironi S, Stark DD, Comptom CC, Hahn PF, Saini S, Wittenberg J, Ferrucci JT. Central scars in primary liver tumours: MR features, specificity and pathologic correlation. *Radiology* 1989;**171**:323-326.
42. Reinig JW, Dwyer AJ, Miller DL, Frank JA, Adams GW, Chang AE. Liver metastases: detection with MR Imaging at 0.5 and 1.5 T. *Radiology* 1989;**170**:149-153.
43. Marchal G, Van Hecke P, Demaerel Ph, Decrop E, Kennis C, Baert ALL, Van der Schueren E. Detection of liver metastases with superparamagnetic iron oxide in 15 patients: results of MR imaging at 1.5T. *Am J Roentgenol* 1989;**152**:771-775.

Recommended Readings

Ferrucci JT, Stark DD (eds). *Liver imaging. International Symposium.* Boston: June 25-27 1990.
Ferrucci JT, Mathieu DG. *Advances in hepatobiliary radiology.* St Louis: CV Mosby Company, 1990.
Friedmann AC (ed). *Radiology of the liver, biliary tract and spleen.* Baltimore:
Williams and Watkins, 1987.
Lee JKT, Siegel SS, Stanley RJ. *Computed body tomography with MRI correlation.* Raven Press, 1989.

High resolution renal anatomy on ultrasound

David Cosgrove
Royal Marsden Hospital, London, UK

Introduction

Renal ultrasound has an important role amongst the other imaging techniques both classical (the intravenous urogram) and new (computed tomography, and nuclear magnetic resonance imaging). Apart from its general advantages of ease of use and immediacy, ultrasound is especially valuable in locating a kidney either because it has not been visualized on the urogram or for biopsy purposes. Its high sensitivity in the demonstration of fluid spaces has made it useful in the evaluation of hydronephrosis and of cysts and in distinguishing these from solid masses. Ultrasound is the most direct way of measuring renal size; this is particularly useful in paediatrics to monitor renal growth and also in acute renal failure because the demonstration that the kidneys are shrunken indicates that the disease is end-stage where biopsy is unrewarding whereas normal-sized or large kidneys suggest an acute process that requires biopsy for diagnosis. The lack of ionizing radiation of ultrasound is a particular advantage in problems during pregnancy and, to a lesser extent, in paediatrics. In urinary tract infections ultrasound is especially valuable in the paediatric age group where it complements both the micturating cystogram and radio-isotope studies so that generally urography is no longer required.

In general, ultrasound does not offer functional information but the addition of Doppler to evaluate the vascular bed is proving increasingly useful.

Embryology

An understanding of the complex embryological changes of the kidneys makes sense of important anatomical features that are otherwise incomprehensible [1,2]. The complexity is partly due to the fact that two primitive renal systems, the pro- and mesonephros develop before the definitive renal tract forms. The definitive renal tract commences with the formation of the metanephric (commonly referred to as 'ureteric') ducts that grow upwards from the primitive bladder. As it grows, each metanephric duct collects a cluster of mesodermal cells from the nephrogenic ridge; these will differentiate into mature nephrons under the stimulus of the growing tips of the metanephric ducts. The end of the duct expands to form the renal pelvis and repeated branching forms the infundibula, calices and collecting tubules.

The development of the nephrons is totally dependent on the stimulus from the tips of the dividing metanephric duct and this defines both the amount and the disposition of the mature renal tissue. Each terminal duct stimulates the formation of some nine nephrons which surround the growing ends of the duct, much as the leaves of a tree surround the smaller branches. Thus the typical renal lobe is formed, each consisting of a layer of nephrons (the cortex) surrounding the central collecting tissue (the medulla) except at the point of entry of the collecting ducts which remains exposed and will form the tip of the papilla. Later the loops of Henle from the deeper nephrons will grow down between the collecting ducts. The increase in bulk of the parenchymal tissue of each lobe indents the end of its calix to form the cup shape that lends its name to the mature calix (calix/chalice). Because there is more branching of the ducts at the upper and lower poles, the renal tissue becomes thickest there.

Within each kidney fourteen or so lobes are thus formed; they are separate in the early fetus, but at about eight months gestation they fuse, leaving only shallow grooves as evidence of their position in the fetus; the residual markings on the renal surface are known as fetal lobation [3]. Because of the way they develop, these grooves are inevitably interlobar in location, overlying the blocks of cortical tissue between the medullary regions (which are known as the cortical septa of Bertin). Adjacent lobes often undergo further fusion, the intervening cortex being absorbed and adjacent calices combined especially at the renal poles. The larger 'compound' lobes that result have a more irregular shape than the pyramidal simple lobes; their calices and papillae are correspondingly larger and more complex in shape. The average mature kidney has some eleven lobes and fewer calices because some drain more than one papilla.

The developing kidneys migrate superiorly along the posterior wall of the abdominal cavity and their axes rotate so that the hila, which originally faced anteriorly, come to face medially. The migrating kidneys are supplied by a series of paired branches from the aorta; these involute sequentially so that usually all but the most superior pair disappear. A similar sequence occurs in the development of the renal veins. Thus, should migration of the kidney be arrested, the vessels also tend to be ectopic, while incomplete atrophy of lower fetal branches results in multiple renal arteries.

Normal Anatomy

General Features

The kidneys are paired retroperitoneal organs lying in the upper abdomen on the muscles of the posterior abdominal wall (Fig. 1) [4-7]. The right kidney is often situated several centimeters inferior to the left (the liver displaces the right kidney downwards), though in practice their positions vary greatly. At one extreme the upper poles may lie up against the diaphragm while at the other, the kidney may lie partly or entirely in the pelvis. They are also freely mobile, descending on inspiration and standing.

Because of the shape of the renal bed (defined by the psoas muscles which thicken inferiorly), they lie somewhat obliquely with their lower poles tilted anteriorly and laterally. Thus, oblique slices are usually required to image the length of the kidney. The renal hila face antero-medially so that the renal vessels and the emerging ureters pass anteriorly as well as medially. Within the hila (or renal sinus) lie the blood vessels and the pelvi-caliceal collecting system together with a variable amount of fat that acts as packing. A strong capsule invests the kidney; at the hilum it blends with the walls of the vessels and collecting system.

The renal bed is formed by the quadratus lumborum muscle posteriorly with psoas postero-medially; the transversus abdominus muscle lies postero-laterally. When the kidney is high lying, its upper

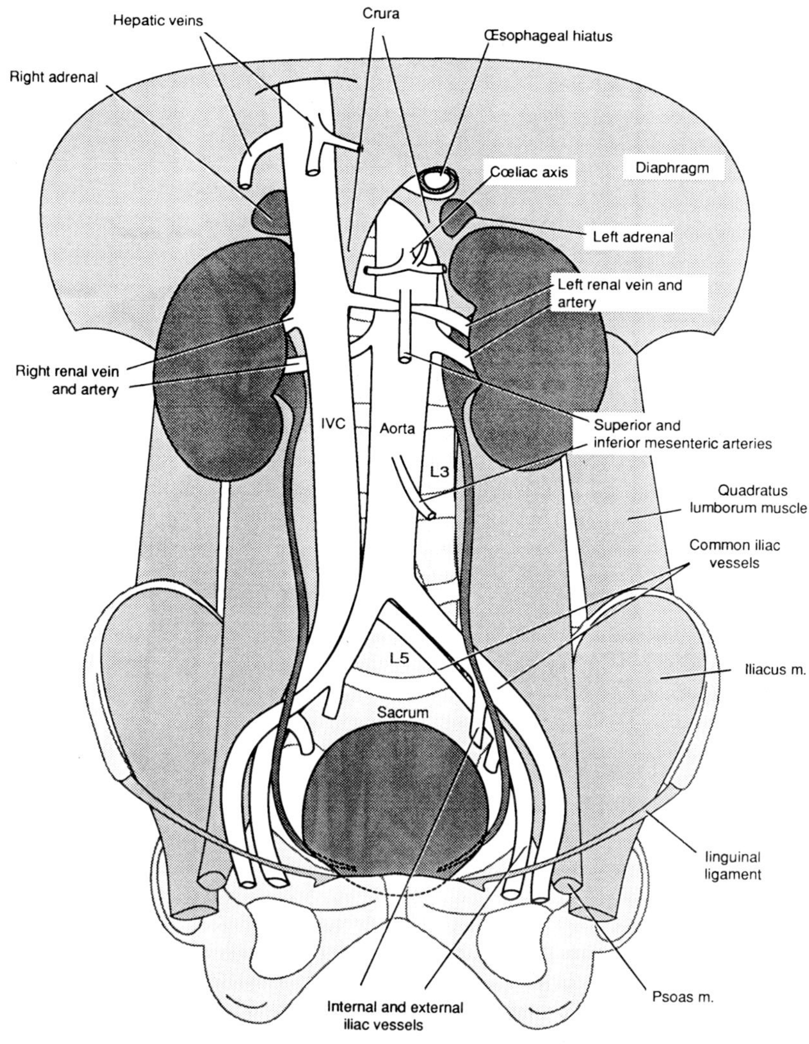

Figure 1. *GENERAL ANATOMY OF THE KIDNEYS. The position of the kidneys in the retroperitoneum is shown to indicate their relations and their lie.*

pole rests on the posterior part of the diaphragm.

The adrenal glands lie adjacent to the upper poles medially, that on the left tending to lie relatively lower so that it often forms a medial relation to the left upper pole. On the right the second and third parts of the duodenum lie against the antero-medial surface of the kidney. The right lobe of the liver is anterior and, depending on its position, the gall-bladder also, both separated from the kidney by peritoneum of the hepato-renal angle (Morrison's pouch). The upper portions of the ascending colon and its hepatic flexure overlie the lower pole and, on the left, the splenic flexure occupies a symmetrical position. The lateral surfaces of both are covered by the peritoneum that forms the paracolic gutters. On the right the peritoneum continues across the anterior surface of the kidney, separating it from the liver, while inferiorly the peritoneum covers the colon.

The spleen overlies the supero-lateral aspect of the left upper pole which is also crossed by the tail of the pancreas anteriorly. The stomach lies anterior and medial to the left kidney, the variable position of both organs determining the extent of the relationship. The peritoneal space of the lesser sac intervenes between the spleen and stomach and the kidney. The arrangement of the peritoneum on the left is more complex than the right because a fold, the lieno-renal ligament, is attached to the posterior abdominal wall across the upper pole; this forms the lateral wall of the lesser sac, so that the medial portion of the kidney is part of the back wall of the lesser sac while the more lateral parts of the kidney are part of the posterior wall of the greater sac.

The blood supply to the kidney is generous, accounting for 20% of the cardiac output via large trunks that arise directly from the aorta (Fig. 2) [8]. The renal arteries usually take origin from the lateral wall of the aorta; they pass postero-laterally and often also somewhat inferiorly, overlying the crura of the diaphragm; the right renal artery crosses posterior to the inferior vena cava. Before entering the renal hilum they typically give off a posterior branch which passes behind the renal pelvis and supplies the posterior mid-portion of the kidney. The larger anterior trunk usually divides into four branches, one supplying each pole and two to the anterior mid-portion. The branching pattern is very variable, but at least partly occurs outside the renal hilum and anterior to the renal pelvis. Supernumerary arteries are also very common.

The renal veins have a similar pattern, with the larger veins lying anterior to the corresponding arteries. The right renal vein has a short course, passing antero-medially to empty directly into the postero-lateral surface of the inferior vena cava. The left renal vein is much longer; it runs antero-medially at first and then curves transversely

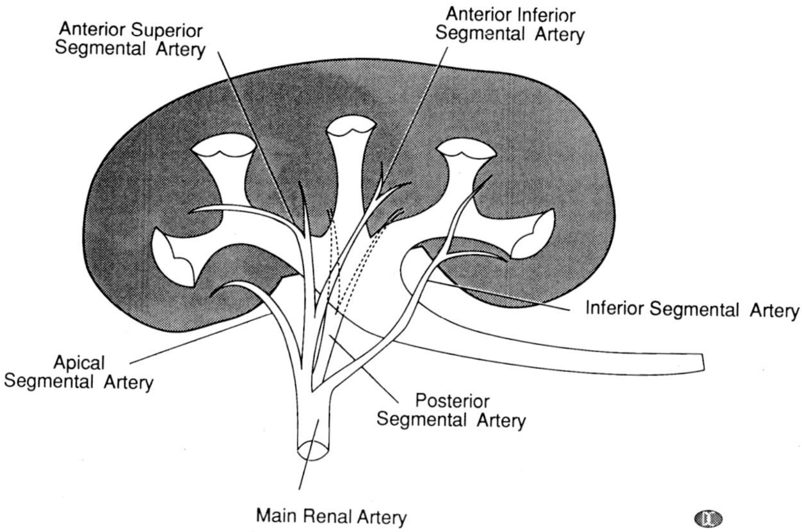

Figure 2. *THE RENAL ARTERIES. Diagram from in front to show the main and segmental arteries with the kidney orientated as for coronal scanning.*

across the aorta. Here it lies posterior to the superior mesenteric artery and at this point is often somewhat narrowed in the antero-posterior direction. This flattening accounts for the fact that it is seen here in transverse section spanning a centimeter or so. There is often also dilatation of the upstream part of this vein which can seem disproportionately large by comparison with the midline portion.

The adult kidney is approximately 4 cm in thickness and 10 cm in length, the latter differing by less than 2 cm between the two sides; their size is related to body size. Radiological measurements are usually about 15% larger than those obtained on ultrasound (due to tube magnification as well as the diuretic effect of intravenous contrast), so that figures derived from X-ray data are misleading. A chart of normal ultrasound values is useful in clinical practice, especially in paediatrics (Fig. 3) [9,10].

The kidneys are surrounded by a layer of fat which is part of the retroperitoneal space but is divided into two portions by the renal fascia (Gerota's fascia). The perirenal fat immediately surrounds the kidneys, while the pararenal fat lies outside the fascia (Fig. 4). The renal fascia itself forms a cap over the kidneys but is open inferiorly.

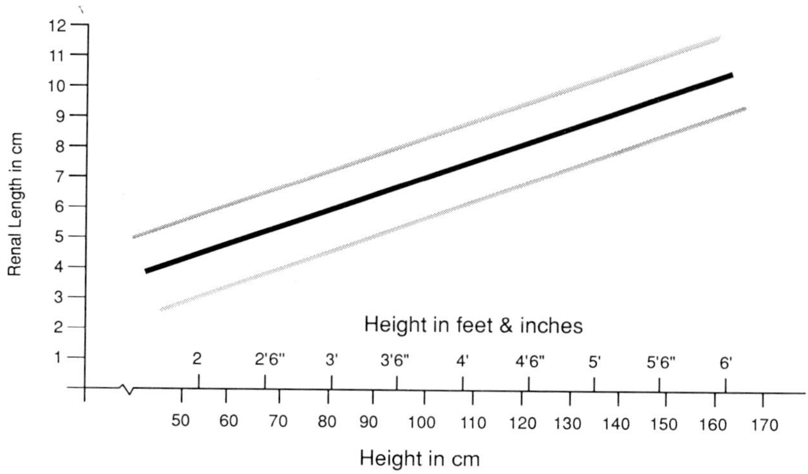

Figure 3. *Chart of renal length with body height.*

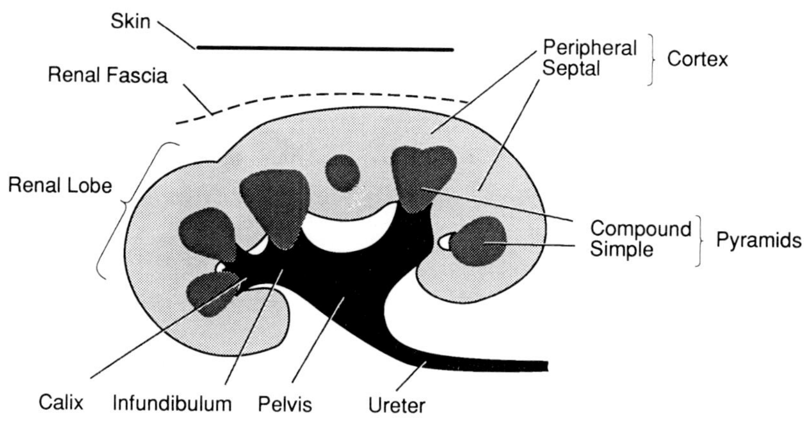

Figure 4. *PERIRENAL TISSUES. Cross and sagittal sections through the right kidney illustrate the tissues around the kidney. The renal (Gerota's) fascia splits the retroperitoneal fat into two layers; it thins and may be absent inferiorly at the pelvic brim.*

It is thickest laterally where it blends with the transversals fascial layer that invests the posterior abdominal muscles. Medially the posterior layer fuses with the psoas fascia, while the anterior layer is continuous across the midline, sometimes fused with the anterior wall of the aorta. The defect in the fascia inferiorly accounts for the relative ease with which urine tracks inferiorly; similarly haematomas and pus can spread down into the pelvis. The adrenals are contained within the perirenal fascia, but lie in separate compartments so that they do not necessarily move with the kidneys.

The Lobar Anatomy of the Kidney

The kidney consists of a series of lobes, each comprising a cortical layer bearing glomerulae surrounding a central medullary layer containing the straight tubules (Fig. 5) [11]. There are typically up to

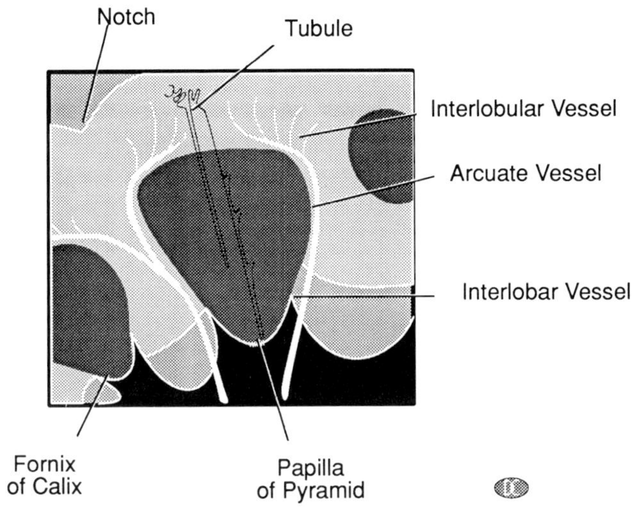

Figure 5. *LOBAR ANATOMY OF THE KIDNEY. The components of the renal parenchyma are shown with the deeper lying medullary pyramids each almost surrounded by a layer of cortex.*

a dozen lobes in each kidney, each having an approximately pyramidal shape, arranged with their apices facing the central hilum. Here, at the papilla, the tip of each medullary pyramid projects a few millimeters into its calix, but everywhere else it is enveloped by a layer of cortex. Thus peripherally the cortex forms the surface of the kidney, covered by the renal capsule. Where adjacent lobes are in contact, the contiguous (septal) layers of cortex blend with each other without an apparent line of demarcation. These intermedullary portions of the cortex are referred to as the septa of Bertin. (They are often termed 'columns' but this term seems inappropriate since they are shaped like curved walls; Bertin's original term in French, '*cloisson*', is more descriptive and is better translated as 'septum'). The peripheral cortex is generally thicker than the septal cortex. The lobar structure is more obvious in the fetal and neonatal kidney as a surface nodularity (so-called fetal lobation) but the grooves tend to be effaced as the renal cortex thickens with maturation of the nephrons so that the lobation is less apparent in the adult though they sometimes persist as a normal variant.

Many of the renal lobes have a simple configuration with a rounded or oval base peripherally, tapering to a single papilla. These simple pyramids have arisen from a single fetal lobe, and when imaged in tomographic sections, have a rounded or pyramidal form. However, the situation is usually complicated by the process of fusion described in the embryology section, whereby two or even three lobes combine. These 'compound lobes' are larger and have a more complex configuration, with an oval or lobulated footprint on the renal capsule. On tomography they often have a lobulated or cardioid shape and taper to large, compound papillae which are oval, in contrast to the conical shape of simple papillae. Compound papillae occur more frequently at the renal poles.

The nephrons of each lobe are confined to that lobe (Fig. 6). The glomeruli lie in the renal cortex, each with its corresponding proximal convoluted tubule close by. These lead into the descending limbs which pass into the medulla and become the loops of Henle. The returning loops (the ascending limbs) cross into the cortex and continue as the distal convoluted tubules. From here they drain into collecting tubules which again pass through the medulla, enlarging as they collect tributaries, to empty into the calix at the tip of the papilla. There are 10 to 20 ducts in each papilla, each draining about eight collecting tubules and, in turn, eight nephrons. Each kidney contains about one million nephrons.

Thus in the cortex the pattern of the glomeruli and the convoluted tubules is multi-directional and contorted. This is emphasized by the associated blood vessels which also form a complex network. In the medulla, however, there is a strong linear pattern of near-parallel tubules passing towards and returning from the papilla with vessels (*vasa recta*) following the same pattern. On ultrasound the complex, omnidirectional pattern of interfaces in the cortex would be expected to generate strong echoes when interrogated from any angle, whereas

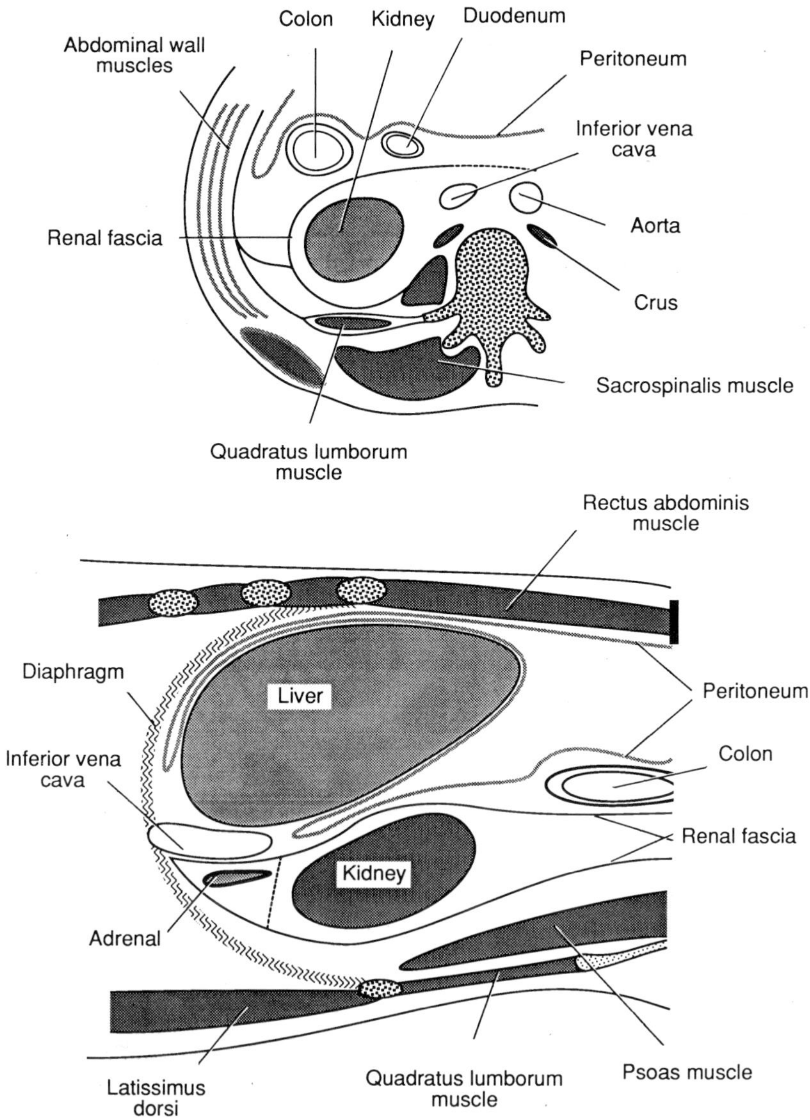

Figure 6. *LOBAR ANATOMY OF THE KIDNEY. A diagram of a magnified renal lobe to indicate the relative positions of the nephron and lobar blood vessels.*

the parallel pattern in the medulla might be expected to give weak echoes unless the ultrasound beam were oriented at right angles across the tubules. This probably accounts for the fact that fewer pyramids are seen on ultrasound scans than are known to be present [12].

The intrarenal blood vessels are also arranged in a lobar fashion (Fig. 6). Branches of the segmental arteries in the hilum divide into interlobar branches which penetrate the renal parenchyma at the junction between the medulla and cortex (i.e. the interlobar cortex or septum of Bertin). Here they are termed the arcuate arteries because of their curved shape as they run round the margins of the pyramids. The arcuate arteries give off numerous small radial interlobular arterioles that pass peripherally within each renal lobe and supply the glomeruli. At the surface of the kidney some of these anastomose with sub-capsular arterioles which derive from retroperitoneal arteries; thus the superficial layer of the cortex has a double arterial supply that may allow it to survive occlusion of the renal artery. Where compound lobes have formed, the embryonic interlobar arteries that originally lay within the interlobar tissue sometimes come to lie within the compound medullary pyramid. The venous drainage follows the same general pattern.

Collecting System

Urine formed by the nephrons is discharged via the papillae into the calices. Usually several papillae empty into each calix, though sometimes a calix only receives one pyramid. Such a simple calix has the shape of an egg-cup, indented peripherally by the papilla. Thus the two-fold layers of the calix (the fornix) are in contact if there is no urine in the collecting system. Where several papillae empty together into a compound calix the arrangement is the same but the overall shape is more complex.

Urine in the calices is passed to the renal pelvis via the infundibula. The exact arrangement varies considerably, the commonest pattern consisting of two or three groups of calices, upper, middle and lower discharging into two or three infundibula. Variations where there are multiple or single calices do occur but are rare. Variations in the length of the infundibula are more common; for example, they may be absent, so that the calices empty directly into an intrarenal pelvis or they may be long so that the pelvis lies mainly or completely outside the renal hilum, a variant known as the 'extra-renal pelvis'. Urine may pool in the less well-supported extra-renal portion of the pelvis and the appearance of this so called 'baggy pelvis' can be confused with hydronephrosis.

Outside the renal hilum the pelvis tapers to a funnel shape towards the pelvi-ureteric junction which continues medially and inferiorly into the upper ureter. Here it crosses the lateral border of the psoas muscle, lifting anteriorly as it does so, and then continues inferiorly. The psoas thus produces a sharp curve in the course of the ureters which makes for difficulties in following them on ultrasound.

Ultrasound of the Normal Kidney

General Ultrasound Principles

Techniques for ultrasound scanning of the kidney are similar to those used for the upper abdomen in general. Frequencies of 3-5 MHz are suitable, the higher frequencies giving better resolution where the kidneys lie sufficiently superficial to allow penetration of the beam. Curvilinear arrays offer the best compromise between the field of view required to accommodate the whole kidney and the need to work through small acoustic windows that limits the usable transducer footprint. No preparation is required, though an allowance for the degree of hydration must be made: the hydrated kidney is larger with better defined pyramids and there may be physiological filling of the pelvi-caliceal system.

The classic window for the right kidney, developed for static scanners, is an anterior sagittal scan through the right lobe of the liver. Best visualization is obtained through a Riedel's lobe. However, the coronal approach from the flank often brings the transducer closer to the kidney, allowing superior detail, and is equally useful on the left. In addition, the scans are in the plane that the pathologist uses to bivalve the kidneys, so that the relations between the parenchyma and the hila are clearly displayed especially useful in disorders of the collecting system. Because of the anterior lie of the pelvis in many patients, an approach from posterior to the true coronal plane is often optimal. In addition, the usual anterior position of the lower pole necessitates a tilted scan to display the full length of the kidney. In some cases these views can be obtained on both sides with the patient supine, otherwise it may be helpful to rotate the patient into the decubitus, placing a pillow under the opposite flank to open the space between the lower ribs and the iliac crest. Transverse views should be part of every routine series since they often clarify an equivocal appearance in the longitudinal scan or clearly demonstrate a lesion that was inapparent.

The kidneys may also be imaged from behind, *via* the paraspinal muscles. In general this gives poorer views than the coronal projection, perhaps because of the diffractive effects of the muscle and fascial layers traversed. In adults this view is not much used except for biopsy guidance but in children it is useful and often convenient since a baby may be held on the parent's chest during the scanning session.

Conventional ultrasound does not offer functional information but the addition of Doppler goes some way to redeem this [13,14]. Because of the depth of the kidney and the anatomical complexity, a duplex system which allows simultaneous real time imaging and Doppler is required so that the anatomical location of a vessel under study can be known. The simplest form of duplex provides a Doppler gate whose position and length can be adjusted so that a vessel that has been imaged can be selectively sampled. The output from such a device encompasses both high velocity signals from the central stream of the vessel, say an artery, and slower flow at the periphery of the vessel, presented as a Doppler-shift spectrum that changes periodically through the cardiac cycle. As well as a graphical presentation, a sound output is provided because the ear is very adept at analyzing the frequency content of complex sounds.

The graphical tracing ('sonogram') plots flow velocity with time (Fig. 7). In a typical renal artery the fast systolic flow is followed by slower but continuous flow throughout diastole, indicating that the vasomotor tone of the resistance vessels (the pre-glomerular arterioles) is sufficiently low that they remain open even at the lower perfusion pressure of diastole. If the resistance to inflow should increased (e.g. in an arteriopathy such as renal transplant rejection) diastolic flow reduces or even stops. In renal artery stenosis, high velocity flow occurs together with turbulence which is depicted as broadening of the Doppler spectrum (i.e. increased flow at low velocities) and even simultaneous reverse flow because of vortices. Venous flow from the kidney is more continuous though it is subject to modulation by cardiac and adjacent arterial activity because of the thin walls and low venous pressure.

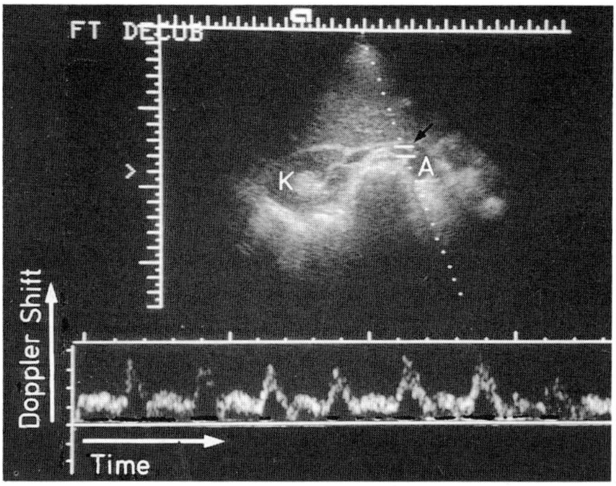

Figure 7. *SPECTRAL DOPPLER SIGNALS FROM A RENAL ARTERY. In this duplex study, the real-time image (a transverse section through the right renal artery in this example) appears at top of the screen with a cursor to indicate the Doppler sensitive gate (arrow). The spectral Doppler tracing or 'sonogram' is shown in the lower part of the screen; it depicts the Doppler shift signals, representing the velocity of blood in the selected vessel, against time. Flow towards the transducer is indicated above the base line, flow away, below. The Doppler shift signals are frequencies (usually in kHz) which can be converted to velocity (m/s) if the transmitted frequency and the angle of insonation are known both usually available. The spread of Doppler shift is attributable to the slower blood flowing at the periphery of the vessel (due to wall drag effects). The amount of blood flowing at any frequency is indicated by the grey scale of the waveform. In this normal tracing the rapid acceleration in systole is shown together with the continued flow throughout diastole that indicates a low resistance to flow.*

A more complex form of Doppler is colour flow imaging (commonly referred to as 'colour Doppler') in which echoes from an area of the ultrasound image are examined for Doppler shift and the signals presented as a colour-coded overlay on the real time anatomical image. Red tints are used to indicate flow towards the transducer and blues for flow away (usually corresponding with arteries and veins). Though no spectral information is available (only the mean flow velocity is presented), the combination of anatomical and functional information is extremely valuable in detecting tissues that are perfused and abnormal vascular patterns as well as to guide the positioning of the gate for spectral Doppler study. In effect, colour Doppler is a form of angiography which is non-invasive, though it is subject to artefacts similar to those that beset ultrasound imaging and there are limitations to its sensitivity to low velocity and volume flow the introduction of suitable ultrasound contrast agents will probably improve these limitations [15].

(a)

(b)

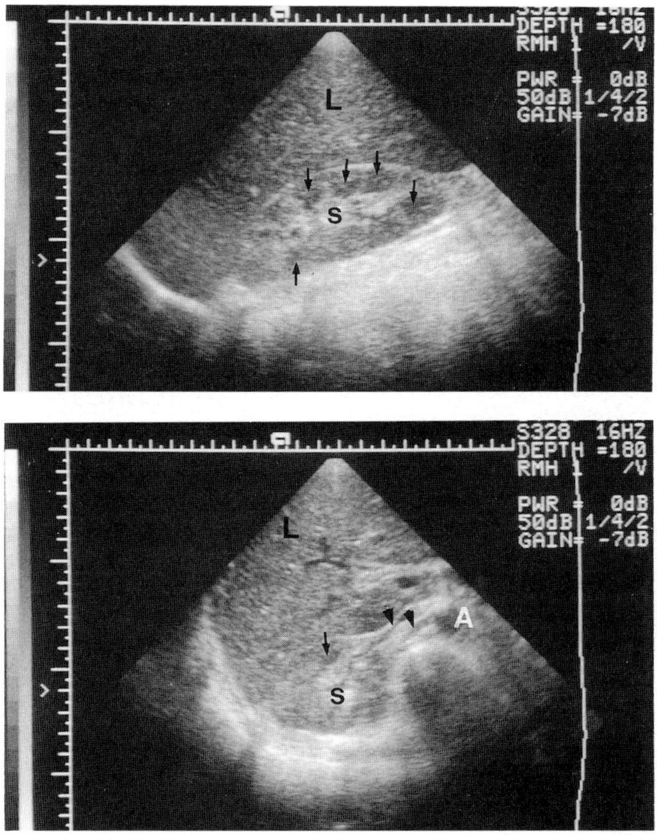

Figure 8. *ULTRASOUND OF THE NORMAL KIDNEY. A longitudinal section of the right kidney (a) showing the echogenic central renal sinus (S) surrounded by parenchyma in which the relatively echo poor pyramids (arrows) can be identified. In transverse section (b) through the hilum, the renal vessels can be identified (arrowheads), with the vein anterior. [L=liver; A=aorta.]*

On ultrasound images the kidneys appear as incomplete layered structures with an overall ovoid shape in longitudinal sections and a rounded shape in transverse sections (Fig. 8) [16]. Their surfaces are usually smooth, but may be scalloped due to fetal lobation the position of the indentations over the interlobar septa distinguishes them from scars which are centred on a lobe. The vessels and fat in the hilum give rise to intense central echoes which usually occupy about one third of the thickness of the kidney at its the mid-portion.

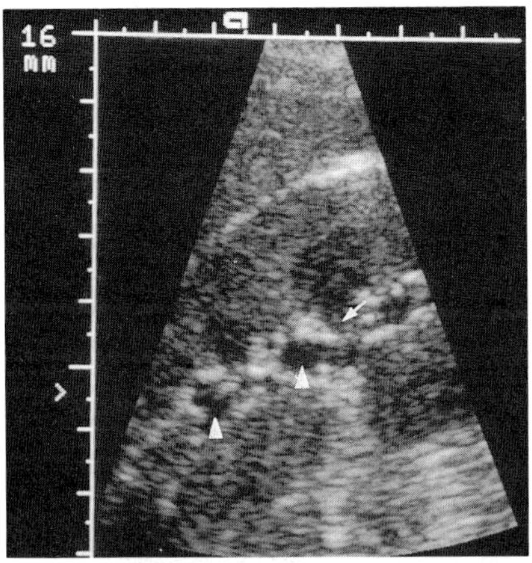

(a)

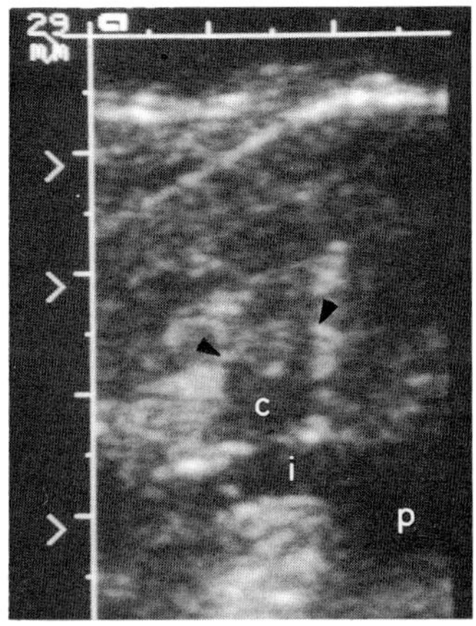

(c)

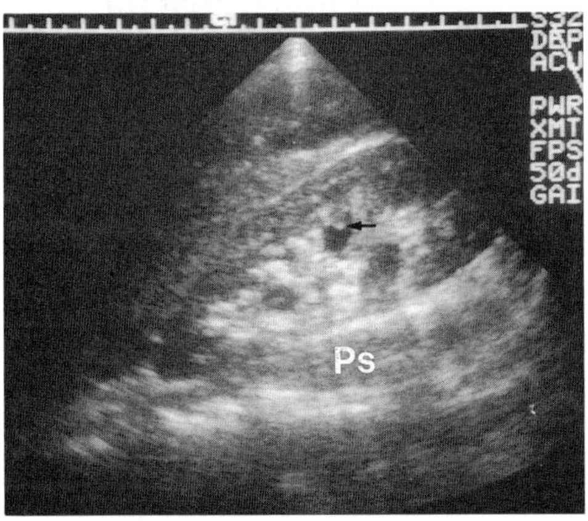

(b)

Figure 9. *LOBAR ANATOMY OF THE KIDNEY ON ULTRASOUND. Detailed views of the kidney show the pyramidal shape of the medulla (a) with the apex (arrow) directed towards the sinus. Vascular structures and portions of the collecting system are seen as echo free spaces in the hilum (arrowheads). The peripheral portions of the pelvi-caliceal system can be identified when it contains some fluid (b & c). The tip of the pyramid (papilla, arrow) indents the calix peripherally so that the pyramid rests in the calix like an egg in an egg cup. Typically the papilla is echogenic and similarly reflective foci may be apparent at the fornices of the calices (arrowheads) (c=calix; i=infundibulum; p=pelvis; Ps=psoas muscle).*

The two components of the parenchyma can be discerned, the more reflective cortical layer enveloping the echo-poor medullary pyramid (Fig. 9). The exact pattern visualized depends on the tomographic projection: the deeper-lying medulla forms pyramidal, oval or rounded regions which are best seen in sagittal or coronal views through the mid-part of the kidney, but are also identified in transverse sections and at the poles. The larger, heart-shaped compound pyramids can be distinguished from the smaller, rounded simple pyramids (Fig. 10) [17]. The interlobar septa of Bertin are seen as blocks of more echogenic tissue, continuous with the peripheral cortex but

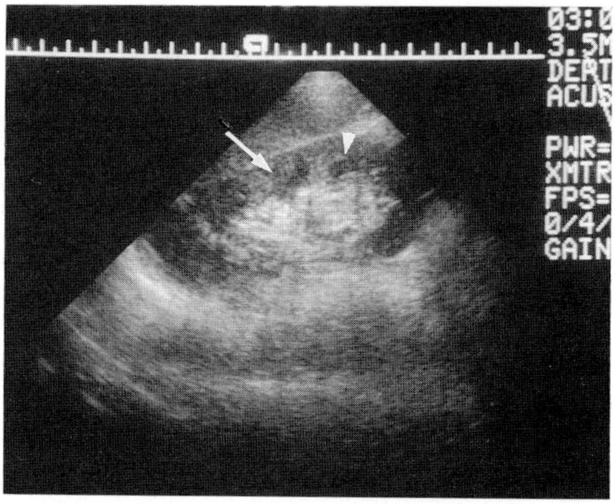

Figure 10. *TYPES OF MEDULLARY PYRAMIDS. The larger, heart-shaped compound pyramids (arrow) can be distinguished from the smaller rounded simple pyramids (arrowhead) in this longitudinal ultrasound scan.*

extending towards the sinus (Fig. 11). The echo intensity and texture of these two cortical regions are identical. The cortex is normally somewhat less intense than the hepatic or splenic echoes though in some normal subjects they may be equally reflective. The sinus is very much more, and the medulla rather less reflective than the cortex.

In the fetus and neonate the kidney has a markedly different appearance with stronger echoes from the cortex and prominent medullary pyramids that produce high contrast between the cortex and medulla (Fig. 12) (Table 1). The cortical echoes are more intense than those of the liver. These differences from the adult are attributable to the immature structure of the still-developing kidney.

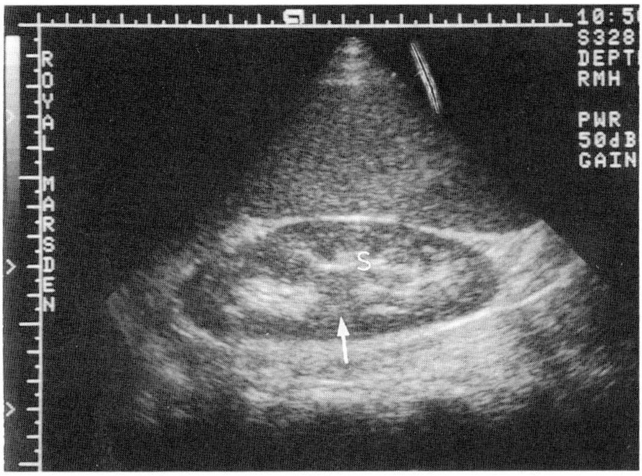

(a)

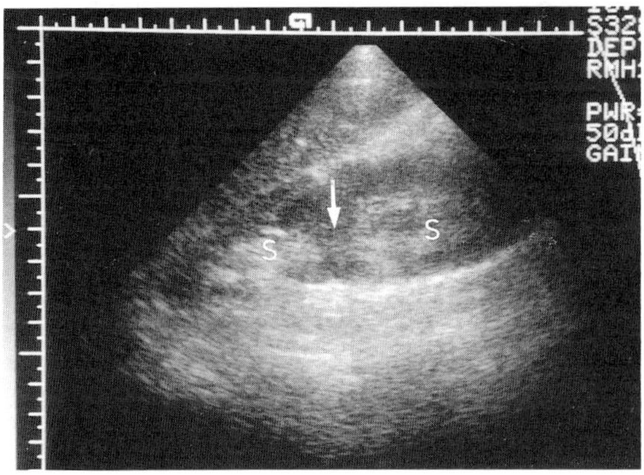

(b)

Figure 11. *SEPTA OF BERTIN. When the interlobar cortical tissue is prominent, blocks of tissue may be demonstrated apparently distorting (a) or even bisecting (b) the renal sinus layer, raising the suspicion of a mass. Their continuity with the peripheral cortex and identical echo pattern indicate their true nature as an anatomical variant. A normal vascular pattern on a colour Doppler study provides further confirmation (S=sinus).*

Although the full complement of nephrons is present by 36 weeks of gestation, the glomeruli are more cellular and are tightly packed together because the intervening tubules have not yet achieved their mature length. As the tubules grow, they separate the glomeruli and the cortex thickens so that the echogenicity falls to the adult level by about four months of age. The prominence of the pyramids is relative; it occurs because they form earliest during nephrogenesis

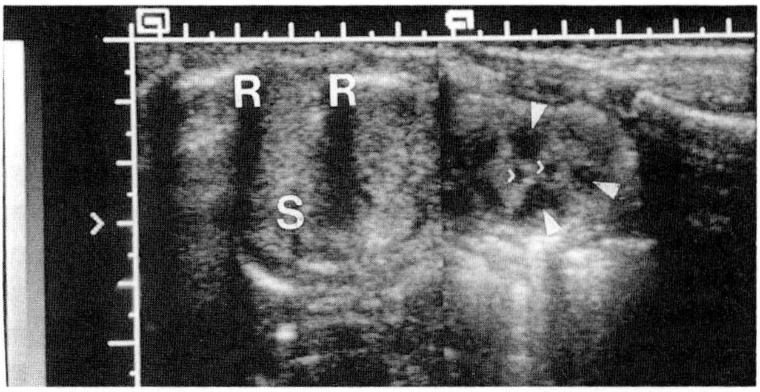

Figure 12. *NEONATAL KIDNEY. The internal anatomy of the neonatal kidney differs markedly from the adult pattern. The cortex is more reflective and the pyramids (arrowheads) are relatively larger and echo poor while the lack of fat within the sinus makes it strikingly inapparent. At the same time, physiological filling of the collecting system renders tubular elements visible in the hilar region (>) (R=ribs; S=spleen).*

Table 1. *Differences between the neonatal and adult kidney*

	Neonatal	Adult
Contour	lobed	smooth usually
Cortex reflectivity	++	+
Medulla size	+ (relatively)	=
echoes	--	-
Sinus	echo poor	echogenic
PCS	often apparent	usually inapparent

and therefore achieve their mature size before the cortex. In the neonate the renal sinus is almost devoid of fat so that it is inconspicuous and much less echogenic than in the mature kidney while the constant diuretic state means that some filling of the collecting system is commonly observed. To these differences must be added the prominence of the fetal lobations in the neonate. Thus it can be appreciated that the neonatal kidney may appear startlingly different from the mature kidney of a child or adult. At first sight it may be considered abnormal, a common error being the misinterpretation of the pyramids as dilated calices.

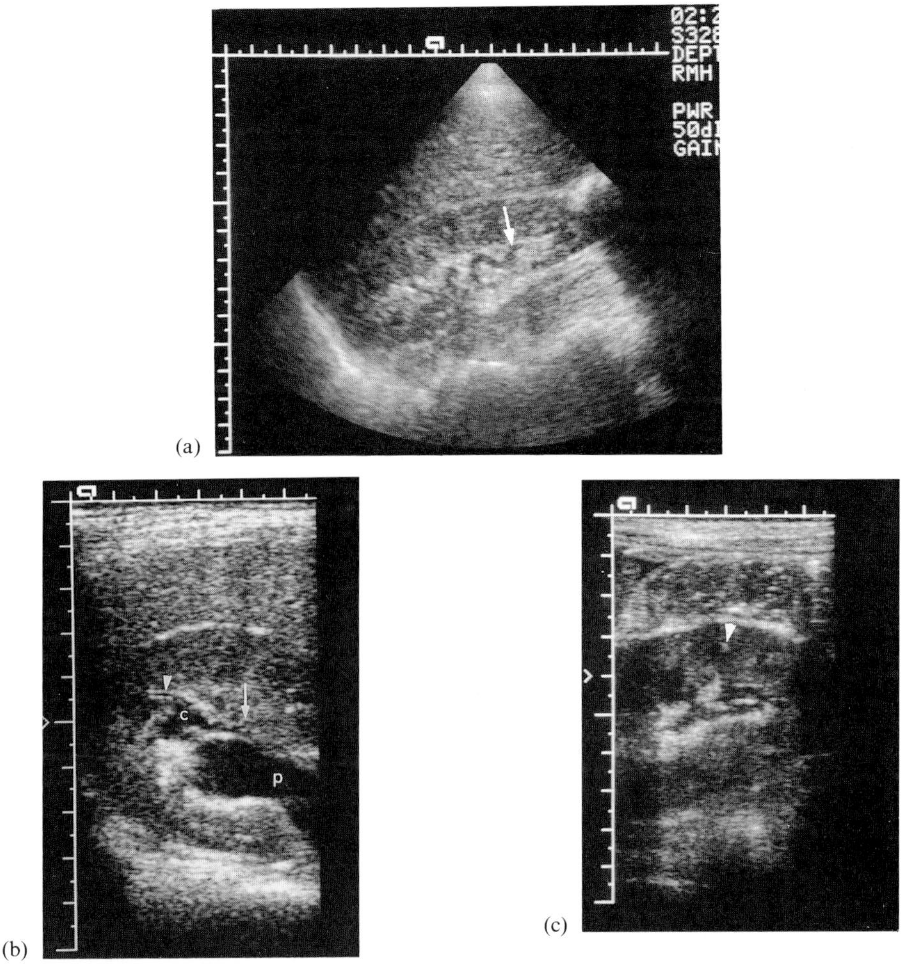

Figure 13. *INTRARENAL VESSELS. Tortuous or branching vessels that can sometimes be discerned in the hilum (arrows in (a) and (b) and parenchyma represent segmental and interlobar branches. Since long infundibula can have a similar appearance, Doppler is required for confirmation.Unless imaging conditions are exceptional, the lumina of the arcuate vessels are too small to be resolved (arrowhead in (b)) but they can usually be identified as echogenic foci at the cortico-medullary junction (arrowhead in (c)) (P=pelvis).*

Using ultrasound, the position of the kidney is readily ascertained, as is the lie of its hilum. When imaging is clear, vascular structures can be made out within the sinus, arteries being distinguishable from veins by the vigorous pulsation of the former and the flowing particles in the latter (Fig. 13) - colour Doppler provides a more direct evaluation. Depending on the quality of imaging, segmental or interlobar vessels may be traced as they divide into arcuates which penetrate the cortical septa and curve around the cortico-medullary junction; usually however, the arcuate vessels are seen only as punctate echogenic foci, one or two at the periphery of each pyramid.

The extra-renal blood vessels may be traced between the aorta or inferior vena cava and the renal hilum. The right renal artery is most readily identified in its typical postcaval position on a sagittal scan through the inferior vena cava as a tubular structure with a diameter of about 5 mm (Fig. 14). It passes postero-laterally over the right crus of the diaphragm which must be separately identified to avoid confusion. When imaging is good, the initial segmental branches can also be detected.

The left renal artery is the most difficult of the four renal vessels and is only sometimes visualized from the epigastrium where it may be seen lying on the crus of diaphragm. Coronal views may reveal it running in an infero-lateral direction from the aorta, looking much like a rose thorn. Occasionally it may be traced out into the kidney.

The short right renal vein may be imaged either from the epigastrium or from the right flank as it passes from the renal hilum directly into the posterior or postero-lateral aspect of the inferior vena cava (Fig. 15). Seen in transverse section at the inferior vena cava it may appear as a beak on the lateral surface of the vein. A similar appearance indicates the termination of the left renal vein, a length of which can usually be traced from just outside the kidney across into the inferior vena cava. This vessel is readily visualized in its characteristic position, sandwiched between the aorta and the superior mesenteric artery while its typical upstream dilatation is easily visible. The 'dilatation' may be so marked as to suggest obstruction and it may be confused with a left para-aortic mass.

Positive identification of the collecting system depends on the presence of at least a trace of urine, otherwise the strong echoes from its walls merge with the sinus so that the collecting system cannot be discerned. Even physiological amounts of urine separating the layers of the pelvi-caliceal system gives an echo-free line or space (Fig. 16).

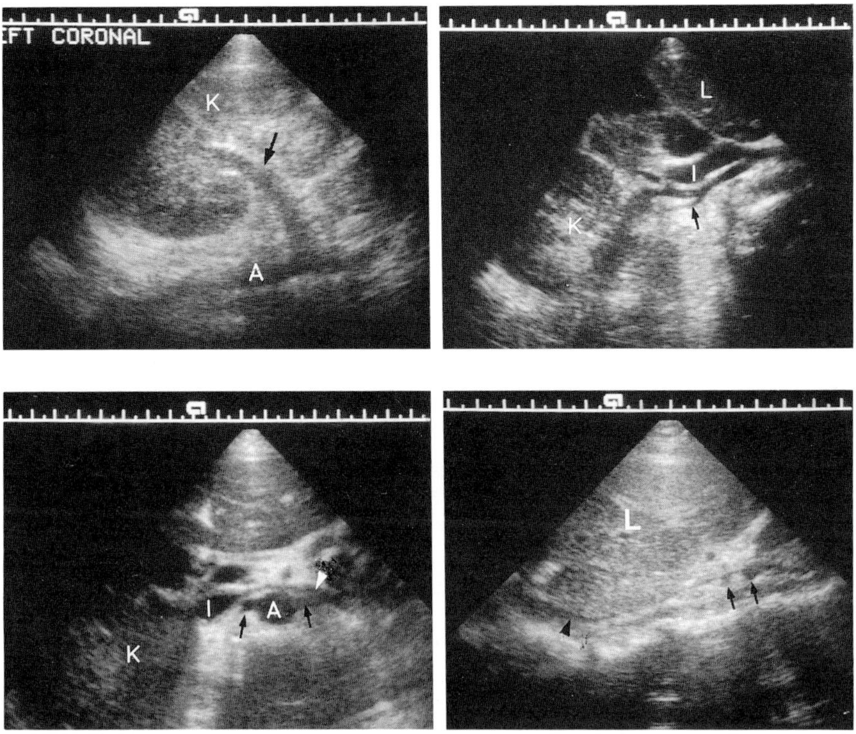

(a) (b) (c) (d)

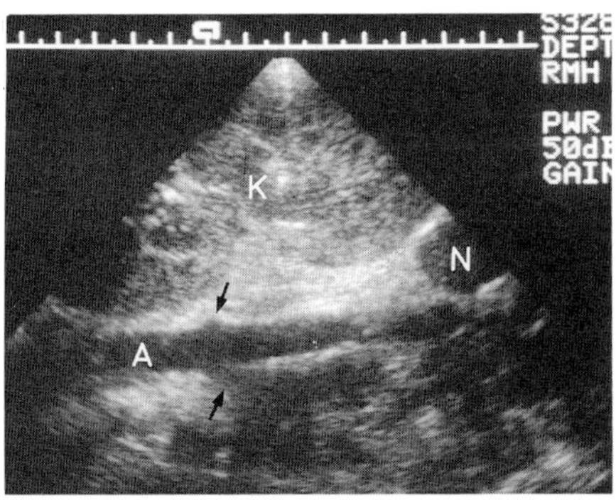

(e)

Figure 14. *RENAL ARTERY. The right renal artery can usually be identified posterior to the inferior vena cava (arrow in (a)) in this example the artery is double (arrowheads). In transverse section through the epigastrium (b) it is often possible to detect the origins of one or both renal arteries (arrows) but they are more readily identified in coronal sections through the flank as thornlike projections from the aorta (arrows in (c)). When superior imaging combine with a fortuitous lie, the length of the artery can be made out (arrow) in (d)) together with segmental branches (arrow in (e)) (A=aorta; I=inferior vena cava; K=kidney; L=liver; N=node, enlarged in this patient with Hodgkin's disease; white arrowhead=left renal vein.*

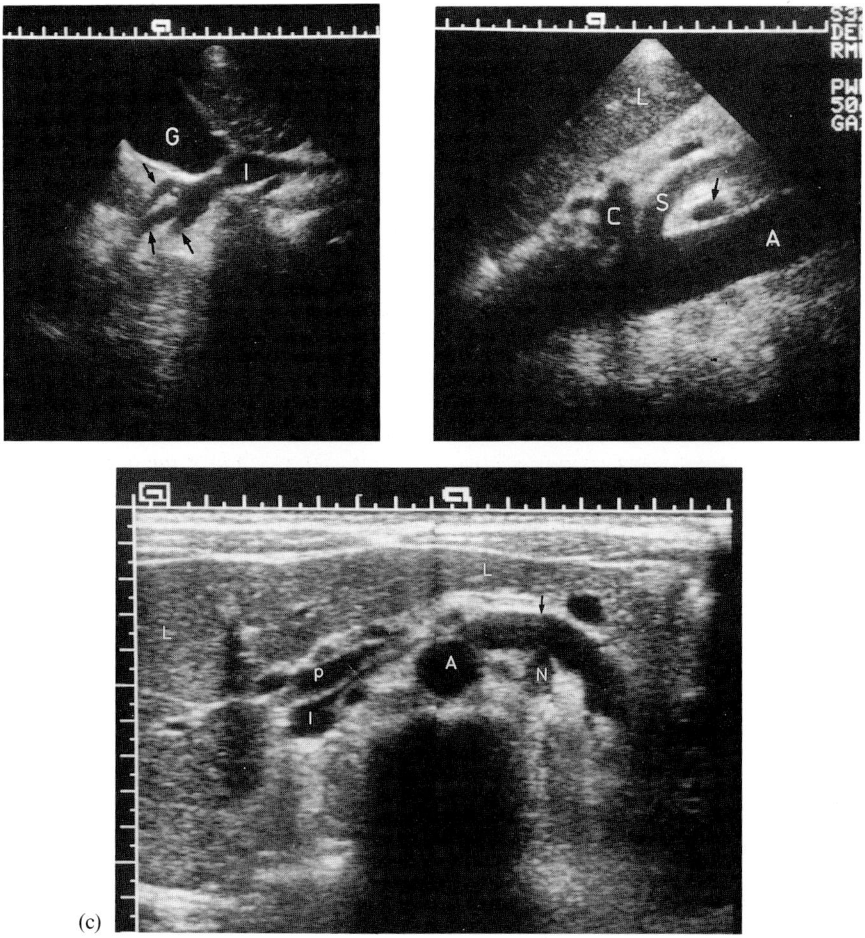

(a) (b) (c)

Figure 15. *RENAL VEINS. The right renal vein is often visualized in transverse sections in the epigastrium as it enters the postero-lateral aspect of the cava. Under favourable imaging conditions, the segmental branches may be demonstrated emerging from the renal hilum (arrows in (a)).The left renal vein is regularly imaged as it crosses the aorta where it lies posterior to the superior mesenteric artery (arrow in (b)); at this point it may be narrowed antero-posteriorly with upstream dilatation that may be so marked as to suggest obstruction (c). This is, in fact, a normal variant (the patient in (c) has para-aortic lymphadenopathy (N)) (A=aorta; G=gall-bladder; I=inferior vena cava; L=liver; S=superior mesenteric artery).*

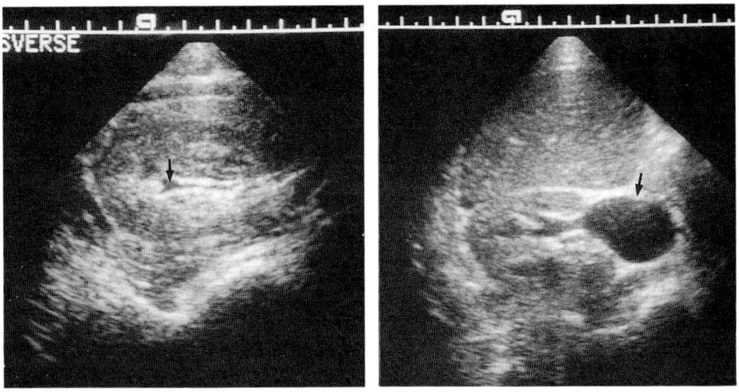

(a) (b)

Figure 16. *PELVIC 'SPLITTING'. Even physiological amounts of urine in the collecting system render it visible with pelvis extending medially in the renal hilum (arrow in (a)). Where the pelvis is baggy (arrow in b)) the filling may be marked but remain within normal limits.*

The pelvis is seen as a linear fluid space within the renal sinus; it may extend medially out of the kidney when there is an extra-renal component. The infundibula may be traced as tubular spaces passing out from the pelvis and expanding into the calices. The calices have a complex pattern, each forming a cup-shape around the tip of its corresponding pyramid (Fig. 17). Often three echogenic spots can be discerned, one at the papilla (presumably from the walls of the larger

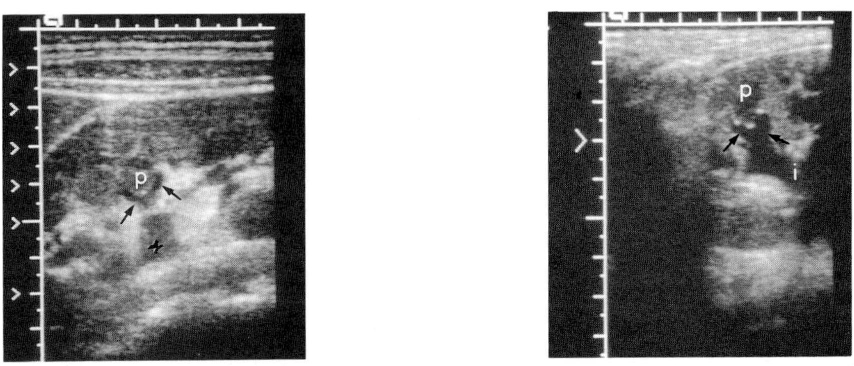

(a) (b)

Figure 17. *THE FILLED CALIX. The cup-shape of the calix is well shown when it is filled, either physiologically (a) or in mild hydronephrosis (b). The arrangement of the papillary tip of the medullary pyramid (p) set in the egg-cup shape of the calix (arrows) is revealed. Note the echogenic foci at the papillary tip and at the fornices of the calix. (i=infundibulum; p=pyramid).*

collecting ducts) and one each of the fornices (perhaps due to the apposed layers of the calix). These form a triple dot pattern that is more clearly seen when the calices are distended.

Physiological filling is attributable to two factors, diuresis and delay in emptying of the pelvis; they may be combined. Increased production of urine occurs in the fluid loaded subject a common situation in abdomino-pelvic ultrasound and whenever the kidney is required to carry an increased amount of fluid, for example in diabetes (both mellitus and insipidus), in the recovery phase of acute tubular necrosis, when there is only one functioning kidney and in response to diuretic drugs. An important instance is the kidney of the newborn whose concentrating power is not fully developed; the neonate is in a constant diuretic state. Delay in emptying is most commonly caused by a very full bladder again a situation commonly encountered in ultrasound scanning and can be eliminated by bladder emptying.

The distinction between physiological filling and pathological dilatation of the collecting system (most often due to obstruction, though other processes such as vesico-ureteric reflux, pyelonephritis and congenital widening must be born in mind) may be difficult, though attention to some details may be helpful. Physiological filling is nearly always symmetrical, affecting both kidneys equally (except where one is damaged or missing) and of minor degree (amounting to no more than 5 mm separation of the layers of the pelvis. There is never any flattening of the tips of the papillae, an early sign of parenchymal damage in hydronephrosis (Fig. 18). Removal of the precipitating cause by rescanning after bladder emptying or in a non-diuretic state (where this is possible) clinches the issue, though not always conveniently because of the delay involved. Two dynamic signs may prove useful: with patient observation it may be possible to observe peristalsis of the upper tract, seen as muscular contractions of the calices or infundibula and sometimes also of the pelvis itself (Fig. 19). In the patient under diuresis, peristalsis can be expected to occur with increased frequency while it is suppressed in a true obstruction. The same information can be acquired by studying the frequency of ureteric jets into the bladder either on real time (by setting the scanner gain sufficiently high) or using colour Doppler. The second change that may prove helpful is the finding that colour flow signals are increased in the acutely obstructed kidney whereas they are normal in physiological filing. At present this is a rather subjective

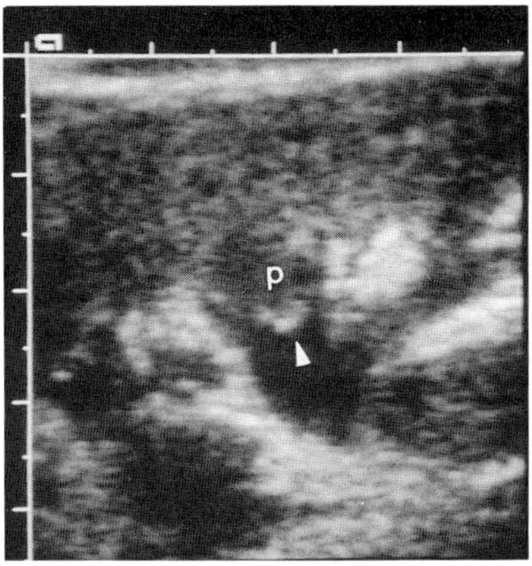

(a)

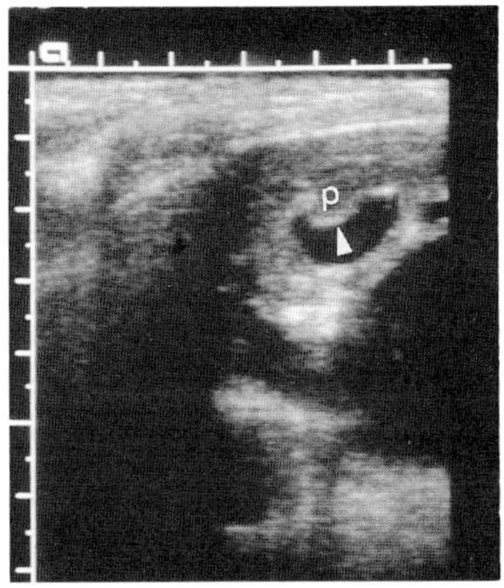

(b)

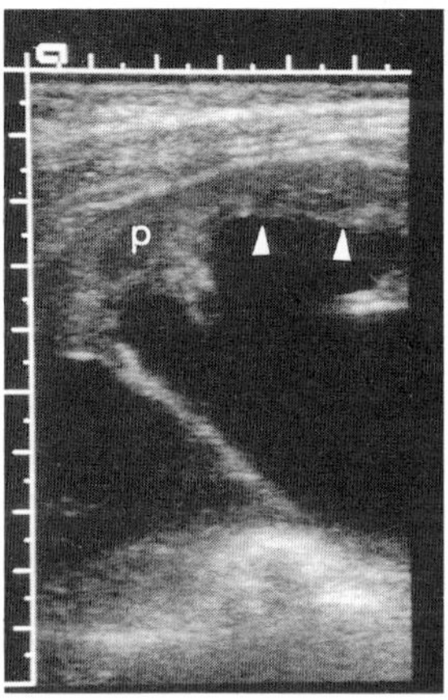

(c)

Figure 18. *PAPILLARY FLATTENING. In physiological filling the papillary tips retain their pointed shape (arrowhead in (a)); flattening (arrowheads in (b) and (c)) signifies parenchymal damage and therefore is always pathological (p=pyramid).*

observation but refinement can be expected with improved technology so that this may become routinely available.

The muscles forming the renal bed are usually obvious, especially psoas, with its characteristic inferior expansion; a positive identification is easily made by observing the movement of the muscle fibres in real-time during hip flexion. Quadratus lumborum is a thinner, strip-like muscle. The diaphragmatic crura are important landmarks, forming echo-poor bands closely applied to the lumbar spine; they must not be confused with the renal arteries, a distinction that can be verified using Doppler.

The fat around the kidneys is usually strongly echogenic and featureless. When high resolution images are obtained, structure may

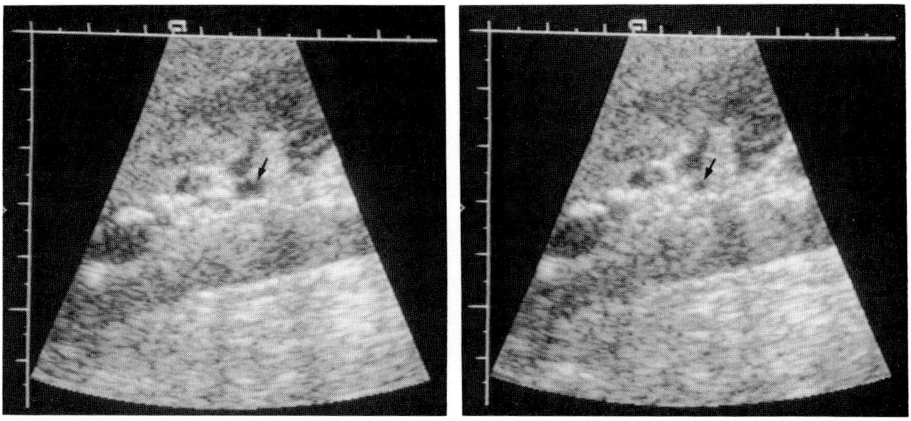

(a) (b)

Figure 19. *PERISTALSIS IN THE INFUNDIBULUM/PELVIS. These two frames taken a few seconds apart from a video recording demonstrate the rapid and rhythmic changes in calibre (arrows) that are typical of active peristalsis in the pelvicaliceal system. The exact nature of the structure examined is uncertain its oval shape suggests that it is an infundibulum seen in cross section.*

be discerned within it, provided the gain levels are not set too high. It is sometimes possible to make out parts of the renal (Gerota's) fascia as an echo-poor line, most readily identified laterally and over the upper pole (Fig. 20). This fascia is not often visualized on ultrasound, presumably because both the fascia and the fat are echogenic.

Variations and Developmental Anomalies

Position

The normal mobility of the kidney with respiration and posture is easily demonstrated with ultrasound [18]. In some patients this gravitational movement may be so extreme that the kidney descends into the pelvis when the patient stands (Fig. 21). This mobility is presumably due to laxity of the suspensory ligaments of the kidney (e.g. the lieno-renal ligament). During such ptosis the kidney takes its blood vessels and ureter with it, in contradistinction to the true ectopic pelvic kidney whose ureter is short and whose vessels tend to

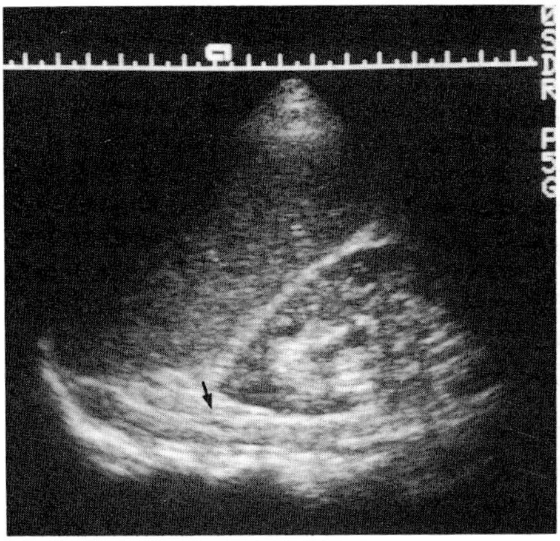
(a)

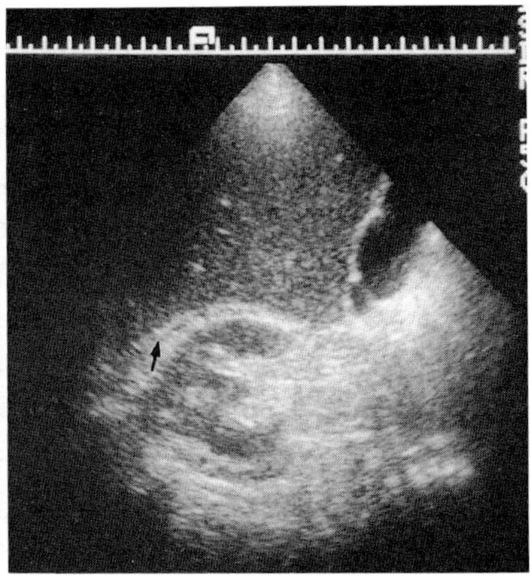
(b)

Figure 20. *PERIRENAL TISSUES. The amount of fat around the kidneys varies with body habitus; it is usually strongly reflective and therefore masks the fascial layers (of Gerota), though occasionally portions can be made out as relatively echo-poor lines (arrows).*

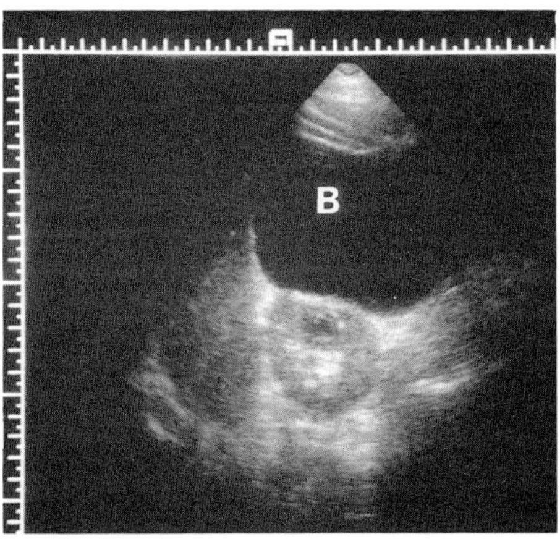

Figure 21. *PELVIC KIDNEY. A pelvic kidney may be most confusing on ultrasound because of its unexpected position and the dilatation of the collecting system due to the anterior rotation of the hilum that is often associated (B=bladder).*

arise from the distal aorta. Pelvic kidneys are particularly difficult to detect on ultrasound since they are obscured by bowel gas.

The kidney may be 'rotated' from its normal position, most commonly with its hilum facing anteriorly. Slight compromise of drainage, producing a mild hydronephrosis, is often associated.

An anomaly of renal ascent may result in one kidney lying in the opposite renal bed (crossed ectopia) [19-22]. The ectopic kidney lies inferior to the normal one and there is usually fusion of the contiguous poles. It retains its own blood supply and its ureter also crosses the midline to insert into the trigone of the bladder on the side of its origin, though the malrotation that commonly coexists may produce mild but chronic obstruction of the pelvis.

A common variant of fusion (1:1000) is the horseshoe kidney in which the two lower poles are joined across the midline. Its ascent is arrested by the first midline aortic branch it encounters; this is usually the inferior mesenteric artery so the renal bridge lies across the aorta, a few centimeters above the umbilicus. The bridge may contain functioning renal parenchyma or may simply be a fibrous band. The arrested ascent interferes with the normal rotation of the kidney so that the lower poles lie medially (often overlying the lumbar vertebra) and the renal sinuses face anteriorly with the pelves and ureters emerging over the front of the kidney where their emptying may be compromised. The renal vessels are low lying, the arteries arising just above the aortic bifurcation or even from the common iliacs. The joining bridge may be difficult to detect on ultrasound because of overlying gas while a fleshy bridge is easily mistaken for pre-aortic lymphadenopathy. The most useful indicator of a horseshoe kidney is the malrotation of the kidneys: a low-lying kidney with its lower pole drawn medially may be the only clue and should prompt a search for the midline bridge.

Number

Renal agenesis is due to a developmental failure of the ureteric duct system so that absence of the kidney is associated with absence both of the ureter and the associated bladder trigone (hemitrigone). In bilateral agenesis no urine is produced resulting in oligohydramnios; since amniotic fluid is essential for lung maturation (without it, surfactant fails to form), the neonate dies with lung hypoplasia. Unilateral agenesis, by contrast, is well compensated for by hypertrophy of the remaining kidney and is compatible with a normal life. Absence of a kidney is difficult to establish with ultrasound because ectopia and extreme atrophy (e.g. involution of a multicystic dysplastic kidney), both of which are commoner, also lead to apparent absence of the kidney from the renal fossa. Urography or isotope renography are more reliable.

Renal hypoplasia, in which the kidney is small with few but normally formed nephrons but a reduced number of renal lobes and calices, is rare (Fig. 22). It presumably arises from a partial developmental failure. Distinguishing this from post-ischaemic or post-infective atrophy depends on the demonstration of the characteristic anatomical features and the absence of scarring; this may be apparent on the urogram but pathological examination is usually required. Ultrasound is unlikely to offer sufficient anatomical resolution to establish these distinctions.

(a) 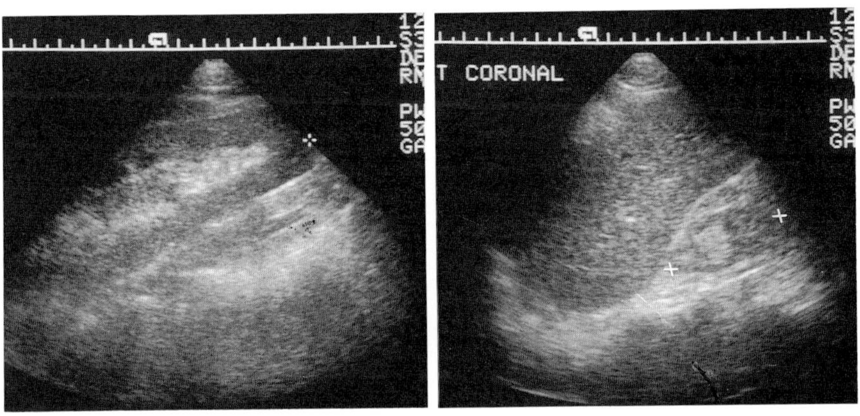 (b)

Figure 22. *HYPOPLASTIC LEFT KIDNEY. This small left kidney was accompanied by a hypertrophied right kidney (15 cm) indicating that the changes were longstanding. The distinction between true developmental hypoplasia and a shrunken diseased kidney may not be possible on ultrasound since it depends on demonstrating normal architecture, and preferably, a reduced number of renal lobes in the small kidney.*

Renal duplication, however, is very common and spans a range from complete to minimal. The various forms result from unusually early division of the ureteric buds so that the arrangement of the collecting system provides the key to the patterns: if the first division of the ureteric bud occurs at the renal pelvis, the standard ('normal') pattern arises with a simple pelvis. A slightly early division gives a bifid or divided pelvis while an earlier division still results in duplication of the ureter, either with fusion at some point along its length or with complete duplication and two separate ureteric orifices (Fig. 23). Even in major divisions on the collecting system, the renal substance remains as a single mass, though the line of fusion of the upper and lower moieties is often evident on the renal surface as an oblique groove (Fig. 24) [23,24]. Often the lower moiety protrudes laterally, forming a hump.

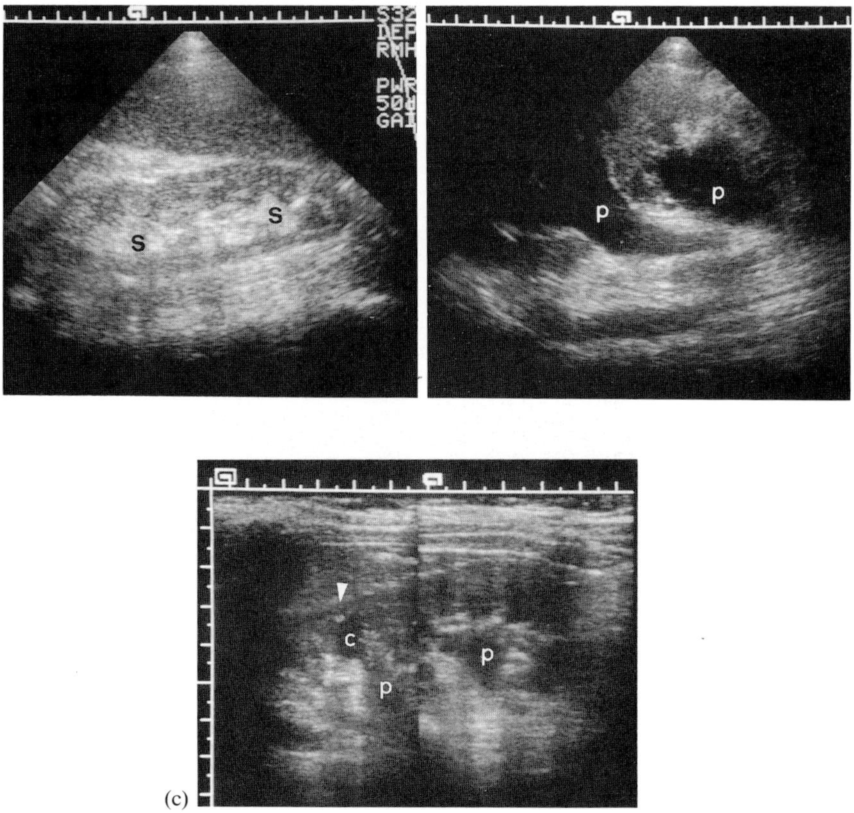

(a) (b) (c)

Figure 23. *DUPLICATED COLLECTING SYSTEM. Often all that can be demonstrated on ultrasound in duplication of the collecting system is an elongated kidney (a) perhaps with separation of the renal sinus (S) into two portions and in many cases even these features are absent. When there is filling of the collecting system, the double pelvis (P) can be visualized (b) together with any parenchymal distortion due to reflux nephropathy (arrowhead indicates thinned cortex, c indicates dilated calix in (c)).*

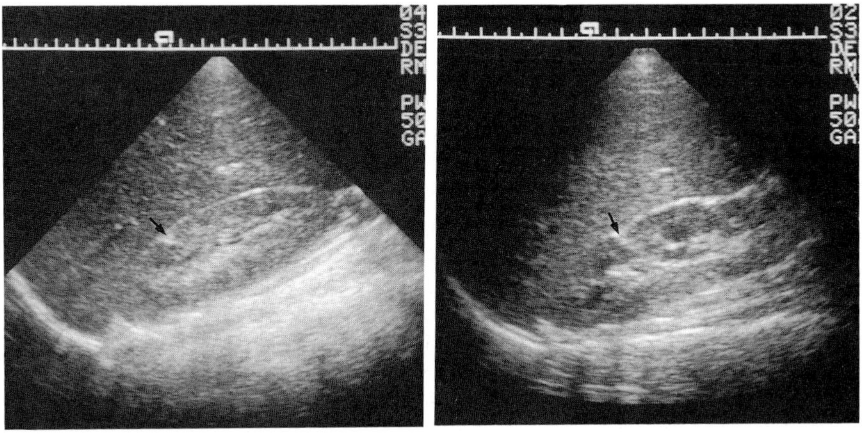

(a) (b)

Figure 24. *INTER-RENUNCULAR FISSURE. An echogenic line (arrows) often marks the junction between two embryonic moieties of the kidney. Its typical position in the upper part of the kidney and its oblique lie help distinguish this normal variant from renal scarring.*

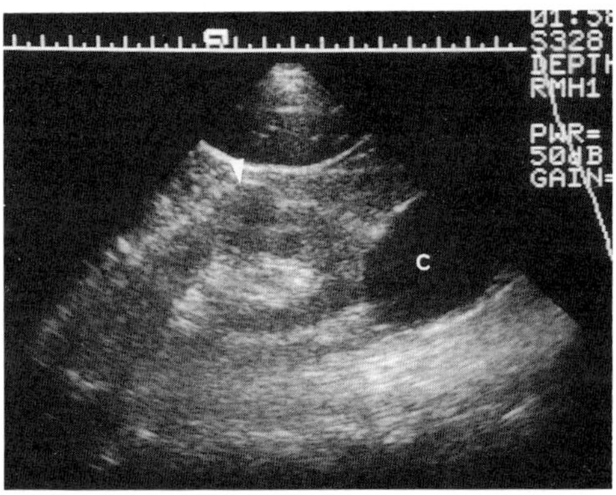

Figure 25. *RENAL HUMP. A protrusion (arrowhead) from the lateral border of the kidney at first sight suggests a tumour mass but the fact that its echoes are the same as those of the surrounding cortex indicate that this is normal tissue. Colour Doppler reveals a normal vascular pattern, providing further reassurance that this is a normal variant and not a tumour mass. (Note the simple cyst, C, at the lower pole).*

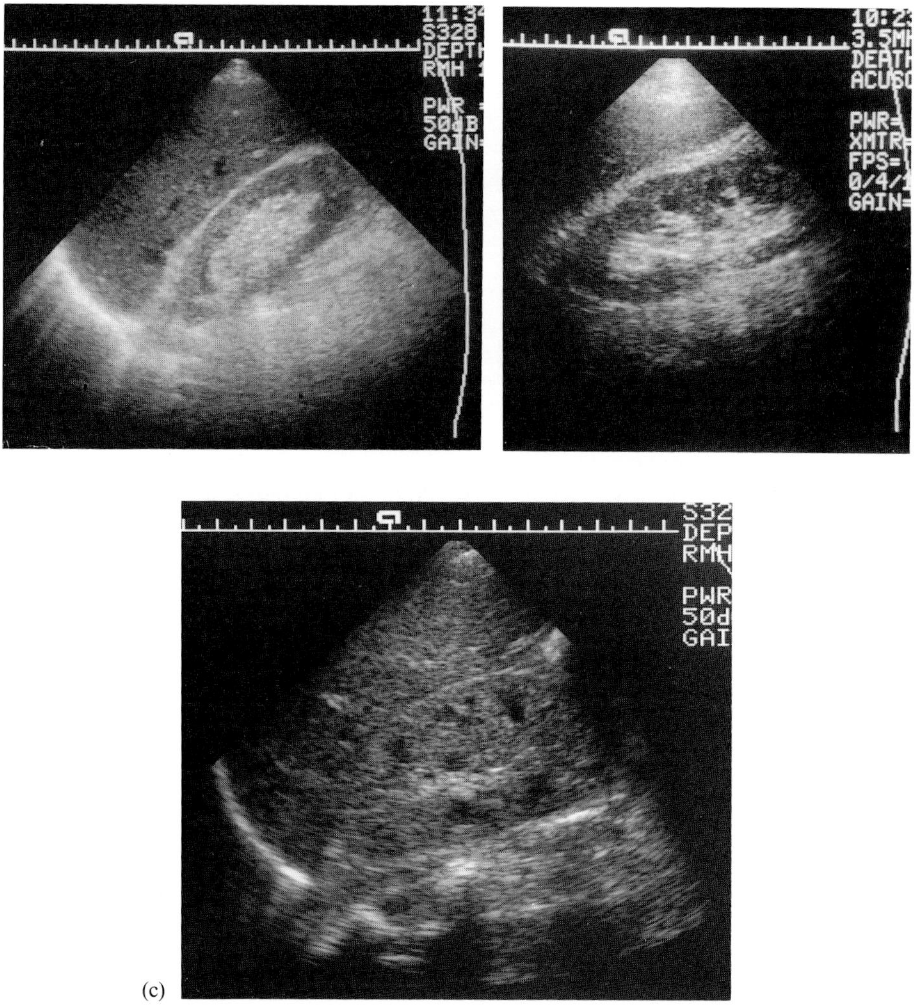

(a) (b) (c)

Figure 26. *VARIATIONS IN RENAL SINUS FAT. The amount of fat in the renal sinus varies within wide limits; excessive fat (a), commonly encountered in obese individuals, widens the sinus layer compared with the 'normal' (b), but the appearance is not confusing. Unusually small amounts of fat (c) changes the overall appearance by removing the striking echogenic layer, so that the kidney may seem abnormal. This pattern is sometimes seen in grossly undernourished patients such as those undergoing chemotherapy.*

These humps form a common variety of renal 'pseudo-tumour', normal variants that mimic mass lesions on the IVU (Fig. 25). They are easily distinguished on CT or ultrasound, as is the other common variety, the so-called 'hypertrophic' septum of Bertin (see Fig. 11).

The amount of fat in the renal sinus is extremely variable; most commonly the sinus is approximately equal in thickness to each parenchymal layer, but in obese subjects an increase in fat thickens the sinus layer (sinus lipomatosis). When there is parenchymal atrophy, additional fat may be laid down in the sinus, in effect replacing the lost renal bulk; this 'replacement sinus lipomatosis' means that conventional measurements of renal size underestimate the loss of functional tissue. Absence of sinus fat is normal in the neonate; it occurs in some disease states, notably in severe renal transplant rejection. Fat free sinus is also encountered in gross cachexia (most often seen in malignancy, especially during chemotherapy) and produces a confusing appearance where the kidney may not be recognizable or at first sight seem to be abnormal (Fig. 26).

Renal Vessels

Variations of the renal arteries are so common that the normal pattern is a statistical concept. Double renal arteries occur in 25% of normal kidneys and are even commoner in ectopic kidneys. Each artery supplies its own part of the kidney without anastomoses. The two arteries usually arise a centimeter or so apart and enter the renal hilum together, though sometimes the additional artery arises more superiorly or inferiorly and enters one of the renal poles directly.

Double renal arteries are usually easy to detect on the right in sagittal sections through the inferior vena cava. Two vessels are seen in cross section lying posterior to the cava (see Fig. 14). Because of the variable level of the arteries, a normal ultrasound appearance does not exclude duplication; angiography remains the definitive technique.

The renal veins are rather less variable than the arteries, though two or more may drain the right kidney, emptying directly into the inferior vena cava (20%). On the left anomalies are rarer, but the vein may pass posterior to the aorta (some 2% of subjects); more commonly the vein is duplicated, with one crossing anterior and the other posterior to the aorta, the so-called circumaortic left renal vein. These variants are difficult to demonstrate on ultrasound.

References

1. Chisholm GD, Williams DI (eds). *Scientific Foundations of Urology*. London: Heineman, 1982.
2. Gosling JA, Dixon JS. Embryology of the Urinary Tract. In Whitfield HN, Hendry WF (eds). *Textbook of Genito-urinary Surgery*, chapter 8. Edinburgh: Churchill Livingstone, 1986.
3. Patriquin H, Lefaivre JF, Lafortune M, Russo P, Boisvert J. Fetal lobation. An anatomo-ultrasonographic correlation. *J Ultrasound Med* 1990;**9:**191-7.
4. Netter FH. *Kidneys, Ureters and Urinary Bladder* (The Ciba Collection of Medical Illustrations. Volume 6). Summit, New Jersey: Ciba-Geigy, 1973.
5. Hollinshead WH. *Anatomy for Surgeons, Volume 2: Thorax, Abdomen and Pelvis*, 3rd edition. New York: Harper and Row, 1985.
6. McMinn RMH, Hutchins RT. *A Colour Atlas of Human Anatomy*. London: Wolfe Medical Publications, 1977.
7. Davidson AJ. *Radiology of the Kidney*. Philadelphia: Saunders, 1985.
8. Resnick MI, Parker MD (Eds). *Surgical Anatomy of the Kidney*. New York: Futura, 1982.
9. Hederstrom E, Forsberg L. Kidney size in children assessed by ultrasonography and urography. *Acta Radiol Diagn* 1985;**26:**85-91.
10. Dinkel E, Ertel M, Dittrich M. Peters H, Berres M, Schulte-Wissermann H. Kidney size in childhood. Sonographical growth charts for kidney length and volume. *Pediatr Radiol* 1985;**15:**38-43.
11. Friedland GW, Filly R, Goris ML (eds). *Uroradiology, An Integrated Approach*. New York: Churchill Livingstone, 1983.
12. Turnbull DH, Wilson SR, Hine AL, Foster FS. Ultrasonic characterization of selected renal tissues. *Ultrasound Med Biol* 1989;**15:**241-53.
13. Wells PN, Blood flow: insights from ultrasound. *Proc Inst Mech Eng H* 1990;**204**:1-20.
14. Martin KW, McAlister WH, Shackelford GD. Acute renal infarction: diagnosis by Doppler ultrasound. *Pediatr Radio* 1988;**18:**373-6.
15. Ophir J, Parker KJ. Contrast agents in diagnostic ultrasound. *Ultrasound Med Biol* 1989;**15:**319-333.
16. Marchal G, Verbeken E, Oyen R, Moerman F, Baert AL, Lauweryns J. Ultrasound of the normal kidney: a sonographic, anatomic and histologic correlation. *Ultrasound Med Biol* 1986;**2:**999-1009.
17. Jones BE, Hoffer FA, Teele RL, Lebowitz RL. The compound renal pyramid. A normal hypoechoic region on the pediatric sonogram. *J Ultrasound Med* 1987;**6:**515-8.
18. Atlas SW, Rochester D, Panella JS, Larson R. The utility of ultrasound in the diagnosis of wandering abdominal viscera. *J Clin Ultrasound* 1985;**13:**275-7.
19. Slovis TL. Pediatric renal anomalies and infections. *Clin Diagn Ultrasound* 1989;**24:**157-85.
20. Saxey R. Sonographic findings in crossed renal ectopia without fusion. *Am J Roentgenol* 1990;**154:**657.
21. Sheih CP, Liu MB, Hung CS, Yang KH, Chen WY, Lin CY. Renal abnormalities in schoolchildren. *Pediatrics* 1989;**84:**1086-90.
22. Goodman JD, Norton KI, Carr L, Yeh HC. Crossed fused renal ectopia: sonographic diagnosis. *Urol Radiol* 1986;**8:**13-6.
23. Hoffer FA, Hanabergh AM, Teele RL. The interrenicular junction: a mimic of renal scarring on normal pediatric sonograms. *Am J Roentgenol* 1985;**145:**1075-8.
24. Carter AR, Horgan JG, Jennings TA, Rosenfield AT. The junctional parenchymal defect: a sonographic variant of renal anatomy. *Radiology* 1985;**154:**499-50.

Radiologic diagnosis of renal tumours

Leif Ekelund
Department of Diagnostic Radiology, University Hospital, Umeå, Sweden

Introduction

Renal carcinoma often presents with unusual and misleading signs and symptoms and has for this reason been called 'the great imitator'. Even though a number of renal carcinomas are not detected before autopsy, the radiologist has a great responsibility in the early detection of renal tumours. Renal masses are usually found on urography and then further evaluated by various imaging techniques. Angiography used to be the common pre-operative diagnostic procedure but the development of ultrasound, computed tomography (CT) and magnetic resonance imaging (MRI) has changed this concept. This chapter reviews these different examination techniques, discusses their individual diagnostic value and finally suggests a practical diagnostic sequence.

As an introduction, the primary symptoms and signs which indicate that radiological examination is required are discussed. Ekelund & Jonsson [1] reviewed the requests for urography in a 10-year sample of 369 patients with renal carcinoma. All cases were confirmed by surgery or autopsy and the frequency of symptoms that indicated the need for a urogram are shown in Table 1.

Gross haematuria as the main symptom was noted in 121 patients (33%). In many cases the haematuria was of short duration and/or had long symptom-free intervals. The classical triad of gross haematuria, flank pain and a palpable mass was noted in only one patient.

Table 1. *Frequency of symptoms and signs indicating the need for primary urography in 369 patients.**

Symptoms	No of patients
Gross haematuria	121
Silent	49
Pain and discomfort in the abdomen	25
Colic pain	13
Signs of malignancy	13
Palpable abdominal tumour	8
Prostatism	8
Trauma	2
Back pain	2
Polycythaemia	1
Microscopic haematuria	14
Incidental finding	3
Pain and discomfort in the abdomen	7
Signs of malignancy	2
Palpable abdominal tumour	1
Raised ESR	1
Pain and discomfort in the abdomen	16
Only symptom	10
Raised ESR	3
Colic pain	3
Back pain	5
Only symptom	3
Raised ESR	2
Palpable abdominal tumour	24
Only symptom	10
Pain and discomfort in the abdomen	7
Gastrointestinal symptoms	3
Raised ESR	2
Prostatic hyperplasia	2

Symptoms	No of patients
Signs of malignancy	76
Only symptom	40
Pain and discomfort in the abdomen	13
Palpable abdominal tumour	8
Raised ESR only	15
Metastases first diagnosed	49
Lungs	14
Skeleton	30
Brain	2
Soft tissue masses	3
Incidental findings	54
At urography because of:	
prostatism	15
cysto-pyelitis	20
hypertension	12
prostatic carcinoma	2
At urography after angiography	2
At GI-examination	3
Other indications	10
Polycythaemia	2
Pathological renography	2
Gastrointestinal symptoms	2
Raised Ca/s	1
Raised creatinine/s	1
At operation	1
Previously operated renal carcinoma	1

Microscopic haematuria was noted in 14 patients (4%). Pain and discomfort in the abdomen was noted in 16 patients (4%) and back pain in five (1%). A palpable abdominal mass with or without other symptoms was found in 24 patients (7%). Clinical signs of malignancy, including tiredness, fever, loss of weight, anaemia and/or elevated erythrocyte sedimentation rate (ESR) were observed in 76 patients (20%). Forty-nine patients presented with metastatic disease: 14 with lung lesions, 30 with skeletal destructions, two with cerebral symptoms and three with soft tissue masses.

Renal tumour confirmed to be a carcinoma was an incidental finding at urography in 49 patients (13%). The indication for the examination in these patients had been prostatism, cystopyelitis, hypertension and prostatic carcinoma.

Renal carcinoma may be symptom-free for a great part of its course and the figures above show that renal carcinoma may be found on urograms in any patient above the age of 30 years. This emphasizes the importance of high quality urograms, enabling the evaluation of both the renal pelvis and the renal contour.

Urographic Techniques

Plain abdominal radiographs including both kidneys and the bladder should be obtained before contrast medium is administrated. Oblique views may be required to check whether a calcification is located within the kidney or ureter or otherwise.

The contrast dose is variable, depending on patient weight and the different routines which can be employed. For most patients, it is usually not necessary to exceed a dose of 20 g of iodine, except for very overweight patients. Most injections of contrast medium are performed by rapidly being completed within 30-60 seconds. The density of the nephrogram relates directly to the plasma level of contrast media. The type of contrast medium used depends on it's cost and the radiologist's preference. Within the next few years, however, current ionic media will probably be largely replaced by safer, new, low osmolar contrast media, which has already been the case, for example, in Sweden.

If there are no contraindications (e.g. obstruction, recent surgery or abdominal aneurysm) abdominal compression should be applied in order to distend the proximal ureters and the pyelocalyceal system, rendering them fully visible. Three tomograms of 25-30° are routinely used when a renal mass is suspected. Routine use of oblique views has largely given way to tomography but it should be stressed that oblique films are necessary in order to demonstrate anteriorly- or posteriorly-located tumours. After the compression has been released radiographs are again obtained including the kidneys, ureters and the bladder. The number of films used for urography varies, but is usually somewhere between eight and twelve.

Ultrasound

Ultrasound is now well established as an accurate, non-invasive means of evaluating patients with a suspected renal neoplasm. Most authorities agree that sonography is optimally utilized as a complement to other imaging techniques. It should probably not be relied upon as an initial screening procedure in the diagnosis of renal masses. Simple cysts are likely to be readily apparent, but neoplasms - particularly small lesions that do not distort the renal contours or pelvicalyceal system - could be easily missed. A high degree of accuracy should result if patients are referred only for further characterization of a renal mass previously documented by urography. One exception is pregnancy with complications suggestive of a renal neoplasm. Due to the lack of ionizing radiation, ultrasound should virtually always be the first diagnostic tool used in the investigation of genito-urinary problems in obstetric cases.

No specific patient preparation is required for renal mass studies. The principles and techniques of ultrasound scanning have been continuously updated as the technology has advanced. Prone scanning was once the standard means of investigating renal masses for diagnosis and biopsy. Compound and sector scanning were usually required with this approach. Real-time units have added a critical new dimension to ultrasound because of the improved resolution and more versatile scanning. The kidneys can now be quickly examined from an anterior approach and the ease and speed of this technique have now made ultrasound more accessible to many patients. Patient co-operation is no longer an issue since prone scans with respiration suspended are no longer required. Patient physique is the single factor determining transducer selection. As a rule, the highest transducer frequency which permits adequate penetration should be used. A routine renal sonogram might consist of anterior scans done with the patient in right and left posterior oblique positions. Additional supine, erect and decubitus views could be obtained as needed, depending on the location of a mass and the information required. In cases where a malignancy is strongly suspected, survey views of the liver, venous structures and the contralateral kidney can be quickly obtained with real-time scans. This serves as a useful, though less accurate, staging procedure than computed tomography. When the diagnosis of a renal neoplasm has been made, the task of evaluating the renal vascular structures poses many problems. The left renal vein is probably the easiest vessel to demonstrate with sonography due to its length, while, in contrast, the right renal vein is more difficult to visualize because it follows a very short path to the inferior vena cava. Every ultrasound examination of a renal mass should always include an attempt to evaluate the renal veins and the inferior vena cava for possible tumour thrombus.

There are three broad sonographic categories of renal masses - cystic, complex and solid. A mass that fulfills the strict criteria for a cyst should be echo-free, smooth, regularly shaped with thin, sharply marginated walls and demonstrate excellent sound transmission (Fig. 1a). A solid ultrasound pattern is characterized by the presence of internal echoes and acoustic impedance of the sonic beam. These masses are often variable in shape, lacking smooth, well-defined borders. The majority of renal neoplasms, regardless of histological type, are solid on sonograms (Fig. 1b). Complex renal masses are mixed, containing cystic and solid components. This type of pattern may result from necrotic or haemorrhagic neoplasms, complicated renal cysts and inflammatory disorders.

Computed tomography

Computed tomography has largely replaced angiography in the pre-operative evaluation of a renal mass. Non-enhanced scans are obtained with contiguous, 1 cm thick slices. Each slice is taken with respiration suspended. Contiguous 5 mm scans are used in children. When the scan is performed to rule out a mass, contrast medium must be injected even though a mass is not seen on the non-enhanced scans, because a small iso-dense intra-renal mass may be present. Bolus or rapid infusion, or a combination of both, may be used in this situation.

The bolus method is preferred when a renal tumour is identified. Properly performed, the renal mass, renal vein and inferior vena cava are all usually clearly demonstrated (Fig. 2). In the pre-operative

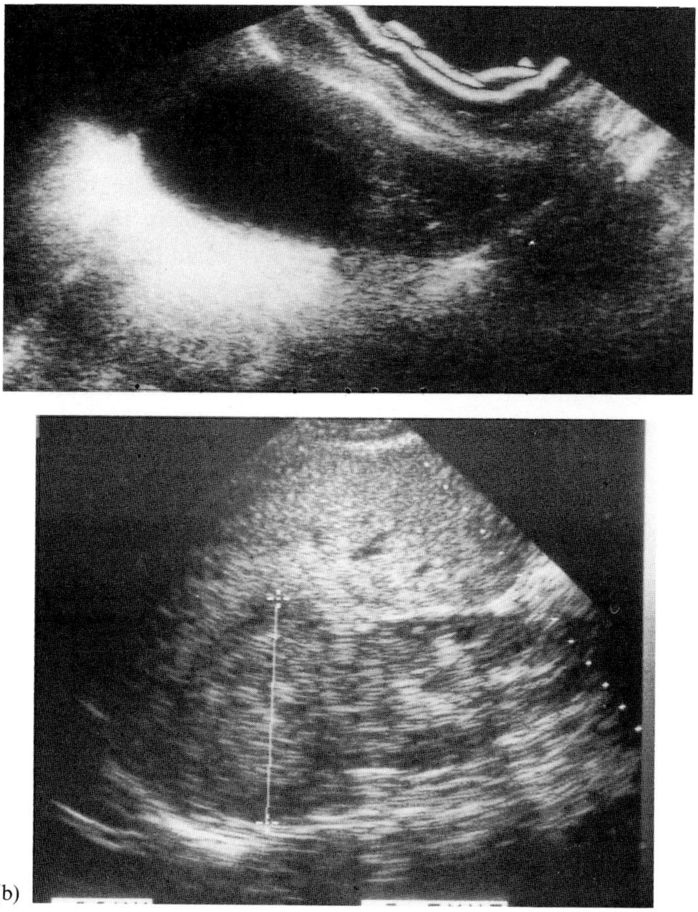

(a)

(b)

Figure 1. *(a) Longitudinal ultrasound scan showing a typical cyst in the upper pole of the kidney. (b) Longitudinal scan showing solid tumour in the upper pole of the kidney.*

examination of a renal malignancy it is the radiologist's responsibility to evaluate the renal veins and the inferior vena cava for possible tumour thrombus as this will influence the pre-operative planning.

A properly performed CT-examination will usually provide sufficient pre-operative information about tumour extent and possible venous involvement. In equivocal cases cavography may still be indicated. Angiography may be helpful in very large neoplasms to

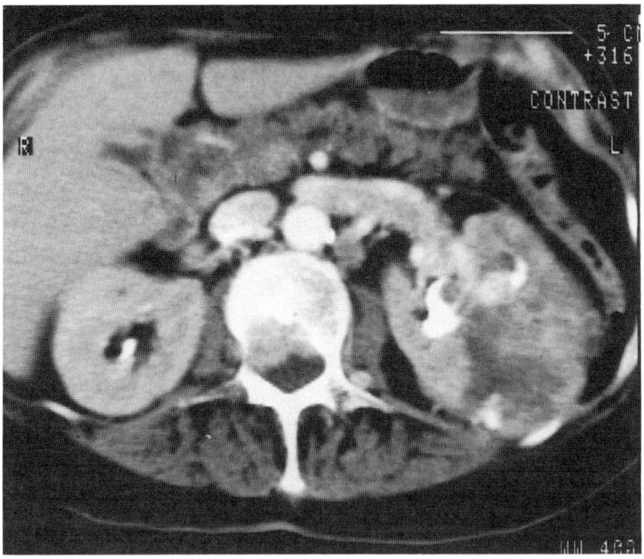

Figure 2. *Contrast-enhanced CT-scan showing large, partly necrotic carcinoma of the left kidney, tumour thrombus of the left renal vein, para-aortic lymph node metastasis and metastatic destruction of the posterior part of the vertebral body.*

demonstrate the vascularization of the mass for the benefit of the surgeon.

Magnetic resonance imaging

The role of MRI in the diagnosis of renal carcinoma has been thoroughly evaluated in two papers, one by Hricak et al [2] and the other by Quint et al [3] and there is also an excellent review by Baumgartner & Chezmar [4]. In the study by Hricak et al, MRI demonstrated 95% of 106 renal cell carcinomas with diameters greater than 3 cm. However, only 62% of the tumours less than 3 cm could be detected. They concluded that MRI can not be used as a screening modality. When, however, renal carcinoma is diagnosed, correct tumour staging is essential for its management. In this regard MRI was excellent, especially in cases where CT-findings were equivocal. In advanced stages, and when large lesions were present, MRI was superior to CT, largely because of direct coronal and sagittal images. In the detection of venous tumour extension into the renal vein and inferior vena cava, MRI had a higher sensitivity and specificity than CT. Also, in depicting lymph node metastases, MRI had a higher accuracy than CT (99% and 83%, respectively). In their opinion, MRI is complementary to CT in the diagnosis of renal tumours but is excellent in staging and eliminates the need for inferior vena cavograms.

The inability of MRI to demonstrate small, especially intra-renal, tumours was investigated by Quint et al [3], both *in vivo* and *in vitro*. They demonstrated that the inherent contrast between tumour and parenchyma is preserved in excised specimens on at least one pulse sequence but is lost during clinical imaging. They suggested that this degradation of *in vivo* images was caused by motion and a relatively poor signal-to-noise ratio obtained with body coils. They concluded that although MRI does not yet compete with CT in renal tumour detection, important technical improvements can be made so that MRI will be capable of depicting small lesions if the imaging conditions can be optimized.

The overall importance of MRI of kidneys and renal masses was thoroughly reviewed by Baumgartner & Chezmar [4]. They extensively reviewed the role of MRI in all of these respects and stressed the possibility of MRI in demonstrating uncomplicated cysts. They also emphasized that cysts complicated by haemorrhage or infection have a variety of signal patterns depending on the amount and age of the blood within the cysts, which sometimes makes a correct diagnosis impossible. They agreed with other investigators that the main role of MRI is not in detection or differential diagnosis of renal carcinoma but in the possibilities of correct staging. Thus MRI is not routinely used in pre-operative evaluation of renal masses, but it may be rather helpful in difficult and equivocal cases.

Ultrasound and CT are established techniques in the diagnosis and staging of renal tumours. This has resulted in a considerable reduction in the number of diagnostic angiographies. The need for angiography today is usually restricted to very large tumours and, of course, in connection with tumour embolization. However, not all radiology departments have access to CT, and if not, angiography will be employed to a greater extent. When performing angiography in renal tumours, the possibility of improvement of the diagnostic quality by the use of pharmaco-angiography should be borne in mind [5].

Urography has been considered the screening procedure of choice for the detection of upper urinary neoplasms for many years.

However, tumours on the anterior and posterior aspects of the kidney may be overlooked at urography but can be detected by cross-sectional methods such as ultrasound and computed tomography. The sensitivity and specificity of these different techniques have been analysed. In one study [6] the ability of urography and ultrasound to detect renal and renal pelvic tumours in a non-selected group of patients referred for urography was compared. Urography and ultrasonography were compared prospectively and blindly in 1306 patients. Renal cell carcinomas were detected in seven patients and carcinomas of the renal pelvis in four patients. Urography detected carcinomas in 10 patients (sensitivity 91%) and falsely suggested malignancy in 52 (specificity 96%). Ultrasound detected carcinomas in 10 patients (sensitivity 91%) and falsely suggested malignancy in 13 (specificity 99%). No difference between the two methods in detecting renal and renal pelvic tumours was observed in the population studied. It is of note that ultrasonography does not provide any information about renal function, as does urography. A common cause of haematuria such as concretions in the urinary tract is also best evaluated by urography.

A similar prospective blind study [7] of 201 patients was performed to determine the relative sensitivities and specificities of urography/linear tomography and ultrasound for the diagnosis of renal parenchymal masses. CT was used as a standard. Urography permitted detection of 10% of CT-confirmed masses (cystic or solid) less than 1 cm, 21% of lesions 1-2 cm, 52% of lesions 2-3 cm and 85% of lesions 3 cm or more in diameter. Ultrasound permitted detection of 26% of CT-confirmed lesions less than 1 cm, 60% of lesions 1-2 cm, 82% of lesions 2-3 cm and 85% of lesions 3 cm or more in size. The results confirm the relative insensitivity of urography/linear tomography for masses less than 3 cm in diameter and of ultrasound for masses less than 2 cm. It was suggested that CT may have a role not only in evaluation of cases in which the urographic or sonographic results are questionable or positive, but also in confirmation of apparently negative urographic findings when clinical suspicion of a lesion is high. This is an important point and signifies that a normal urogram does not exclude the possibility of a small renal carcinoma.

With the advent of CT and ultrasound, small renal tumours are being discovered with increasing frequency. It has sometimes incorrectly been suggested that tumours less than 3 cm should be classified as benign cortical adenomas. Amendola et al [8], however, reported their experience in 39 patients with renal carcinoma smaller than 3 cm in diameter. They found that CT was overall the best imaging procedure for the detection of small renal cell carcinomas (sensitivity 94%); renal ultrasound had a sensitivity of 79% and renal angiography 74%. Of great value in these cases is fine-needle aspiration biopsy, but they found a surprisingly low sensitivity of ultrasound-guided biopsies of 20%, although the CT success rate was 62%. They stressed the importance of the CT-technique in order to avoid partial volume effects and that the section thickness should not exceed half the diameter of the lesion.

To document the earlier discovery and increased detection of renal carcinoma that has occurred since the advent of ultrasound and CT, Smith et al [9] reviewed cases of renal cell carcinoma detected at their institution during the periods 1974-1977 and 1982-1985, with particular emphasis on renal tumours smaller than 3 cm. Only 5.3% of renal carcinomas found in the period 1974-1977 but 25.4% found during the period 1982-1985 were 3 cm or smaller, an increase of almost five times. Of the small tumours in the 1982-1985 group 96.7% (30 of 31) were incidental discoveries and 77.4% (24 of 31) were initially detected with CT or ultrasound. It was concluded that many more small renal tumours are now being detected because of the use of CT and ultrasound. This will undoubtedly increase the cure rate of renal cell carcinoma as these tumours are being detected when they are small and do not produce symptoms.

Of clinical importance is to differentiate the great number of benign cysts from solid lesions or complex or malignant cysts. This problem has been thoroughly discussed in a state of the art review by Bosniak [10]. In this paper he elucidated and clarified the role of sonography, claiming that if the sonogram displays all the criteria for a simple cyst, a confident diagnosis can be made and no further studies are indicated. However, there are a number of potential problems that may necessitate a subsequent CT-investigation. These include clustering of cysts, the suspicion of vascular malformation or aneurysm, some peripelvic cysts that, because of their location, can be hard to prove clearly to be cysts, and lesions that contain calcifications, septations or irregular margins. When CT is performed it is important to obtain both non-enhanced and enhanced scans so that the information concerning possible contrast enhancement of the lesion is available. Enhancement of a renal lesion is one of the most definite radiological findings indicating a vascular mass. Also of great importance is the density of the cyst, which should be between 0 and 20 HU. The problem of a so-called hyper-dense benign cyst is also discussed. Lesions which measure above 20 HU may be cysts, but these lesions require correlation with sonography. Whenever CT reveals a cystic renal mass with a thickened wall which is enhanced after intravenous contrast administration, malignancy should be suspected (Fig. 3).

Pre-operative evaluation of the extent of the renal tumour is of value in determining the prognosis and the most suitable therapy. Comparison of ultrasound, CT and angiography [11] demonstrated that staging of renal tumours with ultrasound is mainly limited by its inability to demonstrate extrarenal infiltration. Both CT and ultrasound proved reliable in the demonstration of tumour spread to the renal vein and inferior vena cava. CT and angiography were equally effective in the evaluation of tumour extension; since CT is easier to perform, less invasive and less time consuming than angiography, it should be the primary method for staging of renal neoplasms. In another correlative clinical and radiological study Hietala et al [12] found that venous extension within the inferior vena cava was correctly identified by CT in 12 of 14 tumours (86%) and within the main renal vein in two of four tumours. Similar results were recently reported by Johnson et al [13]. The false-negative studies are usually found in patients with large infiltrating tumours in which the involved renal vein can not be identified. Improved results can be obtained with dynamic scanning and thin sections. Enlarged renal veins without visible filling defects may lead to a false-positive diagnosis of tumour thrombus. Such enlargement may be due to increased blood flow, however, and does not necessarily imply venous involvement.

Zeman et al [14] also used CT to assess the vascular invasion and tumour vascularity. In 80 patients, the lesion was correctly staged with CT in 90%. With the use of dynamic technique, the ipsilateral renal vein was shown in 99% of the patients. Extension of the tumour into the renal vein or the inferior vena cava was correctly detected in 18 of 19 patients. They concluded that CT is highly accurate in staging renal cell carcinoma but stressed the importance of the technique, using 5 mm thin sections and a bolus injection of contrast medium. Based upon this accumulated experience, the diagnosis and staging of renal masses may be given as shown in Fig. 4.

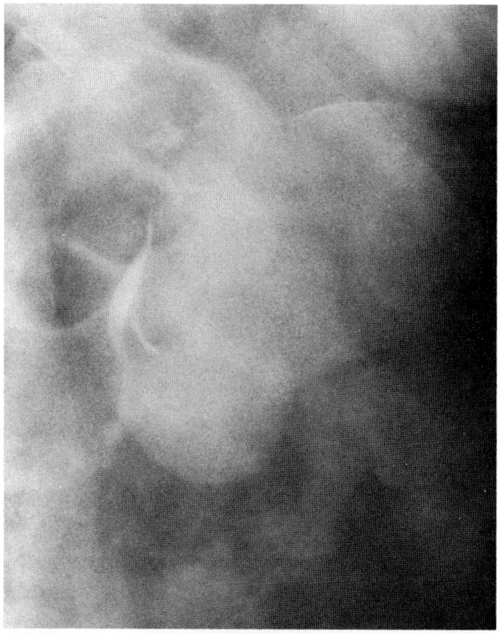

(a)

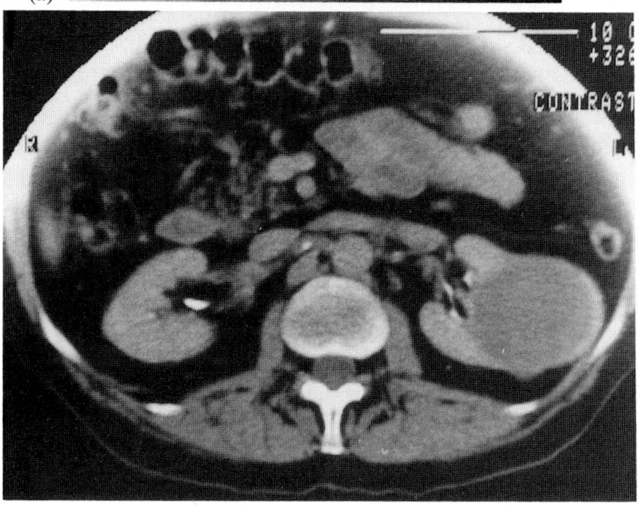

(b)

Figure 3. *(a) Urogram showing a large mass in the lateral portion of the left kidney. A thin rim of calcification is seen in its superior wall. (b) Enhanced CT-scan demonstrating a cystic mass, with thickened wall that showed some contrast accumulation. Note the small nodule posteriorly. This could not be a simple cyst and a necrotic tumour has to be suspected. Differential diagnostic alternatives include infected cyst or abscess. In this particular case, histopathological examination of the excised kidney showed necrotic renal carcinoma.*

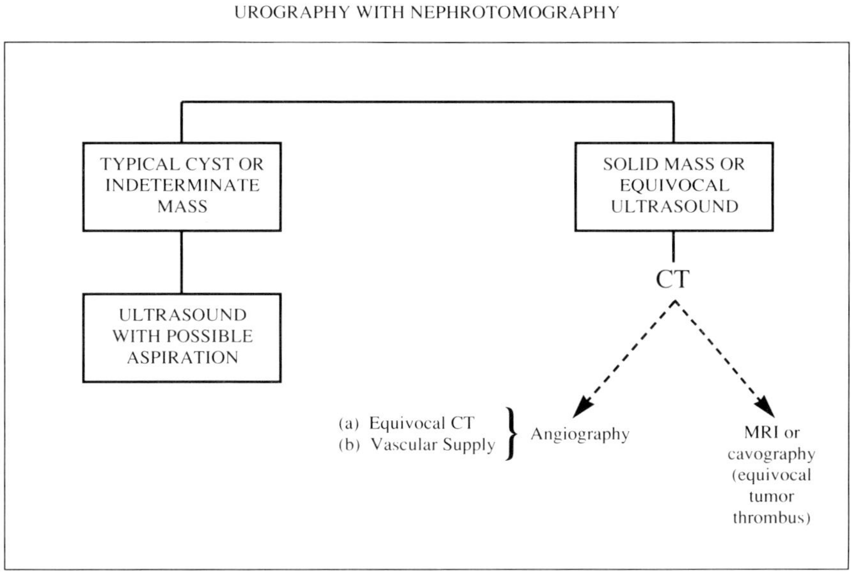

Figure 4. *Diagnosis and staging of renal masses.*

Differential Diagnosis

Renal carcinoma is the most common malignant tumour of the kidney in adults. Transitional cell carcinomas constitute about 20% of malignant tumours of the upper urinary tract and approximately half of those are located in the renal pelvis. Urography in renal pelvic carcinoma will reveal filling defects or calyx amputation, or perhaps a non-functioning kidney (Fig. 5). The diagnosis is confirmed by retrograde pyelography and there is rarely any need for further evaluation with CT pre-operatively.

In a patient with a known primary tumour (particular lung carcinoma), the presence of a small lesion in the kidney could well represent a metastatic deposit. Usually metastatic lesions in the kidney are multiple and bilateral and the diagnosis is suspected because of the history of primary tumour and the distribution of disease. Besides the multiplicity of these small metastases in the kidney, metastatic disease to other organs in the body is usually present. However, occasionally, if the lesion is single, differentiation from a primary tumour of the kidney is not possible and needle biopsy for diagnosis is necessary and often indicated.

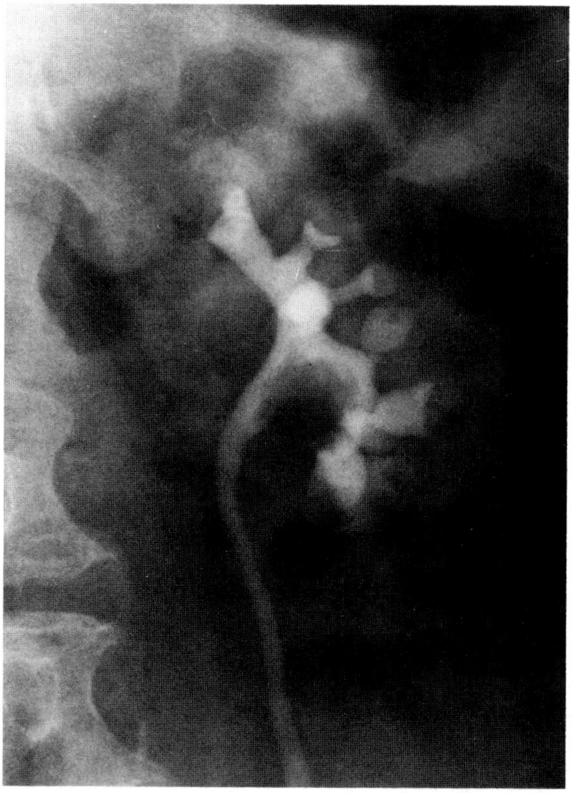

Figure 5. *Urogram in a patient with macroscopic haematuria showing typical contrast defect in the confluence, indicating carcinoma of the renal pelvis, which was confirmed at surgery and subsequent microscopic examination of the specimen.*

Lymphoma of the kidney can also present as a tumour. There are usually multiple foci of the disease when the kidneys are involved and there usually is associated lymphadenopathy. The patients are often known to have lymphoma and therefore there is usually no problem in appreciating the likely diagnosis.

In children, the possibility of a Wilms' tumour must be considered.

There are two types of benign renal tumours with which the radiologist must be familiar. Angiomyolipoma is composed of varying amounts of blood vessels, fat and smooth muscle. Most of these small and asymptomatic lesions are found at autopsy. About

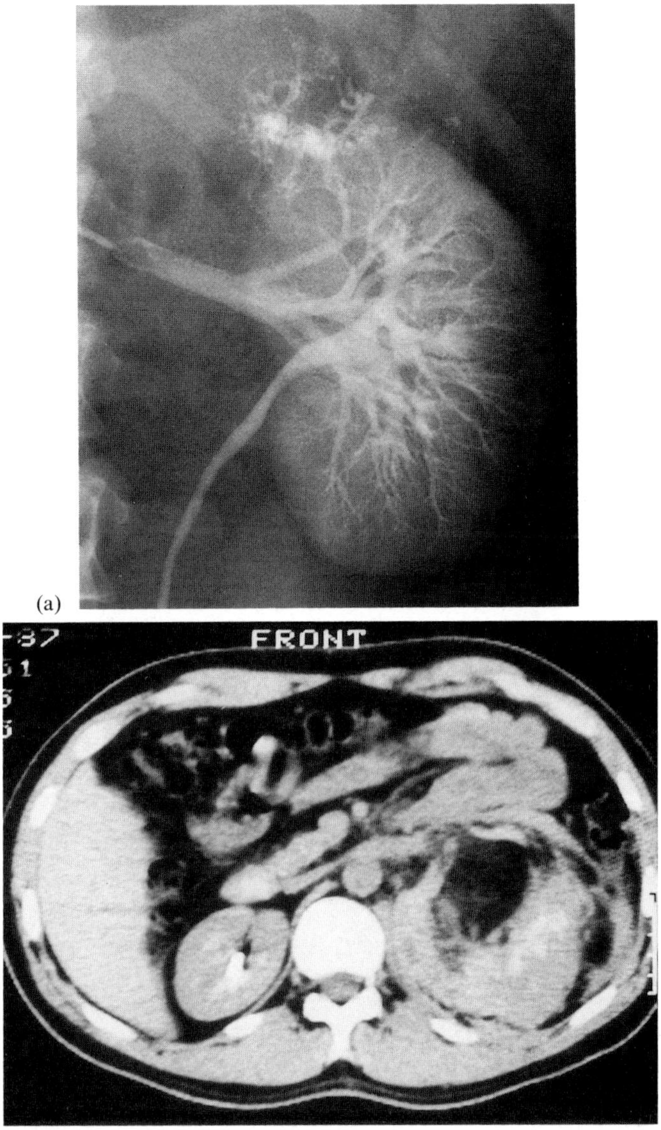

(a)

(b)

Figure 6. *25-year-old man with left flank pain and hypotension. (a) Angiography, performed to reveal a possible source of bleeding, showed vascular tumour in the upper pole of the left kidney. Multi-sacculated aneurysmal dilatation of the vessels is evident. (b) Contrast-enhanced CT-scan demonstrating perirenal haematoma and fat-containing mass in the left kidney with attenuation values of - 80 HU. This is diagnostic of angiomyolipoma. The patient was operated upon because of bleeding and the diagnosis confirmed.*

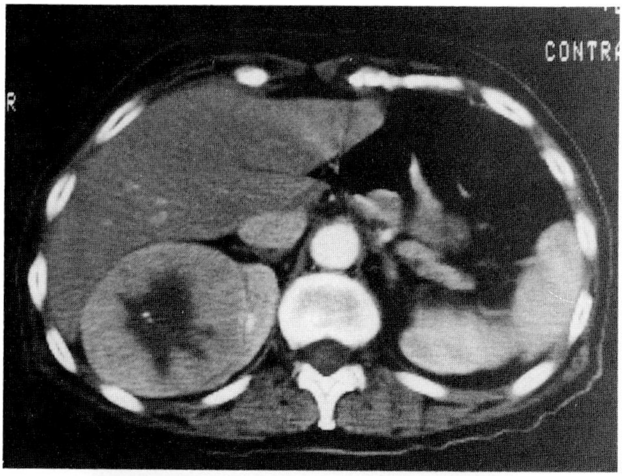

(a)

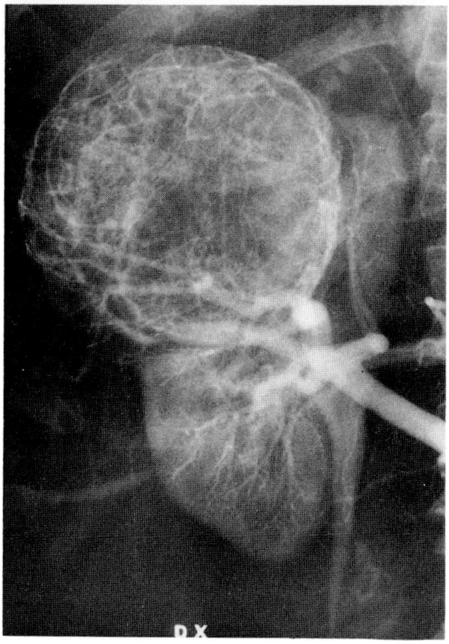

(b)

Figure 7. *63-year-old female in which a tumour of the right kidney was an incidental finding at ultrasound examination of the gallbladder. (a) CT demonstrates a well-defined, rounded and homogeneous mass with a central stellate scar. (b) Angiography, performed on the suspicion of oncocytoma, showing a 'spoke-wheel' configuration of supplying arteries and a homogeneous appearance in the nephrogram phase. Nephrectomy was performed and histopathological examination verified the diagnosis of oncocytoma.*

75% of these are found as isolated, solitary lesions in middle-aged females. An additional 20% are found as part of the tuberous sclerosis complex - these are multiple and bilateral. Many of these lesions are now being found in asymptomatic patients being investigated for other reasons, but they have a tendency to bleed. Diagnosis can occasionally be made on plain films where the fatty material can be recognized as a lucency. On ultrasound, angiomyolipoma is classically described as a highly echogenic tumour. At one time, the angiogram was felt to be virtually pathognomonic for this entity, showing a hyper-vascular mass with large feeding vessels, micro-aneurysms, and multi-sacculated aneurysmal dilatations without arteriovenous shunting. However, this pattern can be clearly mimicked by hyper-vascular renal carcinoma. On the other hand, the CT pattern is usually quite characteristic when showing areas of fat with CT numbers of - 70 HU or less within the tumour (Fig. 6). The importance of detecting small amounts of fat, which can only be made with very thin section CT (5 mm and non-enhanced CT-scan) was recently stressed by Bosniak et al [15]. This increases the spatial and density resolution and decreases susceptibility to partial volume effects, thus allowing a correct diagnosis.

Oncocytoma is another important benign tumour which is also referred to as benign oxyphil adenoma or proximal tubular adenoma. These tumours are often incidental findings, as they rarely bleed or cause pain unless extremely large. On ultrasound, a central stellate scar may be identified and similarly, homogeneous uptake of contrast with a central scar has been reported with CT (Fig. 7a) [16]. At angiography, a spoke2-wheel-like vascular pattern was initially described as characteristic for the diagnosis - unfortunately this pattern can also be seen with renal carcinomas (Fig. 7b). If the tumour is characteristic radiologically and also on gross inspection and surgical biopsy, a partial nephrectomy can be considered because of the excellent prognosis of this neoplasm.

References

1. Ekelund L, Jonsson K. How is renal carcinoma detected? *Int J Urol Nephrol* 1977;**9**:3-10.
2. Hricak H, Thoeni RF, Carroll PR, Demas BE, Marotti M, Tanagho EA. Detection and staging of renal neoplasms: a reassessment of MR imaging. *Radiology* 1983;**166**:643-649.

3. Quint LE, Glazer GM, Chenevert TL, Fechner KP, Gikas PW, Shireman PK, Grossman HB, Li KC. *In vivo* and *in vitro* MR imaging of renal tumors: histopathologic correlations and pulse sequence optimization. *Radiology* 1988;**169**:359-362.
4. Baumgartner BR, Chezmar JL. Magnetic resonance imaging of the kidneys and adrenal glands. *Semin Ultrasound, CT, MR* 1989;**10**:43-62.
5. Ekelund L, Göthlin J, Lunderquist A. Diagnostic improvement with angiotensin in renal angiography. *Radiology* 1972;**105**:33-37.
6. Aslaksen A, Halvorsen OJ, Göthlin JH. Detection of renal and renal pelvic tumours with urography and ultrasonography. *Eur J Radiol* 1990;**11**:54-58.
7. Warshauer DM, McCarthy SM, Steel L, Booklinder MJ, Glückman MG, Richter J, Hammers L, Taylor C, Rosenfield A. Detection of renal masses: Sensitivities and specificities of excretory urography/linear tomography, US and CT. *Radiology* 1988;**169**:363-365.
8. Amendola MA, Bree RL, Pollack HM, Francis JR, Glazer GM, Jafri SZH, Tomaszewski JE. Small renal cell carcinomas: resolving a diagnostic dilemma. *Radiology* 1988;**166**:637-641.
9. Smith SJ, Bosniak MA, Megibow AJ, Hulnick DH, Horii SC, Raghavendra BN. Renal cell carcinoma: earlier discovery and increased detection. *Radiology* 1989;**170**:699-703.
10. Bosniak MA. The current radiological approach to renal cysts. *Radiology* 1986;**158**:1-10.
11. Karp W, Ekelund L, Olafsson G, Olsson A. Computed tomography, angiography and ultrasound in staging of renal carcinoma. *Acta Radiol Diagn* 1981;22:625-633.
12. Hietala SO, Ekelund L, Ljungberg B. Venous invasion in renal cell carcinoma: a correlative clinical and radiologic study. *Urol Radiol* 1988;**9**:210-216.
13. Johnson CD, Dunnick NR, Cohan RH, Illescas FF. Renal adenocarcinoma: CT staging of 100 tumors. *Am J Radiol* 1987;**148**:59-63.
14. Zeman RK, Cronan JJ, Rosenfield AT, Lynch JH, Jaffe MH, Clark LR. Renal cell carcinoma: dynamic thin-section CT assessment of vascular invasion and tumor vascularity. *Radiology* 1988;**167**:393-396.
15. Bosniak MA, Megibow AJ, Hulnick DH, Horii S, Raghavendra BN. CT diagnosis of renal angiomyolipoma: the importance of detecting small amounts of fat. *Am J Radiol* 1988;**151**:497-501.
16. Goldman SM. Benign renal tumors: Diagnosis and treatment. *Urol Radiol* 1989;**11**:203-209.

Imaging of the prostate gland

Howard M. Pollack
University of Pennsylvania School of Medicine and Section of Uroradiology, Department of Radiology, Hospital of the University of Pennsylvania, USA

Introduction

Prior to the advent of modern cross-sectional imaging techniques, the prostate gland could be imaged only indirectly. For many years the intravenous urogram was the only available radiographic modality to permit an estimate of prostatic configuration, but it suffered from gross inaccuracies, especially about the size and shape of the gland. With the advent of cross-sectional imaging it became possible for the first time not only to accurately assess the size of the prostate, but to evaluate for the presence or absence of important prostatic disorders such as carcinoma, benign prostatic hyperplasia (BPH), abscess, etc. This chapter will review the current status of prostatic imaging, with emphasis on ultrasound and magnetic resonance imaging (MRI), but will also attempt to place other less often employed imaging modalities, especially with regard to carcinoma, in their proper perspective.

The Normal Prostate Gland

Ultrasound

Technique

Ultrasonography represented a significant advance in prostatic imaging, and with the development of intrarectal techniques, it became possible to quantify prostatic volume, resulting in more accurate preoperative assessment of prostatic size. In addition, ultrasonography provided a means whereby changes in sonographic texture could be used to differentiate - albeit imperfectly - benign prostatic hyperplasia from carcinoma of the prostate.

Although the prostate gland may be imaged suprapubically and transurethrally, the former approach gives insufficient visualization of the posterior portion of the gland while the latter is too invasive for routine use. The transrectal route (TRUS), therefore, is the one in common clinical usage.

A large variety of equipment is available for transrectal ultrasonic scanning, including transducers that provide purely axial or sagittal depictions of the prostate, and those that provide images in both dimensions (bi-planar scanners) or in a variety of planes (multiplanar scanners). The ability to view the prostate in more than two dimensions is important diagnostically and greatly abets the ability to precisely localize a suspicious area for biopsy. Since bi- and multiplanar instruments provide this capability without the inconvenience of changing rectal probes, they have become quite popular and are currently preferred by many physicians [1]. Other important physical properties of transrectal scanners include the transducer's frequency, beam diameter and focal length. The higher the frequency the greater the resolution, but high frequency transducers produce less depth of penetration than do those of lower frequency. A range of 5 to 7 MHz provides an optimal compromise between resolution and field of view and represents the operating frequencies of most transducers currently in use for TRUS. The width of the beam (transducer aperture) determines the scanner's lateral resolution, while a fixed focus of approximately 2-6 cm will include almost all of the prostate within the high definition field of the transducer. The probe, or its surrounding water-filled balloon, must be held in tight contact with the anterior rectal wall, and the system gain calibrated to ensure that returning low level echoes, as well as the stronger signals, are all recorded. Artefacts from rectal gas and faecal material must be avoided and scrupulous care taken to dispel all trapped air from within the water-filled balloon.

Appearance

The bulk of the normal prostate is comprised of its central and peripheral zones. Both of these areas are uniformly hyperechoic and not always differentiable, although slight differences in their echogenicity can be appreciated in many cases (Fig. 1). In the midline surrounding the urethra, a less echogenic area corresponding to the smooth muscle of the internal sphincter, the transition zone and the periurethral glandular tissue may be identified. With aging, the transition zone - the site of origin of benign prostatic hyperplasia (BPH) - enlarges and eventually may become the dominant part of the gland. The seminal vesicles are identified just superior to the prostate on axial or sagittal images. They are slightly less echogenic than the tissue surrounding them.

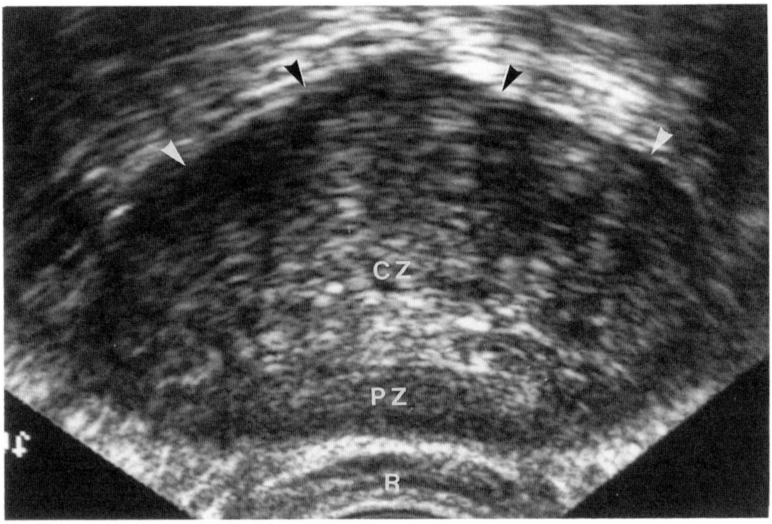

Figure 1. NORMAL PROSTATE. TRUS. *A transrectal ultrasonogram of the prostate. The peripheral zone (PZ) is diffusely echogenic and characterized by the presence of numerous low level echoes of approximately equal intensity. The central gland (CZ) is less homogenous and the echoes are coarser. The boundary between the prostate and the periprostatic fat is readily discernible (arrow heads). R=anterior rectal wall.*

Computed Tomography (CT)

In axial views, the normal adult prostate gland appears as a round, elliptical or sometimes triangular homogeneous structure with a density approaching that of skeletal muscle (Fig. 2). Slight contrast enhancement can be appreciated. The individual zones are not delineated as they are with MRI and the periprostatic and other pelvic fascias are not nearly as well defined. The apical prostate is surrounded by the pubococcygeus muscle, the mid-portion by fat, and the base is bounded by the bladder base anteriorly and the seminal vesicles cranially. Very large prostates may extend to the lateral pelvic wall and abut the obturator internus muscles. Due to its density, the gland does not usually allow clear depiction of the prostatic urethra. Thus, on CT, the prostate gland presents as a uniform, homogeneous structure situated between the bladder and the membranous urethra.

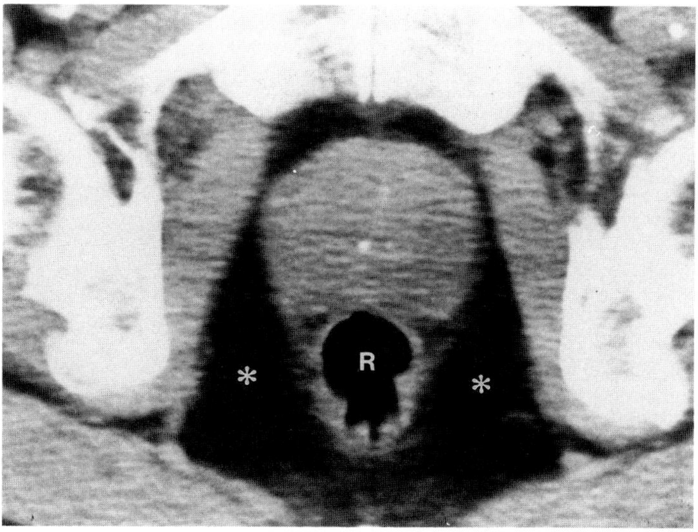

Figure 2. NORMAL PROSTATE. CT. *A CT section through the middle of the prostate gland reveals a homogenous structure isodense with the surrounding skeletal muscle. Several small calcifications are seen in the prostate and the rectum is located dorsal to it. Note that no zonal architecture can be appreciated on this study, and it is not possible to tell whether the prostate is normal, hyperplastic or malignant. R=Rectum, *=ischeorectal fat.*

Magnetic Resonance Imaging (MRI)

Technique

To fully appreciate the MRI appearance of pathological conditions affecting the prostate and seminal vesicles it is important to first understand the normal anatomy of these structures as revealed by

MRI. In most centres, both T_1-weighted (short TR/TE=600/20 milliseconds) and T_2-weighted (long TR/TE=2500/40, 80 milliseconds) spin echo images are included in the examination of the prostate. Gradient echo images and other 'fast scan' techniques have not been found to be very useful. Images are obtained primarily in the axial plane, and are supplemented with coronal or sagittal images as required. The coronal and sagittal images are particularly helpful when the prostate is enlarged. The T_2-weighted images are collected from the superior aspect of the seminal vesicles through the apex of the prostate. The T_1-weighted images are collected to the level of the renal hilum in order to evaluate the pelvic and retroperitoneal lymph nodes. We use a 128×256 matrix with a field of view of 36 cm. The slice thickness is 10 mm on the T_1-weighted images and 5 mm on the T_2-weighted images. We find it helpful to image the patient in the prone position to reduce respiratory motion artifact. We also insufflate the rectum with air and administer 1 mg of glucagon i.m. prior to initiating the scanning.

Normal Anatomy

The normal appearance of the prostate and seminal vesicles on T_1 and T_2-weighted spin echo images is strikingly different. The T_2-weighted images are the most useful in evaluating the internal architecture of the prostate [2-4]. On these images, the appearance of the prostate closely parallels the zonal differentiation described by McNeal [5]. The normal peripheral zone (PZ) has high signal intensity (bright on the images), while the central and transition zones (CZ, TZ respectively) have relatively lower signal intensity, and although well contrasted from the PZ, they cannot ordinarily be distinguished from one another (Fig. 3) [6]. However, since benign prostatic hyperplasia originates in the TZ, the characteristic changes of this disorder, if present, will clearly demarcate the TZ from all other areas of the prostate. For the purposes of MRI, the term central gland is often used to refer to the combination of the CZ and TZ. On T_2-weighted spin echo images the fluid within the tubules of the seminal vesicles has high signal, while their walls have lower signal (Fig. 4). The periprostatic veins and fluid within the bladder also display high signal.

On T_1-weighted images, the prostate, seminal vesicles and periprostatic veins all demonstrate low signal and appear uniform. The internal architecture of the prostate is not visible. In contrast to the

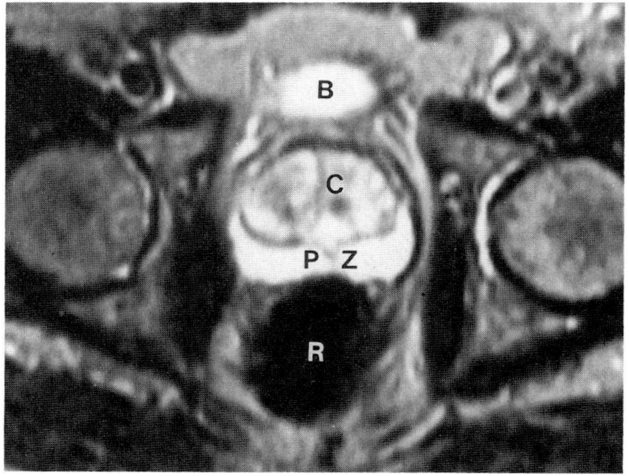

Figure 3. NORMAL PROSTATE. MRI. *T_2-Weighted Spin-Echo Image Tr 2500 msec/TE 80 msec. An axial view through the prostate in a 47 year old man demonstrates significant variations in the signals emanating from various zones of the prostate. The peripheral zone (PZ) is high signal intensity on this T_2-weighted image while the central gland (C) is of a lower and mixed signal suggesting that early prostatic hyperplasia is present. The central gland probably represents an already enlarging transition zone, which is the site of origin if benign prostatic hyperplasia. B=Bladder, R=Rectum.*

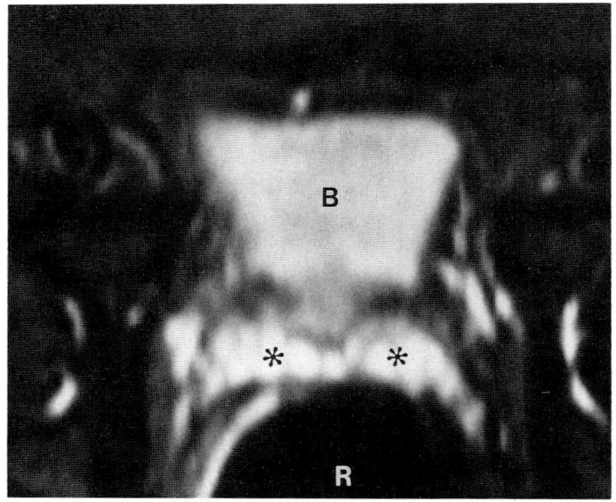

Figure 4. NORMAL SEMINAL VESICLES. MRI. *T_2-Weighted Spin Echo Image Tr 2500 msec/TE 80 msec. An axial view through the seminal vesicles demonstrates them to be symmetrical, normal sized and extremely signal intense on this T_2-weighted pulse sequence (asterisks). This is the typical picture of normal seminal vesicles on T_2-weighted spin-echo images. Any decrease in signal intensity within the ordinarily bright seminal vesicles is indicative of disease. Note the high signal intensity urine within the bladder (B). R=Rectum.*

internal architecture of the prostate is not visible. In contrast to the low signal of these structures, the periprostatic fat has a very high signal, sharply outlining the pelvic soft tissues including, in addition to the prostate itself, important anatomic landmarks such as nerves, muscles, blood vessels, and lymphatics. The neurovascular bundles, located at 5 and 7 o'clock on axial images are particularly important and are usually quite visible on these images, although they are best seen on surface coil images [9a]. These structures run in the triangle of fat in the left and right recto-prostatic angles, and contain the cavernosal nerves which are believed to be responsible for potency [7]. Thus the demonstration of the periprostatic neurovascular bundles is essential in the pre-operative assessment and staging of patients with prostate cancer. The various fascial layers that surround the prostate are also well seen on the short TR/TE images. These include the pubococcygeous muscle and fascia. The true (anatomical) capsule of the prostate and the recto-prostatic interface (Denonvillier's fascia) are not well discriminated on body coil imaging but can be readily identified with surface coil technique.

A balloon based endorectal surface coil has been developed to enhance prostate imaging [8,9]. The increased signal to noise (ratio) and decreased sensitivity profile of the surface coil allow high resolution images of the prostate to be obtained. The use of the balloon is contra-indicated in patients who have had recent rectal surgery, transrectal biopsy in the preceding 24 hours, or prior radiation therapy to the pelvis. The surface coil images are typically obtained with a small (10-12 cm) FOV and a 3-4 mm slice thickness. These images provide significantly more anatomic detail than do body coil images of the prostate and have proved especially helpful in staging prostate carcinoma [9a]. The information obtainable about the prostate and its contiguous structures is far superior to that previously attainable (Fig. 5). While clinical evaluation of this technique is still ongoing, it appears quite promising.

Benign Prostatic Hyperplasia (BPH)

Ultrasound

Benign prostatic hyperplasia (BPH) is an age-related proliferative disorder that is ubiquitous in males over the age of 50. Prostatic

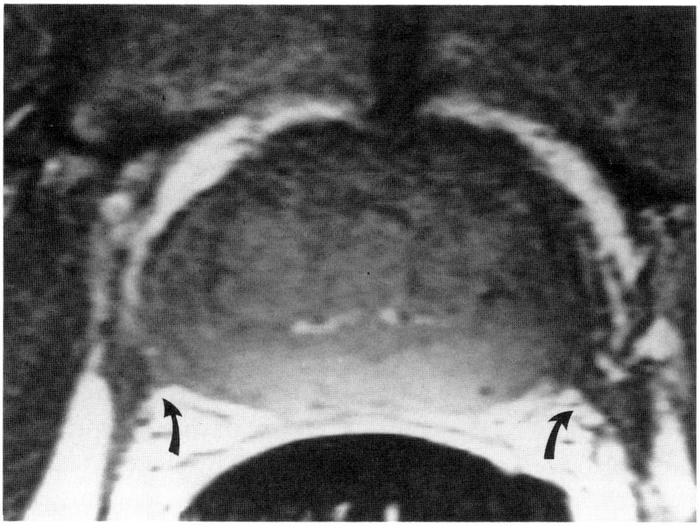

Figure 5. NORMAL PROSTATE GLAND. ENDORECTAL SURFACE COIL TECHNIQUE. *T_1-Weighted Spin-Echo Image TR 600 msec/TE 25 msec. An axial view of a 50 year old man with a normal prostate is performed using an endorectal surface coil. Although the zonal architecture cannot be discriminated on this T_1-weighted image, the periprostatic fat is clearly delineated from the underlying prostate, and the neurovascular bundles are particularly well seen (curved arrows).*

hyperplasia usually occurs in the form of nodules that originate in the transition zone. With age the nodules enlarge in size and number, eventually impinging upon the adjoining central gland, thinning and compressing it. If large enough, these adenomatous masses can also compress and attenuate the peripheral zone.

The sonographic characteristics of the hyperplastic nodules vary. Although they are usually less echogenic than normal peripheral zone tissue (Fig. 6), they may at times be isoechoic or even hyperechoic. The nodules, which are usually multiple, may be surrounded by a thin hypoechoic rim, clearly delineating them. Occasionally, they may be seen extending superiorly, posteriorly or laterally. They may cause bulging of the prostatic capsule, but unlike prostatic carcinoma there will be no capsular disruption.

The volume of the prostate can be estimated from ultrasonographic measurements. Using the formula $V=4/3\pi r_1 * r_2 * r_3$ (where r_1 equals the transverse diameter, r_2 the length and r_3 the height of the prostate,

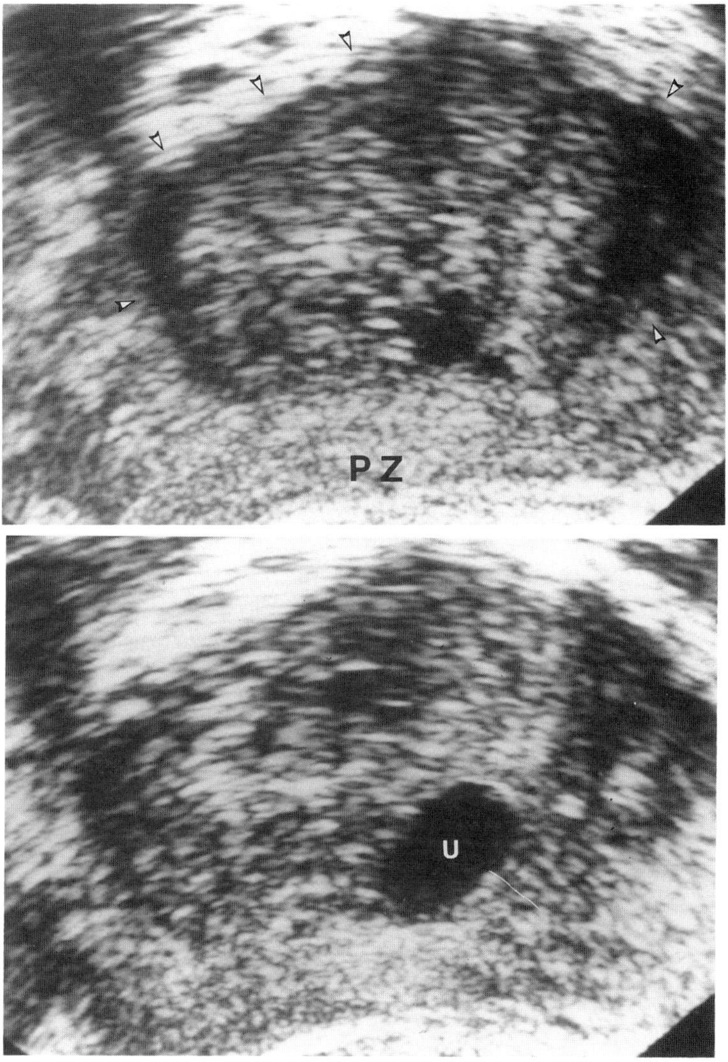

(a)

(b)

Figure 6. BENIGN PROSTATIC HYPERPLASIA. TRUS. *(a) Transrectal ultrasound examination reveals the typical finding of BPH. The peripheral zone demonstrates densely packed homogenous echoes of low to intermediate intensity (PZ), while the centre of the gland is composed of hyperplastic tissue originating in the transition zone. The hyperplastic 'adenoma' contains coarser echoes and is set off from the remaining gland by a hypoechoic rim or pseudocapsule (arrow heads). (b) A more proximal section from the prostate of the same patient demonstrates a cavernous prostatic urethra attributable to a previous transurethral resection. U=Urethra.*

respectively) a reasonably accurate approximation to the true volume can be made. If one assumes the prostate to be spherical, the formula may be simplified to $V=4/3\pi r^3$ or, even further reduced by the approximation $V=d^3/2$. Thus, ultrasonography can be used to assess the prostate's response to various treatment modalities for benign and malignant diseases.

Computed Tomography

Adenomatous hyperplasia appears as a smoothly bordered infravesical mass on CT (Fig. 7a). Not infrequently, polycyclic protrusions into the floor of the bladder can be seen. Like ultrasound, CT can also estimate prostatic volume accurately, but because of its cost, the radiation it produces and the medical resources consumed, it has not found favour as an imaging modality for BPH. CT attenuation values cannot be used to differentiate BPH from prostatic carcinoma, nor can CT depict the internal architecture of the gland. In the absence of frank invasion, therefore, CT is of little value in determining the cause of prostatic enlargement.

Magnetic Resonance Imaging

As previously noted, benign prostatic hyperplasia originates in the TZ of the prostate and often enlarges the TZ until it occupies most or nearly the entire central gland [10]. As the TZ enlarges, it compresses both the CZ and PZ around it, so that the latter forms a pseudo-capsule ('surgical capsule' of the prostate) around the hyperplastic mass of BPH. Histologically, BPH contains both glandular and stromal (smooth muscle; fibrous tissue) elements in variable amounts. On T_2-weighted MR images stomal BPH has intermediate signal, while glandular BPH has high signal (Fig. 7b) [6]. The individual components of BPH are most often not well resolved on body coil images, resulting in a heterogeneous appearing central gland [11,12]. However, large high signal intensity nodules of glandular BPH can occasionally be seen. On T_2-weighted endorectal coil images of the prostate, the individual components of BPH with their characteristic associated fibrous envelope are routinely seen (Fig. 8). On T_1-weighted images, BPH is isointense with the remainder of the prostate.

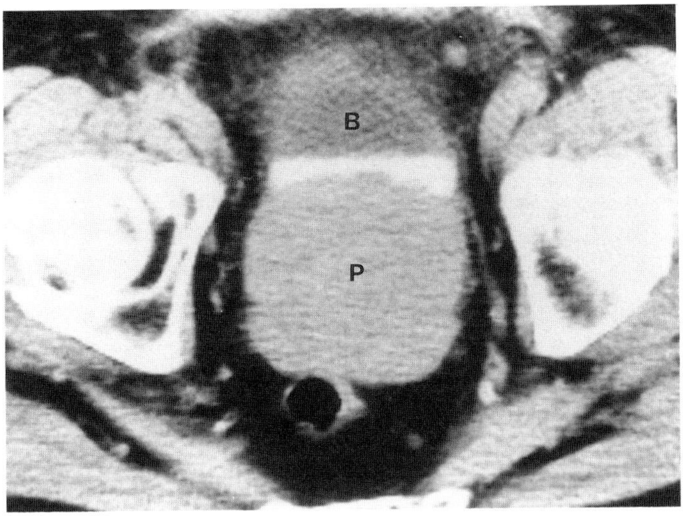

(a)

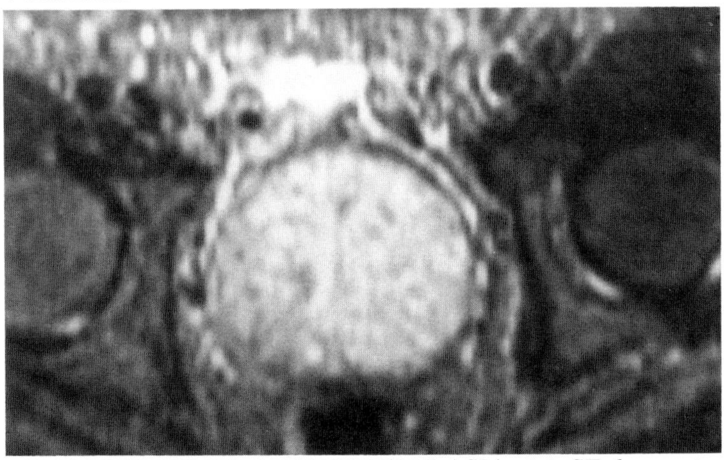

(b)

Figure 7. BENIGN PROSTATIC HYPERPLASIA. *(a) CT demonstration. Computed tomography demonstrates a massively enlarged but smoothly bordered and homogeneously dense prostate gland (P). Anterior to the enlarged prostate is the contrast-containing urinary bladder (B). The prostate weighed 260 grams and was benign. (b) An MRI from the same patient.* T_2*-Weighted spin echo sequence. Tr 2500 msec/TE 80 msec. An axial MRI again demonstrates the massively enlarged gland. The alternating hypo- and hyperintense areas are characteristic of BPH. The high intensity areas represent cystic, glandular hyperplasia while the low signal intensity areas represent fibrous tissue insinuated between the small hyperplastic nodules. The entire gland is surrounded by a low signal intensity fibrous capsule. The massively enlarged transition zone has effectively obscured the peripheral zone and other prostatic landmarks.*

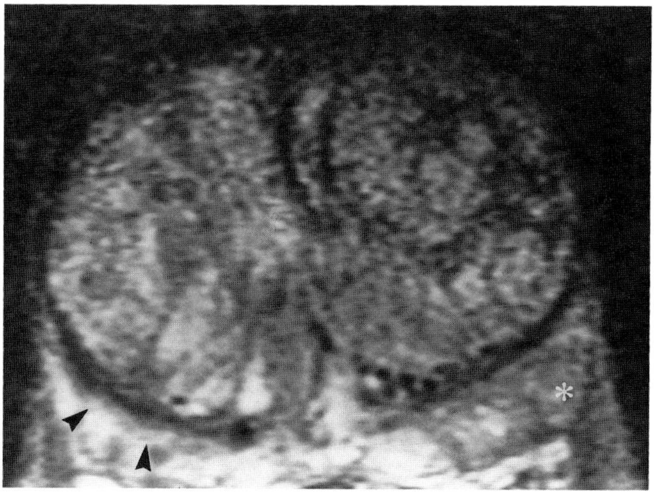

Figure 8. BENIGN PROSTATIC HYPERPLASIA IN A PATIENT WHO ALSO HAS ADENOCARCINOMA OF THE PROSTATE. *MRI demonstration using endorectal surface coil. TR 2500 msec/TE 80 msec. An endorectal surface coil image in the axial plane demonstrates the typical appearance of BPH. The hyperplastic nodules in the transition zone have a heterogeneous appearance. Some are hyperintense and others are hypointense. The hyperplastic nodules are surrounded by a low signal intensity fibrous rim and a more prominent fibrous rim separates the hyperplastic growth from the peripheral zone (arrow heads). While the peripheral zone has a normal high signal intensity on the right side there is a definite hyperintense area on the left (asterisk) corresponding to biopsy-proved adenocarcinoma.*

Adenocarcinoma

Carcinoma of the prostate is the third leading cause of cancer death among males [13]. Advances in the surgical approach to prostate carcinoma concurrent with improvements in imaging technology have raised a flurry of interest in the imaging of this important clinical problem.

While digital rectal examination, prostatic specific antigen and, ultimately, histological examination remain the mainstays in the diagnosis of carcinoma of the prostate, an increasingly important role has evolved for radiological imaging. With the emergence of transrectal ultrasonography (TRUS) and magnetic resonance imaging

(MRI) new vistas have opened in the dual realms of diagnosis and staging of prostatic neoplasms. For the first time, it is now possible to detect prostatic cancer while it is still hidden to both the examining finger and the laboratory, and to stage it non-surgically with a hitherto unattainable accuracy.

Ultrasonography

Approximately 70% of prostatic cancers originate in the peripheral zone, 10-20% in the transition zone, and 5-10% in the central zone [14]. Multicentricity is quite common. Although it is generally acknowledged that most prostatic carcinomas are hypoechoic (Fig. 9), controversy surrounding the prevalence of the more echogenic varieties still exist [15]. Dahnert and co-workers found fully 25% of

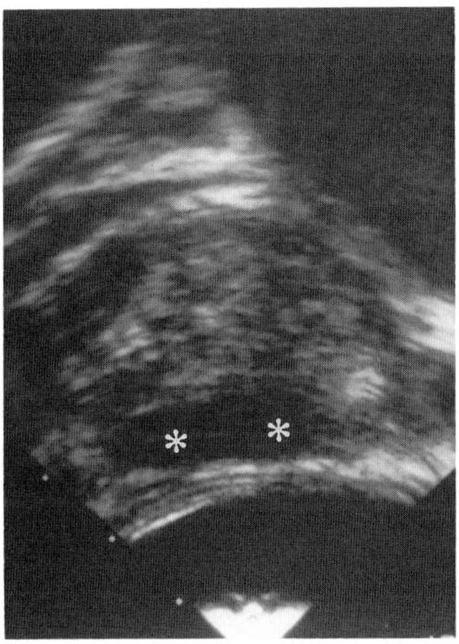

Figure 9. CARCINOMA OF THE PROSTATE. TRUS. *Transrectal ultrasound of the prostate demonstrate a large hypoechoic area (asterisks) occupying almost the entire peripheral zone. The appearance is very suspicious for carcinoma of the prostate which was proved by transrectal biopsy.*

prostatic malignancies to be isoechoic, and thus undetectable by ultrasound [16]. However, Rifkin and associates noted that larger and less well differentiated neoplasms could be mixed in appearance or actually hyperechoic [17]. They suggested that increasing echogenicity is related to the amount of desmoplasia and fibrosis within the tumour, as well as to its degree of cellular differentiation. Lee and colleagues, on the other hand, have emphasized almost exclusively the significance of hypoechoic lesions, while giving less consideration to other ultrasonic types [18]. Thus, the echo characteristics of prostatic cancer are a function of its size and histological grade and may vary based on these considerations.

Hypoechoic prostatic foci are not specific for carcinoma. Prostatic infarcts, prostatitis, benign prostatic hyperplasia, and prostatic cysts are examples of other lesions that may appear hypoechoic and under certain circumstances may mimic carcinoma on TRUS. Thus the specificity of TRUS has been called into question as a fundamental issue regarding its use as a screening modality. The positive predictive value of an isolated hypoechoic area in the prostate reportedly ranges from 0-50%, with the chances of any single hypoechoic lesion representing malignancy generally being placed at 20-25% [15]. Wide variances from these averages may be seen. In the author's experience, only 10% of non-palpable lesions have proved to be malignant, while Lee and associates report 41% [1]. Data on the prevalence of false negative studies are scant, but the work of Dahnert and colleagues - in which 25% of cancers were not detected because of their isoechoic nature - provides some insight into the potential seriousness of the problem [16].

At this time, the question remains whether TRUS is efficacious for screening large populations for non-palpable carcinoma of the prostate. Only large scale, well controlled, prospective studies conducted over many years will determine whether TRUS has the necessary accuracy to fulfil this function. Moreover, much more knowledge about the clinical impact of such early detection on longevity and quality of life remains to be learned before TRUS can be advocated for mass screening. At the moment, the pendulum appears to have swung away from routine screening TRUS [18a].

TRUS has been employed widely to localize both palpable and non-palpable lesions for biopsy. A number of techniques are available including both transrectal and transperineal approaches. Needle guides that fit over the insertable portion of the endorectal probes and direct the needle into the 'line of sight' of the acoustical beam provide added precision to the targeting of prostatic lesions for tissue sampling. Reports differ on the increased effectiveness of the ultrasound-guided technique of prostatic biopsy. Resnick found no added benefit of ultrasound-guided core biopsy when compared to digitally guided biopsy of palpable nodules [19]. Liddell and associates, however, found that their accuracy was improved using sonography [20]. In comparing transrectal digitally guided and sonographically guided transperineal fine needle aspiration biopsies to digitally guided transperineal core biopsy, Goldenberg and co-workers found the latter to be slightly more reliable. They recommended that digitally guided fine needle aspiration biopsy be the initial method of sampling prostatic nodules and that the sonographically directed technique be employed if the first biopsy is negative [21].

There is a paucity of meaningful data on the accuracy of staging prostatic cancer by ultrasound. Periprostatic extension may be suspected at sonography when there is disruption of the capsular echoes (Fig. 9), irregularity, bulging at the capsular margin, or asymmetry of the seminal vesicles, especially when accompanied by the loss of the normal prostato-vesicular angle. Most published studies that address staging, however, have not been based on surgical or pathological assessment. Of those reports that correlate operative findings with pre-operative sonography, the work of Salo and Pontes has been encouraging. Salo and associates found an accuracy of 90% in demonstrating periprostatic tumour infiltration and a 77% accuracy in predicting seminal vesicle invasion [22]. Pontes' group achieved comparable results in cases of gross extension but were unable to detect microscopic capsular invasion [23]. Scardino, however, had better luck achieving 80% accuracy in detecting capsular invasion [24], but Andriole and his co-workers found sonography to be associated with considerable errors in staging clinically localized prostate cancer [25]. All evaluations of TRUS as a means of staging cancer of the prostate must take into account the fact that this technique does not permit lymph node assessment - a deficiency not shared with either CT or MRI.

TRUS may be used to direct the insertion of radioactive sources into the malignant prostate. Holm and associates have used a technique similar to that for guided biopsy to place iodine 125 seeds into the prostate transperineally [26]. After external beam or palliative therapy, TRUS serves as an effective means of surveillance, whereby the effectiveness of treatment may be judged. Changes in size, shape and echo texture of the prostate are readily apparent. Persistent hypoechoic areas raise the possibility that foci of viable tumour may yet be present.

Computed Tomography

Computed tomography brings another dimension to prostatic imaging, in that regional lymph nodes can be imaged in addition to the prostate itself. This is helpful in assessing the presence or absence of metastases from prostatic malignancy. However, CT suffers serious deficiencies with regard to imaging of the primary tumour.

In some patients with carcinoma of the prostate, CT can show gross irregularities in glandular contour, suggesting periprostatic invasion (Fig. 10a), but in others, the examination may fail to disclose clinically obvious extension (Fig. 10b) [27]. Disclosure of gross involvement of adjacent structures such as the bladder and seminal vesicles is a reliable index of stage C disease, as is the demonstration of perirectal extension. Since CT provides images in an axial plane and the vesicoprostatic junction is more oblique than transverse, it may be difficult to appreciate bladder invasion. Both under- and overstaging may result. CT signs of seminal vesicle involvement include enlargement of one or both seminal vesicles, and loss of the normal fat planes between the vesicles and the bladder or prostate (Fig. 10c). These are non-specific findings, however, and can be produced by inflammation or prostatic biopsy.

After a short period of initial enthusiasm, it became apparent that CT had serious shortcomings as an adjunct to the overall evaluation of the patient with carcinoma of the prostate. Its major pitfalls are that, unlike ultrasound and MRI, it cannot differentiate benign from malignant causes of prostatic enlargement, and it does not depict the internal architecture of the prostate. The accuracy of staging with CT has been reported to range between 60% and 75%.

As with any malignancy, CT is useful in demonstrating lymphatic metastases. Pelvic or abdominal lymph nodes greater than 1 cm in diameter are suspicious for nodal tumour deposits, while those greater than 1.5 cm are extremely likely to be malignant (Fig. 11). Small metastases or nodes enlarged because of reactive hyperplasia are common sources for diagnostic inaccuracies. Detection rates are enhanced if a rapid bolus of contrast is injected, thus eliminating potential confusion among lymph nodes, arteries and veins. If no adenopathy is present in the pelvis, the CT scan need not be carried out above the aortic bifurcation, since abdominal adenopathy without pelvic adenopathy is very uncommon in carcinoma of the prostate [29]. The accuracy of detecting lymph node metastases in patients with pelvic malignancies ranges from 80-90% [30]. In Weinerman's series of 32 patients with either carcinoma of the bladder or prostate, which was thought to be surgically curable, 37% had lymphatic

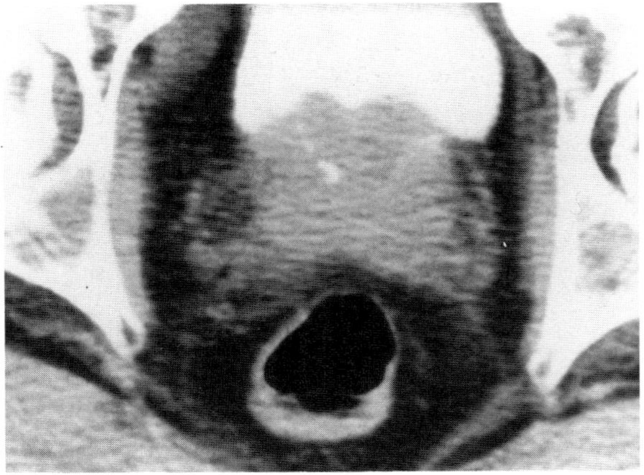

(a)

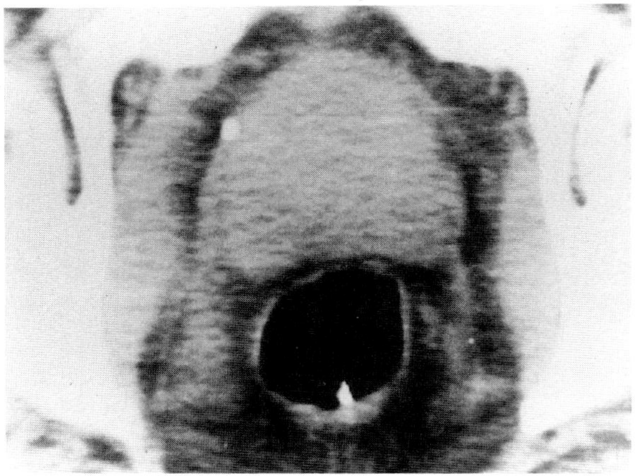

(b)

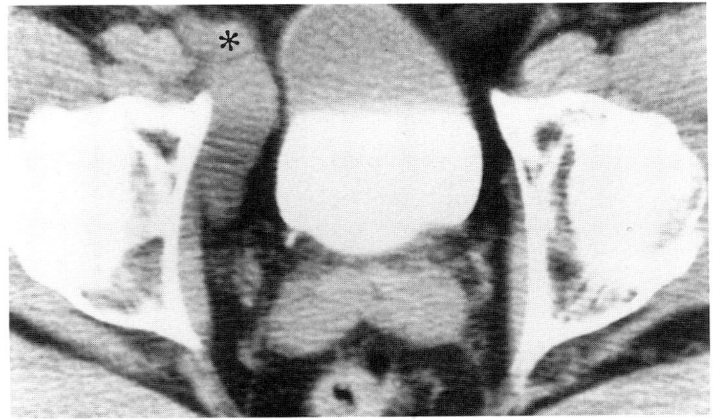

(c)

Figure 10. CARCINOMA OF THE PROSTATE. CT MANIFESTATIONS. *(a) CT in a patient with extensive prostatic carcinoma demonstrates soft tissue extension into the periprostatic fat. Irregularly infiltrating strands of tumour are seen penetrating into the fat surrounding the prostate. Some prostatic calcifications are also present. (b) Minimal evidence of cancer. CT scan of this patient with a Stage C carcinoma of the prostate belies of the existence of, as well as the extent of, the disease. The prostate is homogeneous and aside from a slight prominence posteriorly on the right there is no suggestion of abnormality. (c) CT at a more cranial level, in the patient whose scan is demonstrated in Fig. 10a, demonstrates both seminal vesicles to be markedly enlarged in all likelihood attributable to obstruction of the ejaculatory ducts by tumour. Note the enlarged right external iliac lymph node (asterisk).*

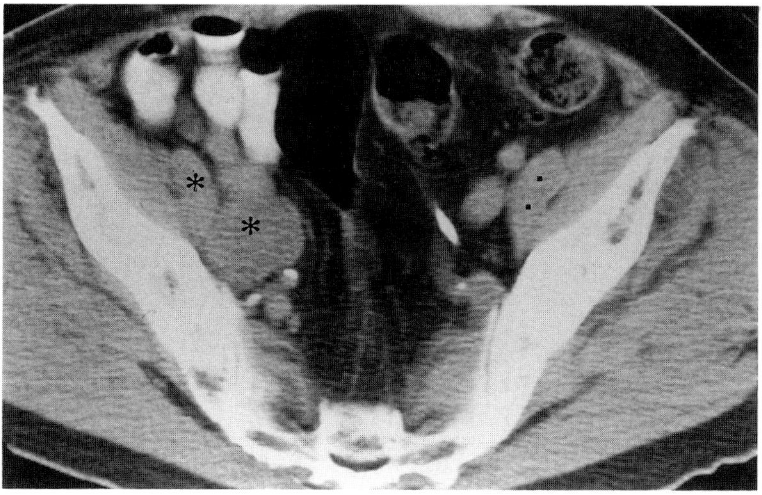

Figure 11. MASSIVE PELVIC ADENOPATHY SECONDARY TO CARCINOMA OF THE PROSTATE. *A CT scan through the pelvis of a patient with carcinoma of the prostate demonstrates unusually bulky adenopathy involving the right common iliac chain (asterisks). Lymphadenopathy is also present on the left, but is much less striking (dots).*

metastases, of which three-quarters were detected by CT [30]. Since reactive hyperplasia may accompany pelvic malignancies, the precise nature of the lymphadenopathy should be confirmed by thin needle biopsy prior to arriving at a firm treatment plan.

More distant sites of metastases from cancer of the prostate - such as lung, liver and bone - are all very clearly and accurately depicted by CT, although a search for bony lesions is more expediently conducted by radionuclide bone scanning and/or radiography. With pre-treatment studies as a baseline, serial CT examinations can provide objective evidence of tumour response to chemotherapy, endocrine manipulation or radiation therapy. Demarcating optimal radiation treatment portals and assessing the geometry of radioactive implants are additional functions that can be nicely fulfilled by CT [31].

In summary, although CT can provide useful information about the patient with carcinoma of the prostate, it is a tool that has recently fallen out of favour as a routine study in these patients. Although evaluation for lymphatic and distant metastases is reasonably accurate, assessment of the primary tumour is hampered by nonspecificity and an inability to obtain consistently accurate results concerning local spread. For these reasons CT is gradually giving way to MRI as a more efficacious way of evaluating patients with prostatic malignancy.

Magnetic Resonance Imaging

Currently, a strong effort is underway to more sharply define the role of MRI in the assessment of prostate cancer. While initially divergent reports led to uncertainty regarding the appearance of prostate carcinoma on T_2-weighted MR images, further investigation has dispelled any controversy and it now appears clear that a decreased signal intensity lesion in the PZ is characteristic of this disease [32,33] (however, isolated cases of carcinoma isointense and h-yperintense to normal PZ have been reported). Histological mapping of prostatectomy specimens has confirmed that the predominant appearance of prostate carcinoma is low signal intensity relative to normal PZ on T_2-weighted images (Fig. 12) [6,12]. However carcinoma in the central gland may be difficult to appreciate since the inherent signal of the central gland prostatic tissue is low, rather than

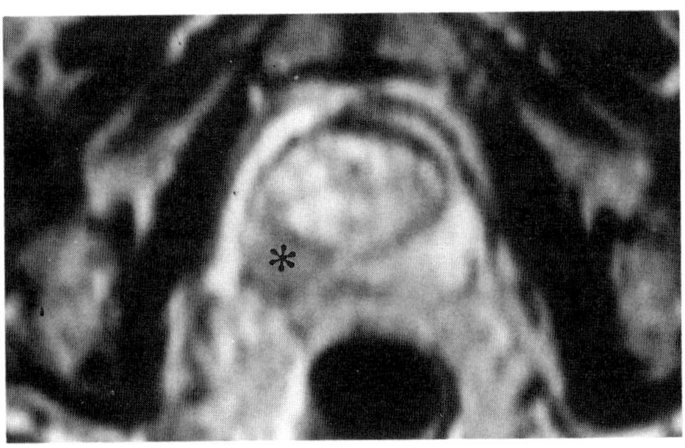

Figure 12. CARCINOMA OF THE PROSTATE (STAGE C). *MRI demonstration. Spin echo T_2-weighted. TR 2500 msec/TE 80 msec. An axial MRI performed with a conventional body coil reveals striking low signal intensity changes in the right half of the peripheral zone (asterisk). The tumour can be seen extending dorsally to the area of the prostatic capsule. while no definite disruption of the capsule or extension beyond it is seen on this image, surgical-pathological staging revealed that there was in fact some extension through the capsule making this a minimal Stage C carcinoma.*

high as is the PZ [34]. Fortunately, 70-80% of the cancers originate in or involve the PZ [35,36]. It now appears that, while MRI can be used to suggest a diagnosis of prostate carcinoma, it cannot at this time be routinely used to make that diagnosis.

The relative abilities of MRI and transrectal sonography to detect prostatic cancer is not yet known. This issue is further clouded by the fact that most comparative studies between the two feature the use of body coil MR images, whereas it seems likely that the high resolution surface coil images will be better in detecting prostate cancer (Fig. 13). Other MR techniques for prostate imaging, such as ultralong TE

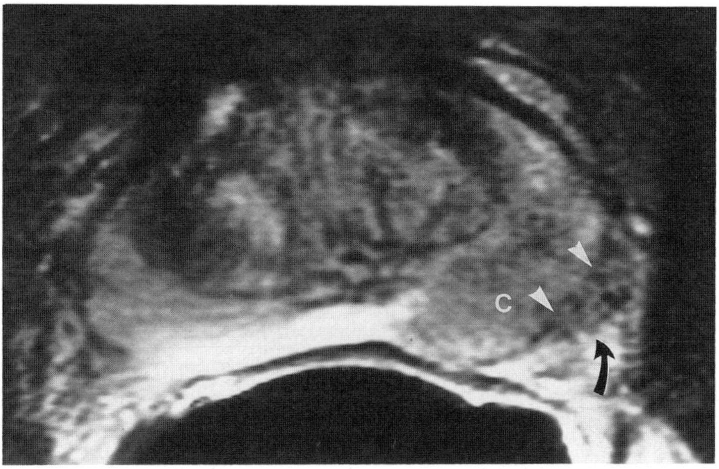

Figure 13. CARCINOMA OF THE PROSTATE WITH LOCAL INVASION (STAGE C). *MRI demonstration. MRI of the prostate using an endorectal surface coil technique reveals the characteristic low signal intensity appearance of carcinoma in the peripheral zone on the left (C=carcinoma). Note how the capsule has been disrupted on the left (arrow heads) and how tumour now appears in the periprostatic fat (curved arrow). Changes of BPH are prominent in the central portion of the gland.*

narrow bandwidth imaging with fat suppression [37] and variable flip-angle spin-echo images [38] need to be evaluated.

Perhaps the most important application of MRI to the prostate is in the staging of prostatic carcinoma. The recent advances in the surgical treatment of carcinoma of the prostate by Walsh et al have placed increased emphasis on pre-operative staging, particularly with reference to the neurovascular bundles which, if uninvolved with tumour, can be surgically spared [39]. In addition, MRI is the only modality to offer the unique opportunity to stage both the pelvic lymph nodes and the local extent of disease with a single study.

The local extent of prostate carcinoma is difficult to assess by any conventional imaging modality. CT for example is notoriously inaccurate in the local staging of prostatic tumours [40,27]. Although endorectal ultrasound provides some information about prostate architecture, it is difficult to judge capsular or seminal vesicle invasion [23,22]. The high soft tissue contrast of MRI is extremely helpful in assessing the spread of prostate cancer into adjacent structures. This is particularly true when evaluating the seminal vesicles. Infiltration of low signal intensity prostate carcinoma into the high signal seminal vesicles on T_2-weighted images can be seen prior to any alteration in the size or contour of the seminal vesicles themselves (Fig. 14). MRI has been reported to be approximately

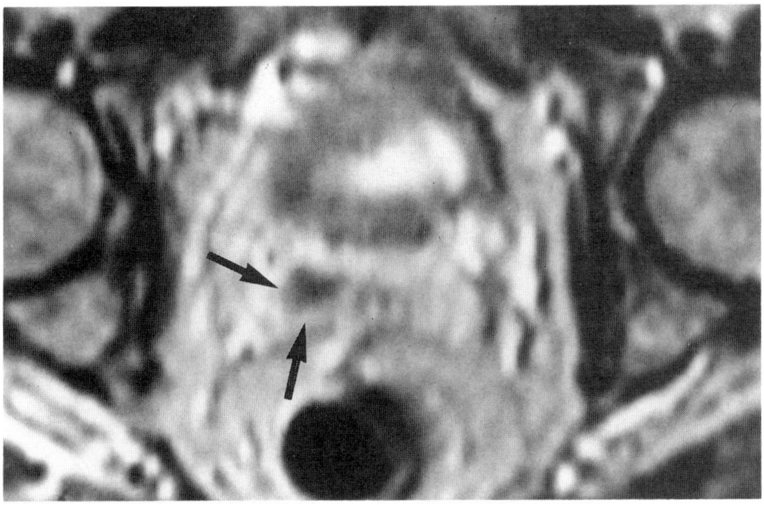

Figure 14. SEMINAL VESICLE EXTENSION FROM CARCINOMA OF THE PROSTATE. MRI. *Spin echo. T_2-Weighted Tr 2500 msec/TE 80 msec. An axial T_2-weighted MRI in a patient with known carcinoma of the prostate demonstrates a discrete low signal intensity area in the right seminal vesicle (arrows). This has a very suggestive appearance of carcinoma and in a patient with known carcinoma it almost certainly represents seminal vesicle involvement.*

87% sensitive in detecting seminal vesicle invasion [36]. Results in detecting direct capsular extension have been less impressive. The prostatic capsule is not reliably seen on the body coil images; therefore, invasion of the periprostatic veins or gross extension into the periprostatic fat must be present before capsular invasion can be identified. The sensitivity of MRI in detecting capsular invasion has been reported to be as low as 44% with body coil technique [36]. The prostatic capsule is, however, reliably seen on the endorectal coil images, and thus a disruption in the capsule can be used as evidence of invasion (Fig. 13). With this technique the staging accuracy of MRI appears to be much higher, having been reported to be 91% accurate in staging 23 patients with clinical (digital rectal exam) stage B carcinoma [9a,41].

When staging prostate carcinoma it is important to recognize biopsy related changes. These are usually manifested by small areas of haemorrhage within or adjacent to the prostate. In the case of a biopsy done less than one month prior to the MRI scan, the haemorrhage will be in the intracellular or extracellular methaemoglobin state. Both of these will be high signal on the T_1-weighted images, while the former will be low signal and the latter high signal on T_2-weighted images [36]. Whenever possible we prefer to perform MRI three or more weeks following biopsy.

When using MRI to evaluate the retroperitoneal and pelvic lymph nodes, nodal enlargement appears to be the best indicator of metastasis. The size criteria are the same as those for CT. Nodes are best evaluated on the short TR/TE images where they are well contrasted against the retroperitoneal fat. The accuracy of MRI for detecting nodal metastasis is similar to that of CT [36,42].

Excretory Urography

Once the backbone of urinary tract imaging for virtually all urinary tract disorders, excretory urography is now little used in the evaluation of patients with prostatic carcinoma. Findings frequently encountered in neoplasms of the prostate, such as hydronephrosis and bladder irregularities (Fig. 15) are reliably shown with other imaging modalities such as ultrasonography, CT, and MRI, all of which provide infinitely more information about the primary tumour as well as the upper urinary tract. The intravenous urogram is best reserved for that subset of patients with carcinoma of the prostate who have, in

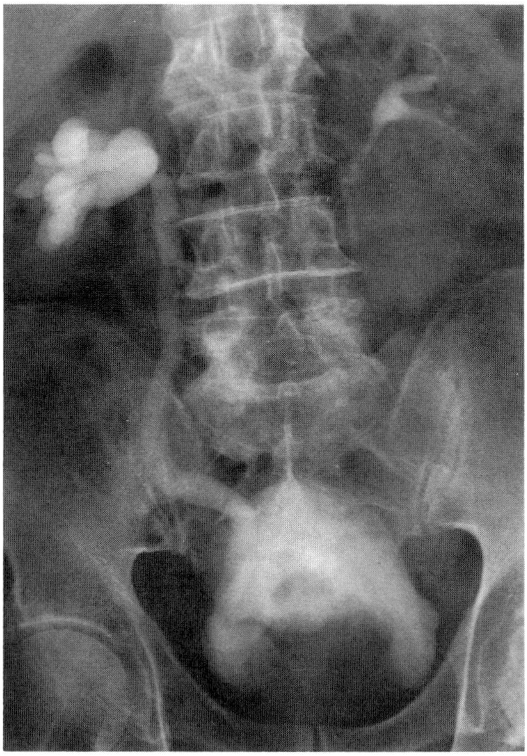

Figure 15. CARCINOMA OF THE PROSTATE (STAGE C). *Intravenous urogram. A 25-minute film from an intravenous urogram performed on a patient with stage C carcinoma of the prostate demonstrates hydroureter and hydronephrosis on the right down to the level of the bladder. When carcinoma of the prostate extends to involve the seminal vesicles the ureter, too, is in jeopardy of being involved. Therefore ureteral obstruction in conjunction with prostatic carcinoma almost certainly indicates stage C disease.*

addition, general urological signs and symptoms such as haematuria, pyuria, etc [29].

Skeletal Radiography

While as many as 85% of patients who die of carcinoma of the prostate demonstrate bony metastases, radionuclide bone scans are more sensitive than radiographs in disclosing these changes, and scintigraphy rather than radiographic bone surveys should be a routine part of the staging process [29]. Skeletal radiographs become important only when scintigraphy is abnormal, so as to allow differentiation between metastases and benign disorders such as degenerative arthritis and Paget's disease. The skeletal lesions of prostatic carcinoma are usually blastic (Fig. 16) but occasionally may be mixed (blastic-lytic) and, in a few cases, purely lytic.

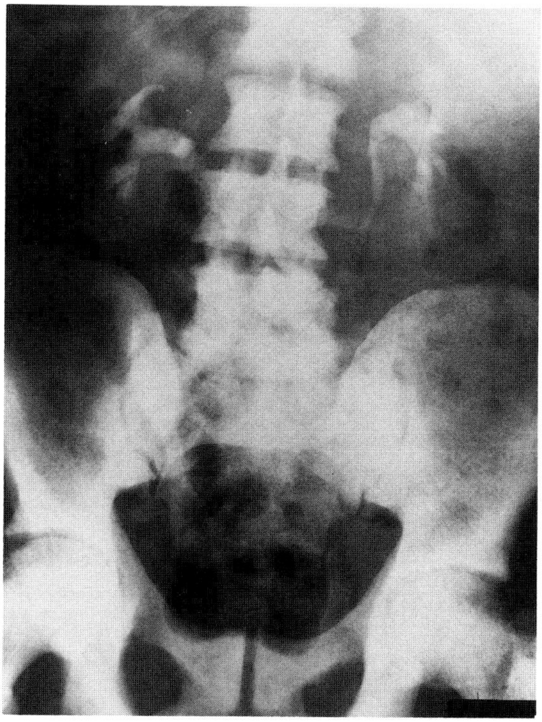

Figure 16. CARCINOMA OF THE PROSTATE. SCLEROTIC BONE METASTASES. *An abdominal radiograph from an intravenous urogram demonstrates diffuse osteoblastic metastases throughout the lumbar spine, pelvis, and hips. While most prostatic carcinoma produces skeletal lesions similar to these illustrated a significant proportion also have mixed blastic-lytic lesions and approximately 3% have lytic lesions only.*

Radionuclide Bone Scanning

Bone scintigraphy with agents such as ^{99m}Tc methylene diphosphonate is the most commonly employed method for detecting bony metastases. The bone scan, however, while extremely sensitive, has little specificity, and abnormal ('hot') areas must be further studied radiographically to confirm that they do indeed represent metastases and not benign foci of osteoblastic activity. Almost one-quarter of bone metastases detected by scintigraphy will go undetected on plain X-ray films, while 16% of patients originally thought to have disease localized within the pelvis will prove after scintigraphy to have metastases to the skeleton.

Only occasionally are bone scans falsely negative in the presence of metastases. The reported prevalence of this association is 8% [29].

An occasional cause of misinterpretation is the so-called 'superscan' (Fig. 17). Here, almost the entire skeleton is the site of metastatic involvement resulting in diffuse, symmetrical uptake of the radionuclide. The absence of a focal 'hot spot' can, at first glance, lead to the impression that the bone scan is normal, but on more detailed inspection of the images, the increased radioactivity in the bones should become apparent. The saturation of the skeleton with the radioisotope results in little or no renal excretion, a further clue that the scintigram is abnormal. Recent work with MRI of skeletal metastasis suggests that it may be even more sensitive than radionuclide scan [42a].

Chest Radiography

The chest radiograph remains one of the essential tools in evaluating the prostatic cancer patient. Six percent of all patients with the disease have intrathoracic metastases when first seen, and 25% of those with stage D disease have spread to the chest. Of the latter, many will evince no evidence of metastases elsewhere [29]. In addition, pulmonary fibrosis, tuberculosis, and cardiovascular disease are quite common in the elderly, and PA and lateral chest radiographs will frequently demonstrate these and other intrathoracic abnormalities which can easily influence the choice of therapy of the underlying prostatic disorder. Whole-lung tomography, as well as chest CT, adds little to the diagnostic yield, and the added expense, radiation, and consumption of scarce resources raises serious questions about the wisdom of their routine employment [29].

Lymphography

Bipedal lymphography is used to evaluate pelvic and para-aortic

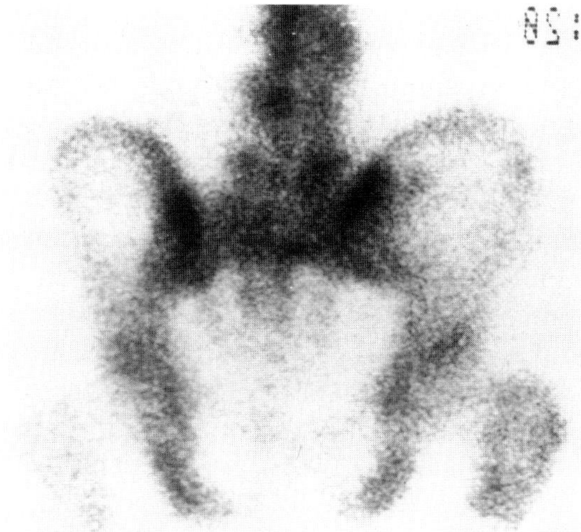

(a)

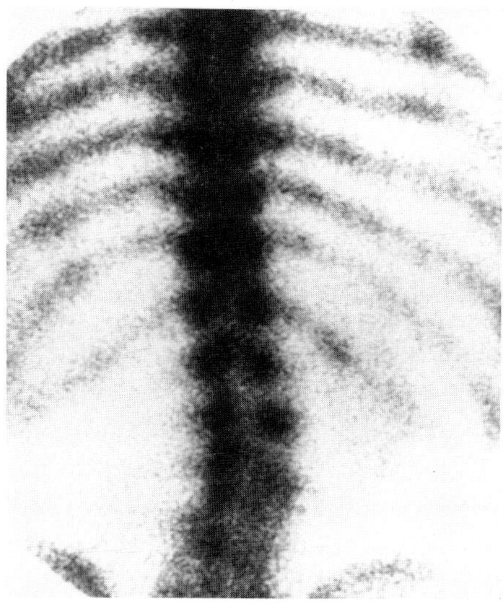

(b)

Figure 17. CARCINOMA OF THE PROSTATE. ^{99m}*Tc diphosphonate bone scan in a patient with carcinoma of the prostate ('Superscan'). (a) Scintigram of ribs, lower thoracic and lumbar spine demonstrates diffusely abnormal and intense uptake throughout the entire visualized skeleton. Note the absence of any excretion by the kidneys. (b) Lumbar spine and pelvis also demonstrate intense uptake as well as the proximal left femur. In view of such diffusely abnormal uptake, scans such as these have occasionally been misinterpreted as normal since there is little or no asymmetry to assist in recognition of any abnormality. Thus the term 'superscan'.*

lymph nodes before instituting therapy. Although the accuracy of lymphography is only approximately 75%, its precision can be markedly improved by routine needle aspiration biopsy of the opacified nodes under fluoroscopic guidance. If sampling of normal appearing as well as abnormal lymph nodes is carried out, the diagnostic yield is further enhanced, as fully 25% of apparently normal nodes will disclose unsuspected metastases [29].

Lymphography with fine needle aspiration biopsy can be carried out easily on outpatients. The combined procedure is cost-effective and may spare many patients from unnecessary staging lymphadenectomies. The obturator nodes - contrary to prevailing opinion - should be opacified in properly performed pedal lymphograms [29].

Other Disorders

Ultrasonography

Prostatic calculi and prostatic cysts are clearly demonstrated by ultrasound (Fig. 18), but are generally of little clinical significance. Prostatic abscess on the other hand may also be readily identified, as

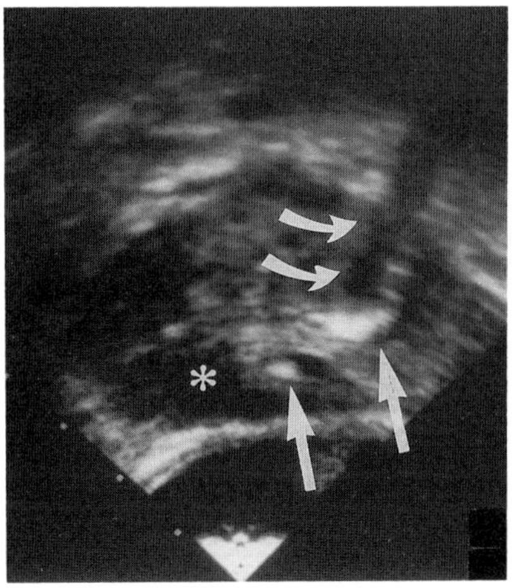

Figure 18. PROSTATIC CALCULI. TRUS. *A transrectal ultrasound examination demonstrates the typical hyperechoic appearance of prostatic calculi (arrows). Note the acoustic shadowing beyond the stones (curved arrows). There is also a hypoechoic focus in the peripheral zone which was later proved to be adenocarcinoma (asterisk).*

well as localized for needle drainage (Fig. 19). Acute prostatitis does not present a pathognomonic picture, but in some cases is associated with diffuse hypoechogenicity. Inflammatory and congenital lesions

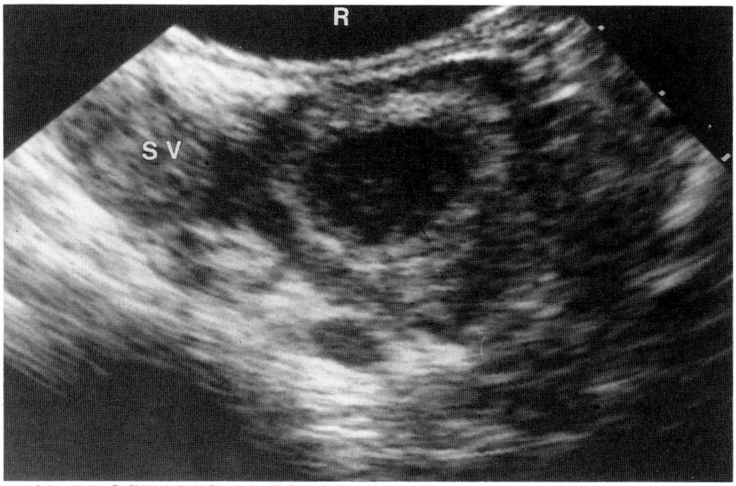

Figure 19. PROSTATIC ABSCESS. TRUS. *TRUS in the sagittal projection demonstrates a hypoechoic focus within the prostate. The area is sharply circumscribed and contains a number of randomly scattered low intensity echoes and is surrounded by a hyperechoic rim. SV=Seminal Vesicle. R=Rectum.*

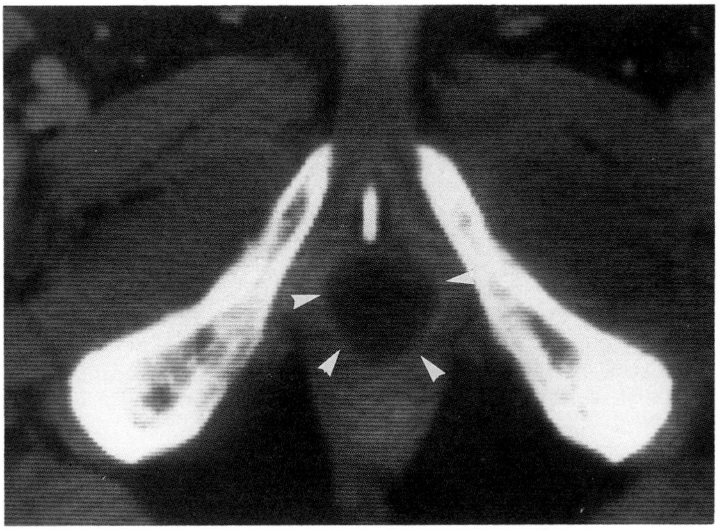

Figure 20. PROSTATIC ABSCESS. CT DEMONSTRATION. *A CT scan through the prostate demonstrates the typical appearance of a prostatic abscess. There is a large, round uniformly hypodense area within the prostate itself. This is very suspicious for a prostatic abscess (arrow heads). There is a very faint suggestion of a hyperintense stain at the periphery of the abscess cavity.*

of the seminal vesicles, such as abscesses and cysts, respectively, may also be recognized.

Computed Tomography

CT has found little practical use in evaluating other prostatic diseases. Prostatic abscess can be recognized as low-attenuation areas, but other inflammatory conditions do not lend themselves readily to assessment (Fig. 20). Prostatic calculi can be well demonstrated by CT, but they rarely have a great deal of clinical significance. Seminal vesicle agenesis, abscess and cyst may be identified.

Magnetic Resonance Imaging

MRI does not appear to have a role in the routine evaluation of acute prostatitis. The MRI in these cases is reported to be normal [43].

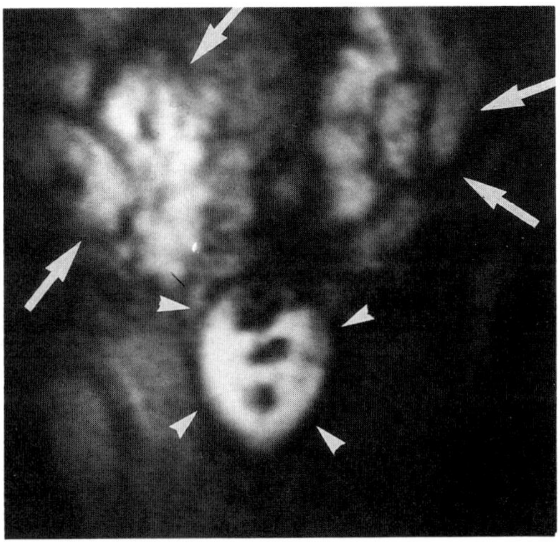

Figure 21. UTRICULAR CYST. MRI WITH ENDORECTAL SURFACE COIL. *Spin echo. T_2-weighted image. Tr 2500 msec/TE 80 msec. A coronal view from a prostatic MRI in a 24 year old man with hypospermia and haematospermia. Endorectal balloon surface coil technique demonstrates an elliptical hyperintense mass in the mid-prostatic urethra (arrow heads). Within the lesion which represents a utricular cyst are seen several hypointense (dark) free floating structures attributable to calculi within the cyst. Both seminal vesicles are extremely dilated secondary to ejaculatory duct obstruction (arrows). The patient was revealed of symptoms following transurethral resection of the cyst.*

However, MRI should be helpful in cases of suspected prostatic and seminal vesicle abscess, since abscesses have a very high signal on T_2-weighted images [44]. The MRI appearance of chronic prostatitis is important since it can mimic carcinoma. Areas of chronic prostatitis are low in signal intensity on long TR/TE images. When they involve the PZ, the appearance is indistinguishable from carcinoma [6]. This is a common cause for false positive MRI scans when evaluating patients suspected of having prostate carcinoma.

Cysts of the prostate may be congenital or acquired. Congenital cysts usually involve the utricle and are of mullarian origin. They may be difficult to differentiate from seminal vesicle or ejaculatory duct cysts, which derive from the wolffian system. Utricular cysts may present with ejaculatory dysfunction, characterized by haematospermia, oligospermia and/or pain on ejaculation. The soft tissue contrast of MRI is ideal for identifying these lesions. The fluid containing cysts will be very high signal on T_2-weighted images (Fig. 21). If the fluid within the cysts is haemorrhagic or has very high protein concentration, it may be high signal on the T_1-weighted images; otherwise it will be low signal on these pulse sequences. The multiplanar capability of MRI is ideal to determine the relationship of the cystic structure to the remainder of the prostate or the seminal tract, an important feature in differential diagnosis. MRI may also be helpful to assess seminal vesicle volume, which may be an indicator of ejaculatory duct obstruction. Early reports on the use of MRI to evaluate males with infertility showed MRI to be helpful in detecting seminal vesicle dilatation and prostatic cysts [45,46]. In the future MRI, especially with surface coil techniques, may play an important role in the primary evaluation of male patients infertility or ejaculatory dysfunction [47].

References

1. Lee F, Torp-Pedersen ST, Siders DB, et al. Transrectal ultrasound in the diagnosis and staging of prostatic carcinoma. *Radiology* 1989;**170:**609-615.
2. Phillips ME, Kressel HY, Spritzer CE, et al. Normal Prostate and Adjacent Structures: MR Imaging at 1.5T. *Radiology* 1987;**164:**381.
3. Sommer GF, McNeal JE, Carrol CL. MR Depiction of Zonal Anatomy of the Prostate at 1.5T. *J Comput Assist Tomogr* 1986;**10:**983.
4. Hricak H, Dooms GC, McNeal JE, et al. MR Imaging of the Prostate Gland: Normal Anatomy. *AJR* 1987;**148:**51.

5. McNeal JE. Regional Morphology and Pathology of the Prostate. *Am J Clin Path* 1967;**49:**347.
6. Schiebler ML, Pollack HM, Tomoszewsky JE, et al. High Resolution of MR Imaging of Prostatic Carcinoma and Benign Prostatic Hypertrophy with Histopathologic Correlation. *Radiology* 1989;**172:**131.
7. Walsh PC, Donker PJ. Impotence Following Radical Prostatectomy: Insight into Etiology and Prevention. *J Urol* 1982;**128:**492.
8. Schnall MD, Lenkinski RL, Pollack HM, Imai Y, Kressel HY. Prostate: MR Imaging with an Endorectal Surface Coil. *Radiology* 1989;**172:**570.
9. Martin JF, Hajek P, Baker L, Gylys-Morin V, Fitzmorris-Glass R, Mattry RR. Inflatable Surface Coil for MR Imaging of the Prostate. *Radiology* 1988;**167:**268.
9a. Schnell MD, Imai Y, Tomaszewski J, Pollack HM, Lenkinski RE, Kressel HY. Prostate cancer; Local staging with endorectal surface coil MR imaging. *Radiology* 1991;178:797-802.
10. McNeal JE. The prostate gland: morphology and pathobiology. In: Stamey TA (ed). monographs in urology. Vol 4. Research Triangle Park, NC: Burroughs Wellcome, 1983:3-33.
11. Phillips ME, Kressel HY, Spritzer CE, Arger PH, Wein AJ, Marinelli D, Axel L, Gefter W, Pollack HM. Prostatic disorders: MR imaging at 1.5T. *Radiology* 1987;**164:**386.
12. Carrol CL, Sommer GF, McNeal JE, Stamey TA. The abnormal prostate: MR imaging at 1.5T with histopathologic correlation. *Radiology* 1987;**163:**521.
13. Silverberg E, Lubera J: Cancer statistics, 1987. *CA* 1987;**37:**2.
14. McClennan BL: Transrectal ultrasound of the prostate: Is the technology leading the science? *Radiology* 1988;**168:**571-575.
15. Rifkin MD: Prostate ultrasound. *Semin Ultrasound CT MR* 1988-9;**9:**352-369.
16. Dahnert WF, Hampter UM, Walsh PC, et al. The echogenic focus in prostatic sonograms with xeroradiographic and histopathologic correlation. *Radiology* 1986;**159:**95-100.
17. Rifkin MD, McGlynn ET, Choi H. Echogenicity of prostate cancer correlated with histologic grade and stromal fibrosis: Endorectal US studies. *Radiology* 1989;**170:**549-552.
18. Lee F, Littrup PJ, Torp-Pedersen ST, et al. Prostate cancer: Comparison of transrectal ultrasound and digital rectal examination for screening. *Radiology* 1988;**168:**389-394.
18a. Hinman FJr. Screening for prostatic carcinoma (ed.). *J Urol* 1991;145:126-130.
19. Resnick MI. Transrectal ultrasound guided versus digitally directed prostatic biopsy: A comparative study. *J Urol* 1988;**139:**754-757.
20. Liddell HT, McDougal WS, Burks DD, et al. Ultrasound versus digitally directed prostatic needle biopsy. *J Urol* 1986;**135:**716-718.
21. Goldenberg SL, Ajzen SA, Allen GJ, et al. Combined biopsy techniques: An approach to the diagnosis of prostatic malignancy. *J Urol* 1989;**141:**870-872.
22. Salo JO, Kivisaari L, Rannikko S, et al. Computerized tomography and transrectal ultrasound in assessment of local extension of prostatic cancer before radical retropubic prostatectomy. *J Urol* 1987;**137:**435-438.
23. Pontes JE, Eisendraft S, Watanabe H, et al. Preoperative evaluation of localized prostatic carcinoma by transrectal ultrasonography. *J Urol* 1985;**134:**289-291.
24. Scardino PT, Shinohara K. *Detection of microscopic extracapsular invasion from prostatic cancer.* Presented at the Third International Symposium on Transrectal Ultrasound in the Diagnosis and Management of Prostate Cancer. Chicago, September 23-24, 1988.
25. Andriole GL, Coplen DE, Mikkelson DJ, Catalona WJ. Sonographic and pathological staging of patients with clinically localized prostate cancer. *J Urol* 1989;**142:**1259-1261.
26. Holm HH, Juul N, Pedersen JF. Transperineal iodine 124 seed implantation in prostatic cancer guided by transrectal ultrasonography. *J Urol* 1983;**130:**283-286.
27. Platt JF, Bree RL, Schwab RE. Accuracy of CT in the staging of carcinoma of the prostate. *AJR* 1987;**149:**315-318.

28. Demas BE. Computed tomography of the prostate gland. *Semin Ultrasound CT MR* 1988;**9**:339-342.
29. Hricak H, Thoeni RF. Neoplasms of the prostate gland. In: Pollack HM (ed). *Clinical Urography*. Philadelphia: WB Saunders Co, 1989: Chapter 47.
30. Weinerman PM, Arger PH, Coleman BG, et al. Pelvic adenopathy from bladder and prostate carcinoma: Detection by rapid sequence computed tomography. *AJR* 1983;**140**:95-99.
31. Pilepich MV, Prasad SC, Perez CA. Computed tomography in definitive radiotherapy of prostatic carcinoma, Part 2: Definition of target volume. *Int J Radiat Oncol Biol Phys* 1982;**8**:235-239.
32. Hricak H, Williams RD, Spring DB, et al. Anatomy and Pathology of the Male Pelvis by Magnetic Resonance Imaging. *AJR* 1983;**141**:1101.
33. Bryan PJ, Butler HE, LiPuma JP, et al. NMR Scanning of the Pelvis: Initial Experience with a .3T System. *AJR* 1983;**141**:1111.
34. Ling D, Lee JKT, Heiken JP, Balfe DM, Glazer HS, McClennan RL. Prostatic Carcinoma and Benign Prostatic Hyperplasia: Inability of MR Imaging to Distinguish Between the Two Diseases. *Radiology* 1986;**158**:103.
35. McNeal J, Redwine E, Freiha M, et al. Zonal Distribution of Prostate Carcinoma: Correlation with Histologic Pattern and Direction of Spread. *Am J Surg Pathol* 1988;**12**:897.
36. Bezzi M, Kressel HY, Allen KS, Schiebler ML, Altman HG, Wein AJ, Pollack HM. Prostatic Carcinoma: Staging with MR at 1.5T. *Radiology* 1988;**169**:339.
37. Mitchell DG, Vinitski S, Rifkin MD, Burk Jr DL. MR Imaging of the Abdomen and Pelvis at 1.5T. *AJR* 1989;**153**:419.
38. Mitchell DG, Vinitski S, Burk Jr. DL, Levy D, Rifkin MD. Variable-flip-angle Spin Echo MR Imaging of the Pelvis:More Versatile T_2-weighted Images. *Radiology* 1989;**171**:525.
39. Walsh PC, Lepor H. The role of Radical Prostatectomy in the Management of Prostatic Cancer. *Cancer* 1987;**60**:526.
40. Golimbu M, Morales P, Al-Askari SA, Shulman Y. CAT Scanning in Staging of Prostatic Cancer. *Urology* 1981;**18**:305.
41. Schnall M, Imai Y, Pollack HM, Lenkinski R, Kressel H. *Local Staging of Prostate Cancer with Endorectal Surface Coil MRI*, (abstract) 75th Annual Meeting of the RSNA 1989, Chicago.
42. Gamori J, Grossman RI, Goldberg HI, et al. Intracranial Hematomas: Imaging by High Field MRI. *Radiology* 1985;**157**:81.
42a. Algra PR, Bloem JL, Tissing H, Falke THM, Arndt JW, Verboom LG. Detection of vertebral metastasis: Comparison between MR imaging and bone scintigraphy. *Radiographics* 1991;11:219-232.
43. Bryon PJ, Butter HE, Nelson AD, et al. Magnetic resonance imaging of the prostate. *AJR* 1986;**146**:5.
44. Sue DE, Chicola C, Scidmore GF, Brant-Zawadslo MN, Hart JB, Hanna JN. MR imaging of seminal vesiculitis. *JCAT* 1989;**13**:662.
45. Zobel B, Tella S, Confalonr D, Passariella R. *Male infertility: MRI assessment* Abstract, 8th annual SMRM meeting. Amsterdam, 1989.
46. Neustein P, Hein PS, Goerger TG. Chronic hematospermia due to mullerian duct cyst: Diagnosis by Magnetic resonance imaging. *J Urol* 1989;**142**:828.
47. Schnell MD, Pollack HM, Van Arsdalen K, Kressel HY. Endorectal surface coil MR imaging of patients with ejaculatory dysfunction (abstract). 76th meeting of the RSNA (1990), Chicago.

Author Index

Keyword Index

M